17. Immune Regulation: Evolution and Biological Significance
Edited by Laurens N. Ruben and M. Eric Gershwin

18. Tumor Immunity in Prognosis: The Role of Mononuclear Cell Infiltration
Edited by Stephen Haskill

19. Immunopharmacology and the Regulation of Leukocyte Function
Edited by David R. Webb

20. Pathogenesis and Immunology of Treponemal Infection
Edited by Ronald F. Schell and Daniel M. Musher

21. Macrophage-Mediated Antibody-Dependent Cellular Cytotoxicity
Edited by Hillel S. Koren

22. Molecular Immunology: A Textbook
Edited by M. Zouhair Atassi, Carel J. van Oss, and Darryl R. Absolom

23. Monoclonal Antibodies and Cancer
Edited by George L. Wright, Jr.

24. Stress, Immunity, and Aging
Edited by Edwin L. Cooper

25. Immune Modulation Agents and Their Mechanisms
Edited by Richard L. Fenichel and Michael A. Chirigos

26. Mononuclear Phagocyte Biology
Edited by Alvin Volkman

27. The Lactoperoxidase System: Chemistry and Biological Significance
Edited by Kenneth M. Pruitt and Jorma O. Tenovuo

28. Introduction to Medical Immunology
Edited by Gabriel Virella, Jean-Michel Goust, H. Hugh Fudenberg, and Christian C. Patrick

29. Handbook of Food Allergies
Edited by James C. Breneman

30. Human Hybridomas: Diagnostic and Therapeutic Applications
Edited by Anthony J. Strelkauskas

31. Aging and the Immune Response: Cellular and Humoral Aspects
Edited by Edmond A. Goidl

32. Complications of Organ Transplantation
Edited by Luis H. Toledo-Pereyra

33. Monoclonal Antibody Production Techniques and Applications
Edited by Lawrence B. Schook

34. Fundamentals of Receptor Molecular Biology
Donald F. H. Wallach

35. Recombinant Lymphokines and Their Receptors
Edited by Steven Gillis

36. Immunology of the Male Reproductive Organs
Edited by Pierre Luigi Bigazzi

37. The Lymphocyte: Structure and Function
Edited by John J. Marchalonis

38. Differentiation Antigens in Lymphohemopoietic Tissues
Edited by Masayuki Miyasaka and Zdenek Trnka

39. Cancer Diagnosis In Vitro Using Monoclonal Antibodies
Edited by Herbert Z. Kupchik

40. Biological Response Modifiers and Cancer Therapy
Edited by J. W. Chiao

41. Cellular Oncogene Activation
Edited by George Klein

42. Interferon and Nonviral Pathogens
Edited by Gerald I. Byrne and Jenifer Turco

43. Human Immunogenetics: Basic Principles and Clinical Relevance
Edited by Stephen D. Litwin, with David W. Scott, Lorraine Flaherty, Ralph A. Reisfeld, and Donald M. Marcus

Additional Volumes in Preparation

CELLULAR ONCOGENE ACTIVATION

edited by

George Klein

KAROLINSKA INSTITUTE
STOCKHOLM, SWEDEN

MARCEL DEKKER, INC. New York and Basel

Library of Congress Cataloging-in-Publication Data

Cellular oncogene activation / edited by George Klein.
p. cm.—(Immunology series; 41)
Inclues bibliographies and index.
ISBN 0-8247-7983-5
1. Oncogenes. 2. Viral carcinogenesis—Genetic aspects.
I. Klein, George. II. Series: Immunology series; v. 41.
RC268.42.C45 1988
616.99'4071—dc 19 88-16149
CIP

MARCEL DEKKER, INC.
270 Madison Avenue, New York, New York 10016

Current printing (last digit):
10 9 8 7 6 5 4 3 2 1

PRINTED IN THE UNITED STATES OF AMERICA

Preface

The oncogene field—an unexpected gift of viral oncology to cellular and cancer biology—has emerged from the largely mistaken notion that tumor viruses owe their oncogenic effects to indigenous viral sequences. This relationship turned out to be true for the DNA but not for the RNA tumor viruses. It was gradually realized that the acute or directly acting retroviruses owe their transforming effect to cellular sequences, which are incorporated into the viral genome by illegitimate recombination and further modified by structural changes during passage and selection for high tumorigenicity. This artificially propagated byproduct of laboratory experimentation has provided an unexpectedly rich source of information. It has revealed the existence of several previously unknown groups of genes that participate in the regulation of cell growth and division. Most authors now accept that the same genes can also contribute to tumor development after various types of in situ activation and without the intervention of viral transduction. Some dissenters, however, would like to draw a sharp dividing line between the virally transduced oncogenes (v-*onc*) and the corresponding cellular protooncogenes. The notion that the latter can act as an "enemy from within" (M. Bishop, *Cell 42*:23, 1985) when activated by mutation, chromosome translocation, or gene amplification has been opposed by postulating the categorical imperative of viral modification as an essential condition for tumorigenicity (P. H. Duesberg, *Science 228*:669, 1985).

The purpose of this book is to assemble the evidence that the cellular proto-oncogenes can play an essential, rate-limiting role in the development of numerous animal and human tumors. They can be activated by a variety of virally mediated or purely cellular mechanisms. The prevalent mechanism of activation differs among the protooncogenes and also among different cell types and animal species. Preneoplastic precedents such as initiation, promotion, or chronic cell proliferation can also influence the probability of a given activation mechanism. In spite of all this diversity, the recurrent themes are more striking than the variations. Oncogenes of the *ras* family are activated by the same point mutations in spontaneous and chemically induced human and animal tumors as are their virally transduced counterparts. The molecular anatomy of viral versus cellular activation shows close analogies for other oncogenes such as *myb, abl, fos,* and *erb*B. The range of transformation of susceptible tissues can be similar or different for the corresponding virally transduced and activated cellular oncogenes, depending on the host cell range of the carrier virus and the impact of the carcinogenic noxa on the cellular target, respectively.

The neoplastic microevolution offers many possibilities, even for a single group of oncogenes. This has been particularly well documented for the *myc* family. The virally transduced avian *myc* gene can transform a wide range of target cells. It can induce hemopoietic, mesenchymal, and epithelial neoplasia in susceptible hosts. Its cellular counterpart, c-*myc*, can also contribute to the development or progression of tumors in all three major tissues in birds and mammals. It can be activated by a variety of mechanisms and can make its impact at an early or late stage in the natural tumor history. Activation by retroviral insertion in chicken B-cell lymphomas or by chromosomal translocation to an immunoglobulin gene region in B-cell-derived human, mouse, and rat tumors is an early event during tumor development. Amplification in human or murine carcinomas, leukemias, or sarcomas is a late, progression-related phenomenon. The v-*abl* oncogene is a fully competent transforming gene for murine pre-B-cells and fibroblasts and can play an accelerating role in murine plasmacytoma induction by mineral oil. Its cellular counterpart fuses with another gene after chromosomal translocation. The resulting *bcr*/c-*abl* fusion protein creates a preleukemic condition, expressed as the Philadelphia chromosome (Ph^1)-positive chronic granulocytic leukemia (CGL) and can also give rise to highly malignant acute leukemia, although in a distinctly different molecular configuration.

Comparison of the Ig/*myc* and the *bcr/abl* translocations provides some interesting parallels and contrasts. The former may activate the normal proto-oncogene by a purely regulatory change whereas the latter truncates the proto-oncogene and links it to cellular sequences that participate in the synthesis of an abnormal protein. The Ig loci provide hot spots for the translocation, as also the less regularly involved T-cell receptor genes, because of their physiological rearrangements and the action of the associated recombination enzymes. The *bcr* gene does not rearrange during normal development and its illegitimate recombination with the proto-oncogene must have other reasons. The *bcr/abl* fusion protein is expressed in parallel with the normal c-*abl* product whereas the high expression of the Ig-activated c-*myc* gene is accompanied by the down-regulation of the normal allele.

The juxtaposition of c-*myc* to an immunoglobulin gene is the clearest example of tissue-specific oncogene activation by a purely cellular mechanism. The risk of what appears as a rare accident of chronic cell division is obviously increased by the pathological stimulation of cell proliferation in the target tissue. The molecular anatomy of the translocation is closely similar in mice, rats, and humans. The wide variation of the breakpoints in and around the c-*myc* gene suggests that breakage occurs at random, but the integrity of the coding sequences must be preserved. This raises the interesting question of why only c-*myc* is involved in the Ig/*myc*-associated tumors. Other oncogene-carrying chromosomes should stand a similar chance of random breakage and illegitimate recombination in the course of chronic cell division. However, the tumorigenic potential of each activated oncogene is restricted to specific "differentiation windows" (for review, see G. Klein and E. Klein, *Cancer Res. 46*:3211, 1986). Activation of other known oncogenes by translocation to the recombination-prone Ig sequences may not affect the relevant precursor cells in the same way. Actually, both the immunoglobulin and the T-cell receptor loci can serve as the recipients of some other putative oncogenes, but these translocations are less frequent and less uniformly associated with specific lymphoma or leukemia types, compared with the Ig/*myc* juxtaposition.

The amplification of cellular proto-oncogenes is without precedence in the field of the virally transduced oncogenes. It has been found in many different types of tumors, but only in a limited fraction of each type (for review see K. Alitalo and M. Schwab, *Adv. in Cancer Res. 47*:235, 1986). Amplication of c–, N- or L-*myc* in small-cell lung carcinomas, N-*myc* in neuroblastomas, and c-*erb*B2 in breast carcinomas is associated with tumor progression. The persistence of the amplified genes in the growing tumors and derived cell lines suggests that they provide their host cells with some growth advantage (J. M. Bishop, *Science 235*:305, 1987). Relaxation of the selective pressure leads to the rapid disappearance of amplified genes in other systems, as particularly well shown for DHFR (dehydrofolate reductase) genes in methotrexate-resistant cells after the removal of the drug.

The activation of cellular protooncogenes in the course of tumor development and progression represents experiments of nature. Their ability to contribute to the carcinogenic process is established beyond doubt by the analytical studies summarized in this volume. The repeated involvement of the same proto-oncogene—such as members of the *ras* or the *myc* family—in many different tumor scenarios emphasizes the unity of cancer biology. The variety of structural and regulatory changes that can activate proto-oncogenes in naturally occurring tumors also shows the direct connection between the activated gene and the cellular phenotype, independently of the mechanism of activation that can include mutation, translocation, retroviral insertion, and amplification.

The role of cellular oncogene activation in tumor development can also be approached experimentally—by examining some of the crucial hypotheses in facsimile tests. Retroviral or tissue-specific enhancer activation of c-*myc* in transgenic and chimeric mice have confirmed the notion that the constitutive expression of the normal oncoprotein can provide an essential step in the tumorigenic process. However, the resulting tumors that arose in cell lineages with a high level of transgene expression were oligo- or monoclonal, showing that at least one additional change was required. Sequential activation of several oncogenes is one possibility; loss of tumor suppressor genes or emerogenes (for review see G. Klein, *Science, 238*:1539, 1987) is another. The latter may or may not belong to the same category as the recessive cancer genes that promote tumor development by their loss (W. Cavenee et al., *Science 228*:501, 1985).

It may be concluded that the widely diversified proto-oncogenes that normally participate in the regulation of normal cell division can contribute to the driving forces of malignant growth, after dysregulation or as a result of specific structural changes. Other, less well known genes can counteract their phenotypic effects. Still others can modify the secondary properties of the neoplastic cell, such as invasiveness, metastasis formation, and immunogenicity. Tumor development is thus probably influenced by a considerable number of gene families. The frequent involvement of the same proto-oncogene (e.g., c-*myc*) in a wide variety of different tumor scenarios suggests, nevertheless, that the number of the most frequently involved genes may be quite limited.

This volume will be of interest to research oncologists, virologists, immunologists, and cellular and molecular biologists.

I would like to express my gratitude to all the contributors for their painstaking work.

George Klein

Contents

Contributors

Jerry M. Adams Molecular Biology Unit, The Walter & Eliza Hall Institute of Medical Research, Melbourne, Australia

Mariano Barbacid Developmental Oncology Section, Basic Research Program, National Cancer Institute, Frederick Cancer Research Facility, Frederick, Maryland

Anton Berns Division of Molecular Genetics, The Netherlands Cancer Institute, and The Department of Biochemistry, The University of Amsterdam, Amsterdan The Netherlands

Hartmut Beug Differentiation Program, European Molecular Biology Laboratory, Heidelberg, Federal Republic of Germany

Georg W. Bornkamm Abteilung Virologie, Institut für Medizinische Mikrobiologie und Hygiene der Universität Freiburg, Freiburg, Federal Republic of Germany

Bruce E. Clurman Laboratory of Molecular Genetics and Oncology, Sloan-Kettering Institute for Cancer Research, New York, New York

Steven J. Collins Molecular Medicine Program, Fred Hutchinson Cancer Research Center, and Department of Medicine, University of Washington School of Medicine, Seattle, Washington

Carlo M. Croce The Wistar Institute of Anatomy and Biology, Philadelphia, Pennsylvania

A. De Klein Department of Cell Biology and Genetics, Erasmus University, Rotterdam, The Netherlands

Dirk Eick Abteilung Virologie, Institut für Medizinische Mikrobiologie und Hygiene der Universität Freiburg, Freiburg, Federal Republic of Germany

J. Groffen Medical Genetics Division, Childrens Hospital of Los Angeles, Los Angeles, California

G. Grosveld Department of Cell Biology and Genetics, Erasmus University, Rotterdam, The Netherlands

Mark Groudine Division of Basic Sciences, Fred Hutchinson Cancer Research Center, and Department of Radiation Oncology, University of Washington School of Medicine, Seattle, Washington

Frank G. Haluska The Wistar Institute of Anatomy and Biology, Philadelphia, Pennsylvania

Willaim S. Hayward Laboratory of Molecular Genetics and Oncology, Sloan-Kettering Institute for Cancer Research, New York, New York

N. Heisterkamp Molecular Genetics Division, Childrens Hospital of Los Angeles, Los Angeles, California

Carl-Henrik Heldin Ludwig Institute for Cancer Research, Uppsala, Sweden

A. Hermans Department of Cell Biology and Genetics, Erasmus University, Rotterdam, The Netherlands

Karl-Heinz Klempnauer Zentrum für Molekulare Biologie der Universität Heidelberg, Heidelberg, Federal Republic of Germany

Karin Moelling Max Planck Institute für Molekulare Genetik, Berlin, Federal Republic of Germany

Herbert C. Morse, III Laboratory of Immunopathology, National Institute of Allergy and Infectious Diseases, National Institutes of Health, Bethesda, Maryland

Rolf Müller European Molecular Biology Laboratory, Heidelberg, Federal Republic of Germany

J. Frederic Mushinski Laboratory of Genetics, National Cancer Institute, National Institutes of Health, Bethesda, Maryland

Roel Nusse Division of Molecular Biology, The Netherlands Cancer Institute, Amsterdam, The Netherlands

Axel Polack Abteilung Virologie, Institut für Medizinische Mikrobiologie und Hygiene der Universität Freiburg, Freiburg, Federal Republic of Germany

Ulf R. Rapp Viral Pathology Section, Laboratory of Viral Carcinogenes, National Cancer Institute, Frederick Cancer Research Facility, Frederick, Maryland

Yoshihide Tsujimoto The Wistar Institute of Anatomy and Biology, Philadelphia, Pennsylvania

Björn Vennström European Molecular Biology Laboratory, Heidelberg, Federal Republic of Germany

Bengt Westermark Department of Pathology, University of Uppsala, Uppsala, Sweden.

ONE

Cellular Oncogenes Encoding Nuclear Proteins: *fos*, *myb*, *myc*, and *erb*A

Rolf Müller
European Molecular Biology Laboratory
Heidelberg, Federal Republic of Germany

Karl-Heinz Klempnauer
Zentrum für Molekulare Biologie der Universität Heidelberg
Heidelberg, Federal Republic of Germany

Karin Moelling
Max Planck Institut für Molekulare Genetik
Berlin, Federal Republic of Germany

Hartmut Beug and Björn Vennström
European Molecular Biology Laboratory
Heidelberg, Federal Republic of Germany

THE *fos* GENE

Role of c-*fos* in Biological Processes

The *fos* oncogene has been detected in two different mouse osteosarcoma viruses, in the Finkel-Biskis-Jinkins mouse osteosarcoma virus (FBJ-MSV), isolated from a spontaneous osteosarcoma-like tumor in a CF-1 mouse, and in the Finkel-Biskis-Reilly mouse osteosarcoma virus (FBR-MSV), and recovered from a radiation ^{90}Sr-induced osteosarcoma in a X/Gf mouse (Finkel et al. 1966, 1975). Both retroviruses induce chondro-osseous neoplasms and fibrosarcomas upon inoculation into newborn rodents. In the past years, the function of the viral *fos* genes and their cellular progenitor, the c-*fos* proto-oncogene, have been the subject of intense research efforts. The function of the c-*fos* proto-oncogene product in biological processes has been addressed by mainly two approaches.

First, it has been analyzed in which tissues and cell types and in which conditions (e.g., state of differentiation or proliferation) the c-*fos* gene is expressed. In the second approach, the phenotypic effects (e.g., on the differentiation state of the cell) of exogenous c-*fos* genes introduced into suitable recipient cells have been investigated. The results of these studies (for a more detailed review, see Müller, 1986) strongly suggest multifunctional properties for the c-*fos* gene product. This is based on several observations. A role for c-*fos* in cellular differentiation has been proposed because of its high, specific expression in certain types of terminally differentiated cells (i.e., blood granulocytes and late gestation amnion cells), and because of its differentiation-promoting effect upon introduction into certain teratocarcinoma cell lines. On the other hand, c-*fos* seems to play a role in the induction of DNA synthesis in quiescent fibroblasts. This is based on the observation that the c-*fos* gene is rapidly and transiently induced by treatment of quiescent fibroblasts with growth factors (e.g., platelet-derived growth factor, PDGF) or other proliferative stimuli (such as the wounding of a confluent monolayer) (reviewed in Müller, 1986). This hypothesis was lent strong support by the intriguing observation of Nishikura and Murray (1987) who used antisense *fos* RNA to analyze the role of c-*fos* protein in quiescent fibroblasts. These authors reported that the abrogation of c-*fos* protein induction rendered the cells unable to reenter the cell cycle upon growth factor stimulation, whereas no significant effect on DNA synthesis in normally cycling cells was observed. The latter finding, however, needs to be verified since it is in apparent contrast with the findings of another study (Holt et al., 1986). A role for c-*fos* proliferation and differentiation is also strongly suggested by its apparent involvement in bone development. While physiologically the c-*fos* gene is expressed at high levels specifically in the cartilaginous growth zone of fetal bone (Dony and Gruss, 1987), its deregulated expression in transgenic mice interferes with normal bone development by perturbing the bone remodelling process (Rüther et al., 1987). Finally, a function of c-*fos* protein in signal processing in neuronal cells is suggested by the induction of c-*fos* by nerve growth factor and its modulation by a variety of neurotropic drugs affecting, for instance, chloride or calcium channels (Curran and Morgan, 1985; Greenberg et al., 1985, 1986; Kruijer et al., 1985; Morgan and Curran, 1986).

The fact that c-*fos* plays a role in a variety of biological processes could be explained by the hypothesis that c-*fos* protein figures in the regulation of other genes and may thus modulate the expression of different (sets of) genes in different cell types with the consequence of different biological effects. As discussed below, the available data of the molecular and biochemical properties of *fos* protein are compatible with such a proposed transregulatory function.

Regulation of c-*fos* by External Signals

In a wide variety of cell types transcription of the c-*fos* gene is inducible by external signals mediated, for example, by trophic factors, hormones, and neurotransmitters. Induction of c-*fos* is usually rapid (reaching maximum levels of messenger ribonucleic acid, mRNA, after 15–30 min) and transient (decreasing to the level found in nonstimulated cells within 2 hrs). Examples of this type of induction are fibroblasts stimulated with PDGF, epithelial cells treated with epidermal growth factor, neuronal cells exposed to nerve growth factor, NGF, or acetyl choline and macrophages stimulated with colony-stimulating factor 1 (e.g., Curran et al., 1985, 1986; Greenberg and Ziff, 1984; Greenberg et al., 1985, 1986; Kruijer et al., 1985, 1986; Müller et al., 1984, 1986). Dependent on the system analyzed different intracellular signal transduction pathways seem to be involved in the transient induction of c-*fos* transcription, including the activation of protein kinase C, the release of calcium from intracellular pools, and the influx of potassium ions (Bravo et al., 1987; Curran and Morgan 1985; Greenberg et al., 1986). Another induction mechanism seems to exist in macrophages where cyclic adenosine monophosphate mediates a rapid, but relatively stable (i.e., for >12 hrs) induction of c-*fos* transcription. Also in amnion cells, where c-*fos* expression appears to be constitutive, transcription of the c-*fos* gene is apparently under control of external signals generated by placenta- or embryo-derived factor(s) (Müller et al., 1986). These findings suggest that expression of the c-*fos* gene may be controlled by extracellular signals in most, if not in all, cell types.

The rapid induction of c-*fos* by growth factors is reminiscent of the stress response of heat shock genes (for a review see Nover, 1984). It was indeed possible to show that raising the temperature to 42 °C led to a three- to five-fold increase in the level of c-*fos* mRNA in quiescent NIH3T3 cells (R. Wallich and R.M., unpublished observation). Interestingly, the heat shock induction of c-*fos* is not transient, and thus differs from the kinetics observed after growth factor stimulation. In the presence of the protein synthesis inhibitor cycloheximide, a much more dramatic induction of c-*fos* is observed 15–60 min after heat shock, presumably due to stabilization of the induced c-*fos* mRNA. A strong induction—similar to that observed with fetal calf serum—was also found with heavy metal ions (Cd^{2+} or Zn^{2+}) and with hydrogen peroxide. A variety of other compounds previously found to induce certain heat shock genes proved negative with regard to c-*fos* induction, including NaN_3, ethanol, dexamethasone, arsenite, puromycin, and 2,4-dinitrophenol. These results are thus compatible with the classification of c-*fos* as a heat shock gene showing a specific response to defined stress-inducing agents.

Anatomy of the c-*fos* Promoter Region

Transcription of the c-*fos* gene is subject to complex regulatory mechanisms. The c-*fos* 5′ flanking region contains several sequence elements that are required for transcription and/or represent protein-binding sites and partly coincide with nuclease hypersensitive sites and topoisomerase cleavage sites in vitro (see Fig. 1). A region that is crucial for serum induction of the human c-*fos* gene following its transfection into HeLa cells has been identified some 300 bp 5′ to the cap site (Deschanps et al., 1985; Renz et al., 1987; Treisman, 1985). A 22-bp element of dyad symmetry located in this region (serum response element, SRE) plays a crucial role in the function of the c-*fos* enhancer, since it not only represents a protein binding site (Gilman et al., 1986; Greenberg et al., 1987; Prywes and Roeder, 1986; Treisman, 1986), but is also sufficient to confer serum-

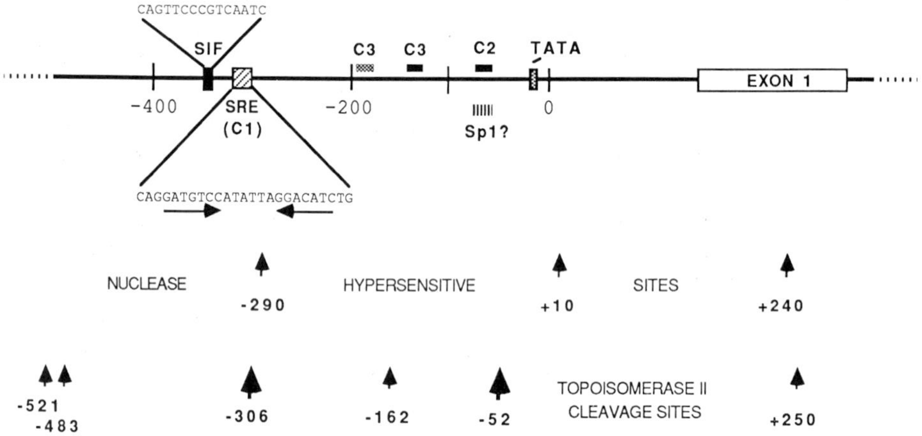

Figure 1 Structure of the c-*fos* promoter region. Indicated are regulatory elements and protein-binding sites (filled boxes), nuclease-hypersensitive regions (±40 nucleotides) in mouse c-*fos* (Renz et al., 1985) and VP16-induced topoisomerase II cleavage sites in human c-*fos* (Darby et al., 1986). Numbers indicate positions (nucleotides) relative to the putative cap site. TATA: TATA-box; C1, C2, C3: binding sites for protein complexes 1, 2, and 3 in mouse c-*fos* (the black box indicates a primary binding site for complex 3, the dotted box a secondary site); SRE: serum response element (enhancer) in human c-*fos* with the region of dyad symmetry indicated below; SIF: binding site for serum-inducible factor in human c-*fos* (the sequence represents an oligonucleotide shown to bind SIF); Spl: region in the mouse gene that matches the SPI recognition sequence (not conserved in human); see text for details. The bold arrows indicate clusters of topoisomerase II cleavage sites (five sites in the "-306-cluster" and three sites in the "-52-cluster").

inducibility on c-*fos* genes lacking all sequences upstream of nucleotide-261 (Treisman, 1986). The factor (SRF) binding to the SRE is present in both uninduced and induced HeLa cells, suggesting that serum induction involves modification or complex formation with other proteins of the SRF rather than changes in the level of its expression. This seems to be different in A431 cells where a factor binding to the same dyad symmetry element is inducible by epidermal growth factor, EGF (Prywes and Roeder, 1986). It is likely that this factor is identical to the SRF identified by Treisman (1986). Interestingly, although efficient inducers of the c-*fos* gene, neither the tumor promoter TPA nor the calcium ionophore A23187 induced an increased level of protein binding to the SRE or another region of the c-*fos* enhancer (Prywes and Roeder, 1986). Inducible binding to a different region of the c-*fos* enhancer has been reported by Hayes et al. (1987). These authors could demonstrate a binding activity in serum- or PDFG-stimulated BALB/c-3T3 cells that was not detectable in quiescent cells. This factor (serum-inducible factor; SIF) was found to interact with a binding site approximately 346 bp upstream of the cap site; i.e., a short distance 5 ′ to the SRE (Fig. 1). In contrast to the results obtained with SRF in A431 cells, binding of SIF was not induced by EGF. In addition, no induction was found with TPA or insulin.

Gilman et al. (1986) have identified in extracts from the mouse B-lymphoma cell line WEHI231 three protein complexes binding to the c-*fos* promoter/enhancer region. Complex 1 (C1 in Fig. 1) binds to SRE, and is thus presumably identical to SRF. Complex 2 (C2 in Fig. 1) binds to a region some 140 bp 5 ′ to the cap site and, with a reduced affinity, to another region about 40 bp further upstream. A third complex (C3 in Fig. 1) was found to interact with a sequence element approximately 65 bp upstream from the cap site. It is possible that complexes 2 and 3 interact with regions required for basal level promoter activity. In the mouse c-*fos* gene the sequence interacting with complex 3 is located in a region harboring a potential binding site for the transcription factor Sp1. This site, however is not conserved in humans (Renz et al., 1987).

Regulation of c-*fos* expression seems to be even more complex, since it apparently involves also negatively acting factors. This is suggested by competition experiments where increasing amounts of the c-*fos* flanking region (-711 to -100) transfected into quiescent 3T3 fibroblasts (Sassone-Corsi and Verma, 1987) lead to the induction of a cotransfected c-*fos*–CAT fusion gene presumably due to competition with a repressor molecule binding to the c-*fos* promoter/enhancer. In stimulated cells, on the contrary, transfection of the same upstream sequence resulted in a decreased induction of c-*fos*. This is consistent with the results reported by Treisman (1986) that serum induction is abolished by cotransfer of SRE competitor deoxyribonucleic acid (DNA). Serum stimulation may thus lead to both removal or inactivation of negative transacting factor(s) and the induction of DNA binding of transactivating protein complexes.

In the context of transacting factors modulating expression of the c-*fos*, it is interesting to note that the adenovirus Ela product transactivates both the c-*fos* and c-*myc* gene (Sassone-Corsi and Borelli, 1987). It has previously been shown that Ela transactivates a variety of cellular and viral genes while repressing expression of others (Moran and Mathews, 1987). The Ela protein does not bind to DNA, and there is no specific DNA sequence requirement for its transregulatory action, suggesting that it exerts its effect on gene transcription by a more general mechanism. Interestingly, the c-*fos* gene is stimulated—as is the c-*myc* gene—by c-*fos* protein (I. Verma, personal communication). Although this observation is suggestive of an autoregulatory function of c-*fos* protein, this is not required for the induction of c-*fos* by growth factors, which is even increased in the presence of protein synthesis inhibitors.

A Role for *fos* Protein in Gene Transcription?

The c-*fos* gene encodes an acidic phosphoprotein of 380 amino acids with a highly charged center region and a potential Zn-finger–like structure at the C-terminal (see Fig. 2) (Van Beveren et al., 1983). Both cellular and viral *fos* gene products form a complex with a group of basic proteins (p39) in fibroblasts (Curran et al., 1985; Franza et al., 1987; Müller et al., 1987). In

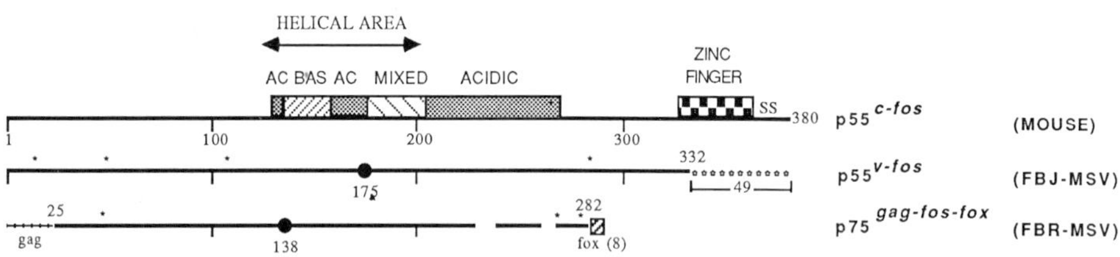

Figure 2 Structure of cellular and viral *fos* gene products. Indicated are the highly charged clusters of amino acids in the center (ac: acids; bas: basic) and the potential Zn-finger structure at the C-terminal of c-*fos*. Mutations (at the amino acid level) in the viral genes are indicated by asterisks, deletions, and truncations by open spaces (relative to c-*fos*) and fusion with heterologous sequences in $p75^{gag\text{-}fos\text{-}fox}$ by boxes. Biologically important amino acid substitutions are shown by filled circles: The change from V to E at position 138 has activated the immortalizing potential of the FBR-MSV gene product, whereas the change from E to K at position 175 resulted in a decreased transforming capacity of the FBJ-MSV *fos* protein. (Jenuwein et al., 1987, and unpublished observations.)

the pheochromocytoma cell line PC12, where c-*fos* is inducible by NGF and other compounds, c-*fos* protein seems to form a complex with another acid protein (p40) rather than with the basic p39 (Franza et al., 1987). The function of these complex-forming proteins is not known. While the c-*fos* gene product of FBJ-MSV ($p55^{v\text{-}fos}$) is similar to c-*fos* (except for a different C-terminal), the FBR-MSV–transforming protein ($p75^{gag\text{-}fos\text{-}fox}$) is much more different from c-*fos* owing to mutations, deletions, and fusions with heterologous sequences (see Fig. 2). Both viral proteins thus lack the Zn-finger motif present in c-*fos* (Fig. 2).

The subnuclear localization of *fos* gene products has been studied in serum-stimulated and virus-transformed murine fibroblasts and in NGF-treated PC12 cells (Renz et al., 1987; Sambucetti et al., 1986). The c-*fos* protein complex is almost quantitatively released from intact nuclei by DNase I or micrococcus nuclease treatment under conditions where only a minor fraction of DNA and other nuclear proteins is released. In gel filtration experiments, the c-*fos* protein complex cofractionates with chromatin and seems to be associated with regions of increased deoxyribonuclease I (DNase I) accessibility. In vitro, the c-*fos* protein-complex binds to double- and single-stranded calf thymus DNA, suggesting that its association with chromatin is at least in part due to an interaction with DNA. In agreement with this conclusion, part of the c-*fos* protein complex is released from nuclei by incubation with transfer ribonucleic acid (tRNA), presumably due to competition for binding sites. It has to be stressed, however, that in all these experiments the role of other nuclear proteins (such as p39 and p40) remains to be clarified. It is thus not clear whether *fos* protein binds to DNA directly, or whether its apparent affinity to DNA is due to its interaction with other DNA-binding proteins present in the nuclear extract used for the binding studies.

More direct evidence for a role of c-*fos* in gene transcription has recently been obtained by several investigators. It has been shown that both transfected and endogenous α_1(III) collagen gene promoters as well as a transfected Rous sarcoma virus long terminal repeat are stimulated in cells expressing a v-*fos* oncogene (Setoyama et al., 1986a,b). Based on this observation, it has been suggested that c-*fos* protein participates in the transactivation of the α_1(III) collagen gene. In addition, as mentioned above, c-*fos* protein can transactivate both the c-*fos* and c-*myc* gene (I.M. Verma, personal communication). Interestingly, in contrast to transactivation of the α_1(III) collagen gene, transactivation of c-*fos* and c-*myc* is not observed with v-*fos* gene product, suggesting that at least in this case the Zn-finger–like structure at the C-terminal may play a role in transactivation.

An intriguing result is the recent observation made with the aP2 (adipocyte lipid–binding protein P2) gene which is induced during the differentiation of preadipocytes to adipocytes (Distel et al., 1987). The aP2 gene contains a regulatory element (FSE2) 124 bp upstream from the cap site. The FSE2 represents a binding site for a protein complex in both preadipocytes and adipocytes, but the pattern of protein binding in a gel retardation assay changes dramatically during differentiation, suggesting a negative regulatory role for the FSE-2 binding complex in preadipocytes. The c-*fos* protein seems to be a pivotal constituent of this protein complex, since *fos*-specific antibodies disrupt the binding of the protein complex to FSE2 DNA. Most significantly, protein complexes cross-linked by UV to the FSE2 element are immunoprecipitated by antibodies against *fos* protein. These observations strongly suggest that the *fos* gene product is part of a transcription complex albeit its precise role remains to be investigated.

Activation of the Transforming Potential of the *fos* Gene

Analysis of cloned viral and cellular *fos* genes indicated that the former has the capacity to transform fibroblast cell lines, whereas the latter does not (Miller et al., 1985). The molecular mechanisms involved in the activation of the c-*fos* proto-oncogene have been extensively analyzed using v-*fos*/c-*fos* chimeric molecules. These studies clearly showed that a plasmid (MMV), containing all 5′ and coding sequences from c-*fos* and the 3′-noncoding region from FBJ-MSV efficiently induces transformation in vitro and sarcomas in newborn mice (Miller et al., 1985). This finding demonstrates that no structural alterations in the coding region of c-*fos* are required to activate its transforming potential. The presence of a long terminal repeat (LTR), however, is not sufficient for the activation of c-*fos*. In addition, a 67-bp element in the 3′-noncoding region (123–189 bp upstream from the poly A addition site) must be deleted. It has also been shown that deletion of a 130-bp region of the C-terminal coding sequence has the same effect as the removal of the 67-bp element (Meijlink et al., 1985). The mechanism by which the latter region inhibits *fos* mRNA and protein expression may involve the formation of a mRNA hairpin structure.

c-*fos* expression is under stringent control not only at the transcriptional level (see earlier section on the anatomy of the c-*fos* promoter region), but also posttranscriptionally (Fort et al., 1987; Rahmsdorf et al., 1987). In serum-stimulated fibroblasts degradation of c-*fos* mRNA occurs extremely rapidly (half-life < 10 min), but is prevented by the protein synthesis inhibitor cycloheximide, suggesting that a labile protein (probably a nuclease) is involved in regulating c-*fos* mRNA turnover. The signal for c-*fos* mRNA degradation is located in the 3′-noncoding region containing AU-rich stretches previously identified as a RNA-destabilizing motif (Shaw and Kamen, 1986). Removal of this region from the c-*fos* gene significantly increases the half-life of its mRNA, thus leading to greatly increased steady-state levels of expression from constitutively transcribed *fos* genes (such as LTR-activated genes). Activation of the transforming potential of c-*fos* thus requires two alterations: (a) deregulation of transcription by addition of a constitutively active promoter/enhancer element (e.g., an LTR), and (b) the elimination of the recognition signal for RNA degradation. It would now be interesting to investigate whether the RNA-degrading mechanism is equally efficient in all cell types, since there are examples of cells which show a high constitutive expression of c-*fos* mRNA (Bravo et al., 1987; Müller et al., 1986).

Normally, as described above, c-*fos* is expressed at very low levels in fibroblasts, but is inducible by growth factors. This induction, however, does not lead to transformation, indicating that activation of the transforming potential of c-*fos* by disrupting the 3′ interaction is the result of a deregulation of *fos* expression. In addition, it has been shown that the induced c-*fos* protein is subject to more extensive posttranslational modification (mainly phosphorylation of serine residues) than the proteins expressed from transforming viral and cellular *fos* genes (Curran et al., 1984; Müller et al., 1987). It is possible, therefore, that the posttranslational modification of c-*fos* protein is part of a regulatory mechanism controlling its transforming potential. An intriguing finding in this context is the apparently inhibitory effect of phosphorylation on the binding of *fos* protein to DNA cellulose (Müller et al., 1987). This raises the possibility that phosphorylation may modulate the transforming potential (and perhaps other biological properties) of *fos* protein by interferring with its interaction with DNA or DNA-protein complexes.

Identification of Functional Domains in *fos* Protein

The analysis of a variety of terminal deletion mutants showed that rather long stretches at both the NH_2- and the COOH-terminal are functionally dispensable in the FBR-MSV *fos* protein (Jenuwein and Müller, 1987; Fig. 3). Thus, truncation of 39 NH_2-terminal amino acids did not detectably alter the biological properties of the protein, and truncation of 110 amino acids from the NH_2-terminal yielded a protein with strongly decreased but still detectable transforming activity. Likewise, truncation of 161 amino acids from the COOH-terminal of a FBJ-FBR hybrid caused an only relatively small reduction in biological activity. The truncation of further COOH-terminal sequences rendered the protein inactive. The functionally indispensable sequences in the protein can therefore be reduced to a region encompassing amino acids 111 to 219, representing 28% of the entire *fos* protein (Fig. 3). Such a truncated protein is, however, not functional, apparently—at least in part—due to lack of stability. The fusion with either

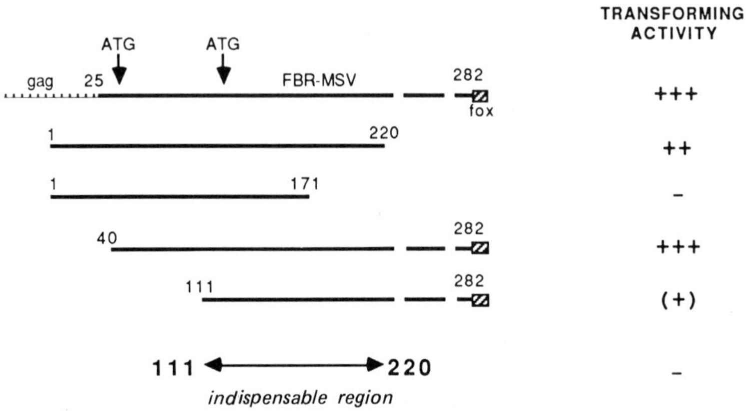

Figure 3 Deletion analyses of *fos* protein. The FBR-MSV protein was terminally truncated as indicated (using internal ATGs as start codons in the case of N-terminal truncations) and analyzed for focus induction and morphological transformation in 208F rat fibroblasts. + + +: Efficiency as wild type; + +: Efficiency reduced to approximately 30%; ±: No focus induction, but morphologically transformed colonies detectable after selection for G418-resistant cells (following transfer of constructs containing both the mutated *fos* gene and the *neo* gene); −: neither *fos* nor transformed G418-resistant colonies detectable. (Data from Jenuwein et al., 1987.)

NH_2- or COOH-terminal *fos* sequences is required for stable expression and biological activity. The functional importance of the center region in *fos* protein is emphasized by the evolutionary conservation of just this domain (see Fig. 4), which is identical between the mouse and the human, and 98% homologous between the mouse and the chicken (H. Mölders and R. Müller, in preparation). There are structurally interesting features in this region, including an acidic, a mixed-charged, and a strongly basic cluster of amino acids, leading to the prediction of a marked α-helical domain (Fig. 4).

The *fos* oncogenes of FBJ-MSV and FBR-MSV exhibit marked differences with respect to their biological properties. First, the *fos* gene product of FBR-MuSV ($p75^{gag\text{-}fos}$) is more efficient at inducing transformation in mouse connective tissue cells in vitro compared with the FBJ-MuSV gene product ($p55^{v\text{-}fos}$), and second, only $p75^{gag\text{-}fos}$ can trigger the immortalization of nonestablished cells (Jenuwein et al., 1985). Since $p55^{v\text{-}fos}$ and $p75^{gag\text{-}fos}$ are expressed at similar levels and show comparable turnover rates, the biological properties of the FBR-MuSV gene product appear to be directly related to its structural alterations. The analysis of a variety of $p55^{v\text{-}fos}/p75^{gag\text{-}fos}$ hybrid genes confirmed this conclusion (Jenuwein and Müller, 1987). Two rather subtle structural alterations were found to be largely responsible for the increased biological potential of the FBR-MSV gene

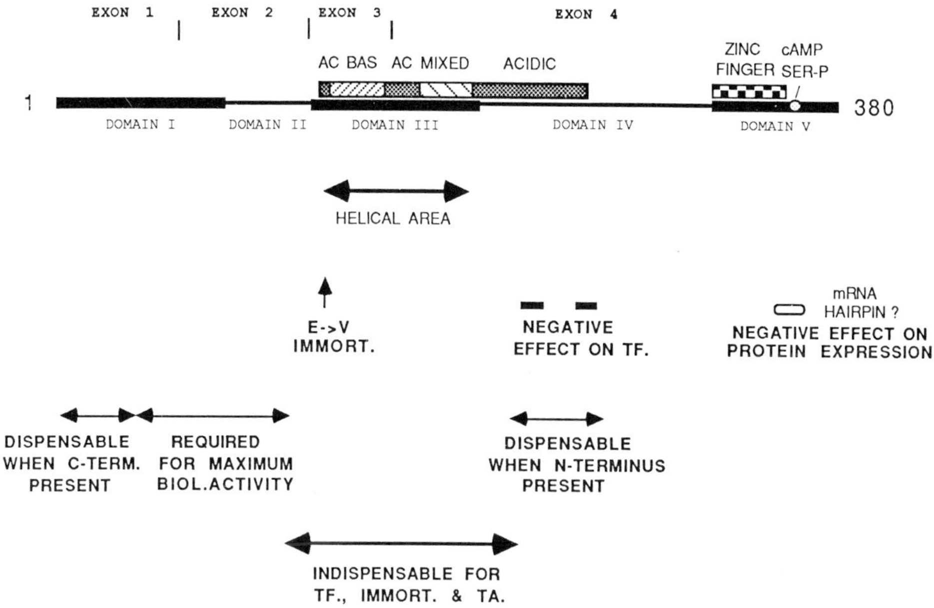

Figure 4 Structure-function analysis of *fos* protein. The top part of the figure shows the position of charged regions in *fos* protein (ac: acidic; bas: basic; mixed: mixed-charged), the Zn-finger motif and a potential serine phosphorylation site for a cAMP-dependent protein kinase, the α-helical stretch in the center, and the evolutionarily conserved domains. In the middle of the scheme, functionally important regions are indicated, including the position of E-138 where a substitution with valine activates the immortalizing potential of v-*fos* protein, sequences required for nuclear transport of *fos* protein, the position of the deletions in the FBR-MSV gene product which increase the transforming potential of *fos* and the potential mRNA hairpin structure at the C-terminal. At the bottom of the figure, functionally dispensable and indispensable regions are depicted as derived from the deletion analysis shown in Fig. 3. See text for details. Tf: transformation; TA: transactivation.

product: a single amino acid exchange (Glu to Val at position 138; Fig. 4) activates the immortalizing potential of v-*fos*, whereas two small internal in-frame deletions in the COOH-terminal half (Fig. 4) contribute to the increased transforming capacity of p75$^{gag\text{-}fos}$. The two internal deletions are located in a nonconserved region of the protein that is dispensable for its biological activity (Fig. 4), so that the significance of this observation is hard to assess. In contrast, the single amino acid change which activates the immortalizing potential of v-*fos* is located in a conspicuous region of the protein, where an acidic cluster of amino acids (Glu-Glu-Glu-Glu) is directly followed by a strongly basic region (Lys-Arg-Arg-Ile-Arg-Arg-Glu-Arg-Asp-Lys). The point mutation changes the last Glu (position 138) in the acidic cluster to Val. It is tempting to speculate that the Arg/Lys–rich region may interact with a substrate or cofactor, and that the point mutation changes these binding properties. Because of its basic character, this domain of *fos* protein represents a potential DNA-binding site, a hypothesis that remains to be investigated.

The functional importance of the highly charged, helical center region in *fos* protein is not only suggested by its evolutionary conservation, by the results of the deletion analysis, and the role of amino acid 138 in the activation of the immortalizing potential of *fos*, but also by the presence of sequences required for nuclear transport. (T. Jenuwein and R. Müller, in preparation). In addition, a limited homology of the center region with the yeast transcriptional activator protein GCN4 (Vogt et al., 1987) suggests that this domain is involved in the putative transregulatory function of *fos*.

THE *myb* GENE

Cell Transformation by v-*myb*

The v-*myb* gene has been identified as the oncogene of two independent isolates of chicken retroviruses, avian myeloblastosis virus (AMV), and avian leukemia virus E26 (E26) (Gonda et al., 1981; Leprince et al., 1983; Nunn et al., 1983; Roussel et al., 1979; Souza et al., 1980). Based on the isolation of transformation-defective temperature-sensitive mutants of both viruses (Beug et al., 1984; Moscovici and Moscovici, 1983), v-*myb* is thought to be responsible for the ability of AMV and E26 to transform myeloid cells in vivo and in vitro. The oncogenicity of v-*myb* appears to be restricted to myeloid cells, since AMV has not been observed to transform other cell types (Beug et al., 1979; Moscovici et al., 1975). E26 has a broader oncogenic spectrum and also transforms erythroid cells and fibroblasts (Graf et al., 1979; Moscovici et al., 1981, 1983; Radke et al., 1982); however, transformation of nonmyeloid cells by E26 is generally attributed to the v-*ets* sequences residing in the E26 genome (Leprince et al., 1983; Nunn et al., 1983). The molecular basis of the cell-type specificity of the transforming activity of v-*myb* is not known. The specificity does not seem to be due to an inability of AMV to infect nonmyeloid cells or express the v-*myb* protein in such cells. For example, it has been demonstrated that AMV can infect chicken fibroblasts and express the transforming protein in these cells (Klempnauer et al., 1984). There is also no correlation between cell transformation and the expression of the cellular progenitor (c-*myb*) of the viral *myb* genes. All major hematopoietic lineages express c-*myb* (see below), yet only myeloid cells are transformed.

c-*myb* Structure and Expression

In the past years, the c-*myb* gene has been cloned from several vertebrate species and from *Drosophila melanogaster* (Castle and Sheiness, 1985; Gonda and Bishop, 1983; Katzen et al., 1985; Lavu and Reddy, 1986; Majello et al., 1986). The architecture of the gene appears to be quite complex. In the mouse, where it has been characterized most thoroughly, the *myb* gene occupies approximately 40 kb and consists of at least 11 coding and an unknown number of noncoding exons (Lavu and Reddy, 1986). Mouse c-*myb* mRNA shows considerable heterogeneity at the 5′ end. The gene lacks a unique mRNA cap site; instead the RNAs start at one of a number of individual start sites clustered in a 1-kb region at the 5′ end of the gene (Bender and Kuehl, 1986; Watson et al., 1987). The structural analysis of c-*myb* and its oncogenic derivatives has allowed important insight into the mechanisms by which c-*myb* acquires transforming properties. In the transduced v-*myb* genes of AMV and E26 as well as in several murine tumors of myeloid origin, in which c-*myb* is altered by proviral integration, oncogenic activation of c-*myb* is accompanied by truncation of the coding region (Klempnauer et al., 1982; Nunn et al., 1983; Rosson et al., 1986; Shen-Ong et al., 1986; Weinstein et al., 1986). Interestingly, in the two independent viral isolates and in several of the murine tumors similar stretches of coding sequences have been deleted. It therefore appears likely that these truncations are important for the oncogenic activation of the *myb* gene.

c-*myb* is expressed at high levels in immature cells of various lineages of the hematopoietic system, including lymphoid, erythroid, and myeloid cells (Gonda et al., 1982; Sheiness and Gardinier, 1984; Westin et al., 1982a). In general, the most mature cells in these lineages express the lowest levels of c-*myb* mRNA. Consistent with this observation, a decrease in c-*myb* expression occurs in immature cells upon induction of differentiation by treatment with various agents (Craig and Block, 1984; Gonda and Metcalf, 1984; Westin et al., 1982). These observations suggest a role for c-*myb* in the proliferation of hematopoietic cells. The cell cycle dependence of c-*myb* has been studied in a number of cells. In some cells c-*myb* steady-state levels appear to be correlated with the cell cycle, presumably as a result of post-transcriptional control mechanisms (Thompson et al., 1986). For example, c-*myb* mRNA levels are highest in the late G1 and the early S phase of the cell cycle in a transformed chicken T-lymphoma cell line and in normal B lymphocytes. By contrast, in normal chicken thymocytes, which exhibit very high levels of c-*myb* mRNA, c-*myb* expression appears to be controlled at the transcriptional level and is independent of the cell cycle. The different patterns of c-*myb* expression suggest that c-*myb* may have multiple functions in the hematopoietic cell system.

For some time it was thought that c-*myb* functions exclusively in hematopoietic cells. Recently, however, expression of c-*myb* was also observed in quiescent fibroblasts following serum stimulation (Thompson et al., 1986). This observation raises the possibility that c-*myb* function is not restricted to hematopoietic cells. This view is also supported by the recent identification of a c-*myb* homologue in *Drosophila melanogaster* (Katzen et al., 1985). If c-*myb* had a function only in hematopoietic cells, the presence of a *myb* gene in vertebrates and insects would pose conceptual problems because the hematopoietic systems of these organisms differ substantially. It is therefore likely that, in addition to performing a specific role(s) in hematopoietic cells, c-*myb* is involved in cell proliferation in general.

The Proteins Encoded by v-*myb* and c-*myb*

The products of the v-*myb* genes of AMV and E26 and the chicken c-*myb* gene have been identified and their structural organization is well understood (Bister et al., 1982; Boyle et al., 1983; Klempnauer et al., 1982, 1983; Nunn et al., 1983). As indicated in Fig. 5, both v-*myb* genes encode extensively truncated versions of the 75,000-M_r c-*myb* protein. In the two viral gene products a central *myb* domain, lacking amino acid sequences from both the N-terminal and the C-terminal of c-*myb* protein, is fused to

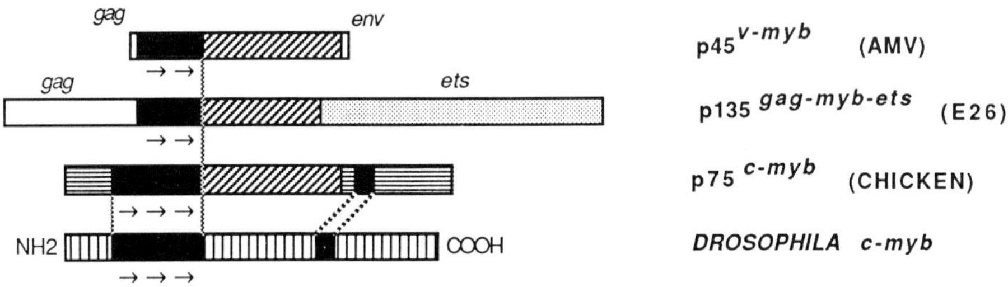

Figure 5 Comparison of v-*myb* proteins encoded by AMV ($p45^{v\text{-}myb}$) and E26 ($p135^{gag\text{-}myb\text{-}ets}$) and of proteins encoded by chicken c-*myb* ($p75^{c\text{-}myb}$) and *Drosophila* c-*myb*. Different regions of the proteins are represented by bars marked as follows:
- (solid) regions conserved between vertebrate and *Drosophila myb* proteins
- (hatched) chicken c-*myb* sequences transduced into retroviral genomes
- (horizontal lines) chicken c-*myb* sequences absent from retroviral genomes,
- (open) regions encoded by viral genes (*gag* or *env*),
- (stippled) region of $p135^{gag\text{-}myb\text{-}ets}$ encoded by v-*ets* sequences,
- (vertical lines) *Drosophila* c-*myb* sequences not homologous to vertebrate c-*myb* proteins

The arrows indicate the tandem repeats present in *myb* proteins.

different amino acid stretches derived from the retroviral *gag* or *env* genes (in the case of the 45-kd v-*myb* protein of AMV, p45$^{v\text{-}myb}$) or from the retroviral *gag* gene and the cell-derived v-*ets* gene (in the case of the 135-kd v-*myb* protein of E26, p135$^{gag\text{-}myb\text{-}ets}$) (Klempnauer et al., 1982, 1983; Nunn et al., 1983). The deletion of similar c-*myb* coding sequences in the two independent viral isolates provides strong evidence for a role of these truncations in the activation of the oncogenic potential of c-*myb*. In addition to the truncations, both v-*myb* proteins have undergone a number of amino acid substitutions. However, there are no substitutions common to AMV and E26. In contrast to the truncations described above, there is no evidence for a role of these substitutions in the oncogenic activation of c-*myb*.

Comparison of the amino acid sequences of the chicken, mouse, and human c-*myb* proteins (Gerondakis and Bishop, 1986; Gonda et al., 1985; Majello et al., 1986; Rosson and Reddy, 1986; Slamon et al., 1986) showed that these proteins, besides having a similar size and overall hydrophilic character, share a highly conserved region of approximately 200 amino acids located close to the N-terminal (see Fig. 5). This conserved domain, which presumably plays an important role in *myb* function, is composed of an interesting repetitive structure consisting of three imperfect tandem repeats of about 60 amino acids each (see Fig. 6). As indicated in Fig. 5, most of this conserved region (except the first half of the first of the three repeats) is present in both v-*myb* proteins. The importance of this conserved domain was further stressed by the recent identification of a *D. melanogaster* homologue of c-*myb* (Katzen et al., 1985). The *Drosophila myb* gene shows 73% homology with the repeat structure described above, whereas the surrounding sequences share no detectable homology to vertebrate *myb* proteins. The recent isolation and characterization of a

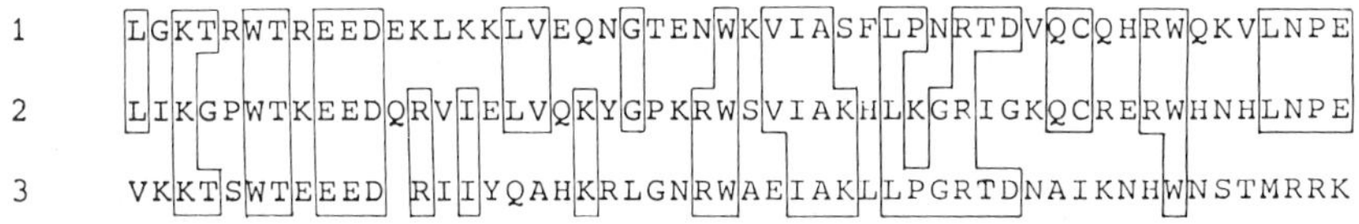

Figure 6 Tandem repeats at the N-terminal of the chicken c-*myb* protein. The amino acid sequence of the highly conserved N-terminal domain of the chicken c-*myb* protein (containing three tandem repeats) is shown in the single-letter amino acid code. Numbers mark the individual repeats. Amino acids identical in two or three of the repeats are boxed. A gap in repeat 3 was introduced to maximize the alignment.

Drosophila myb complementary deoxyribonucleic acid (cDNA) clone has revealed the presence of an additional short region of homology to vertebrate *myb* proteins, located close to the carboxyterminal of the protein (see Fig. 5) (C. Peters, A.E. Sippel, M. Vingron, and K.-H. Klempnauer, in press). Interestingly, this region of homology is absent from the two v-*myb* proteins. The possible role of C-terminal truncations in the oncogenic activation of c-*myb* suggests that the conserved carboxyterminal region is involved in an as yet unknown function of the protein required to control of the oncogenic potential of the protein.

Investigation of the biochemical properties of *myb* proteins has shown that despite the structural differences between v-*myb* and c-*myb* proteins, all *myb* gene products are located in the cell nucleus (Boyle et al., 1984; Klempnauer et al., 1984). The nucleotropism of these proteins is presumably determined by as yet unidentified sequences present in the 30,000-M_r central domain of c-*myb* shared by all *myb* gene products. A single case of nonnuclear location of a *myb* protein has been reported (Klempnauer et al., 1984a,b). Induction of differentiation of AMV-transformed myeloblasts by treatment with LPS and TPA is accompanied by transit of the v-*myb* protein from the cell nucleus to a perinuclear location. This observation is consistent with the view that nuclear location of v-*myb* proteins is required for transformation. The presence of the protein in the nucleus, however, is not sufficient for transformation to occur, since $p45^{v\text{-}myb}$ is expressed in the nuclei of AMV-infected chicken fibroblasts (Klempnauer et al., 1984), yet these cells are not transformed. Moreover, loss of nuclear location is no prerequisite for the temperature-induced differentiation of myeloblasts transformed by temperature-sensitive *myb* mutants of E26 (Moelling et al., 1985).

Subnuclear localization experiments have shown that v-*myb* and c-*myb* proteins are associated with several nuclear compartments such as nuclear matrix, chromatin, and nucleoplasm (Boyle et al., 1985; Klempnauer and Sippel, 1986). This might indicate that *myb* proteins have several nuclear targets and perform more than one function. However, the extent of association with various nuclear substructures varies substantially, depending on the exact conditions used to prepare nuclei. For example, the variations in the extent of nuclear matrix association seen by different investigators appear to be caused by a temperature-dependent insolubilization effect, also observed with *myc* proteins (Evan and Hancock, 1985). It is therefore presently difficult to give a precise picture of the subnuclear distribution of *myb* protein.

All known *myb* proteins have relatively short half-lives of approximately 30–60 min (Klempnauer et al., 1986). Metabolic instability seems to be a characteristic feature of a number of nuclear-transforming proteins, such as the products of c-*myc* (Hann and Eisenman, 1984), the adenovirus E1A region (Spindler and Berk, 1984) and the p53 gene (Reich et al., 1983) and suggests that these nuclear oncoproteins may be involved in regulatory processes.

DNA-Binding Properties of *myb* Proteins

v-*myb* and c-*myb* proteins exhibit DNA-binding activity in vitro (Klempnauer and Sippel, 1986; Klempnauer et al., 1986; Moelling et al., 1985). Since DNA binding was demonstrated for *myb* proteins purified by immunoaffinity chromatography (Moelling et al., 1985) or expressed in bacteria (Klempnauer and Sippel, in press), it is likely that DNA-binding activity is an intrinsic property of *myb* proteins and does not require interaction with other proteins.

Two additional lines of evidence suggest that *myb* protein function involves an interaction with DNA. First, it was observed that $p135^{gag\text{-}myb\text{-}ets}$ proteins encoded by transformation-defective temperature-sensitive mutants of E26 either lack DNA-binding activity in vitro or lose this activity at the nonpermissive temperature (Moelling et al., 1985). Second, inhibition of DNA binding by monoclonal antibodies to known epitopes of $p45^{v\text{-}myb}$ (Fig. 7) and analysis of DNA-binding activites of partially deleted v-*myb* proteins expressed in bacteria (Fig. 8) showed that the highly conserved sequences located at the aminoterminal of $p45^{v\text{-}myb}$ function as a DNA-binding domain (Klempnauer and Sippel, in press). By similar methods it was demonstrated that the corresponding region of the Drosophila *myb* protein also encodes a DNA-binding domain (C. Peters, A.E. Sippel, M. Vingron, and K.-H. Klempnauer, in press). The conservation of this region between *myb* proteins of different species and its ability to function as a DNA-binding domain lends strong support to the notion that *myb* proteins interact with DNA in vivo.

The precise role of DNA binding of *myb* function remains to be investigated. *myb* protein–DNA interaction might occur at specific sites in the genome, caused either by sequence-specific binding of the *myb* proteins themselves or by association of *myb* proteins with other factors which confer sequence specificity. In this respect, it is interesting that *myb* proteins can interact with specific regions on phage λ DNA which presumably contains degenerate versions of a binding site for *myb* protein (Bading et al., 1987; H. Biedenkapp, A.E. Sippel, and K.-H. Klempnauer, unpublished results). Alternatively, it is also possible that *myb* proteins do not interact with specific sites in the genome, but rather function as part of a DNA-traversing machinery (e.g., the replication or transcription complex). A detailed analysis of the DNA-binding properties of *myb* proteins and the identification of genes, whose expression changes in response to *myb*, will be crucial to distinguish between these possibilities.

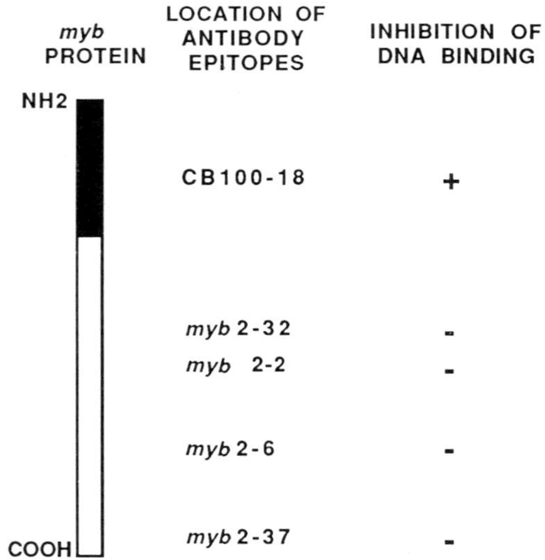

Figure 7 Inhibition of DNA binding of p45$^{v\text{-}myb}$ by monoclonal antibodies. The location of the epitopes of several *myb*-specific monoclonal antibodies (Evan et al., 1984; Klempnauer et al., 1986) and their ability to inhibit DNA-binding of p45$^{v\text{-}myb}$. The region shown as a black bar represents the highly conserved amino terminal doman of the v-*myb* protein.

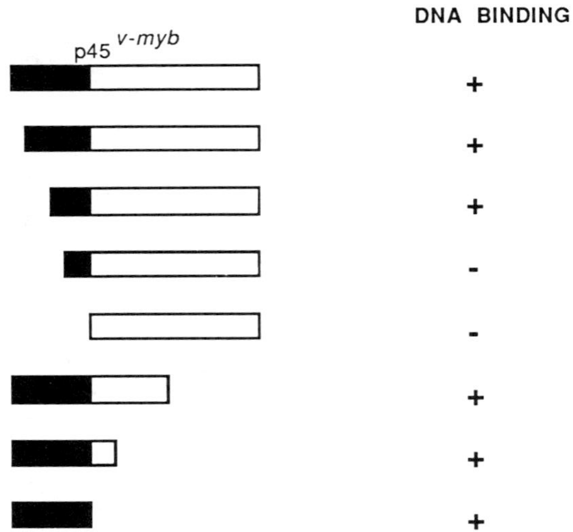

Figure 8 DNA-binding activity of deleted v-*myb* proteins. Full-length or deleted forms of p45$^{v\text{-}myb}$ are shown as horizontal bars. The region shown as a black bar represents the highly conserved N-terminal domain of p45$^{v\text{-}myb}$. All proteins were produced by bacterial expression and their ability to bind to DNA was analyzed by the "Southwestern" blotting technique.

THE *myc* GENE

Genomic Organization of Viral and Cellular *myc* Genes

The v-*myc* oncogene has been detected in four acute avian leukemia virus isolates, the myelocytomatosis virus MC29, originating from Bulgaria, the cytomatosis virus CMII from Germany, the OK10 strain found in Finland by Oker-Blom, and the Mill-Hill strain MH2 isolated in England. All of them induce a broad spectrum of malignancies, including myelocytomatosis, endotheliomas, liver and kidney carcinomas, and erythroblastosis in chickens and other fowl (Graf and Beug, 1978). A high incidence of liver carcinomas is observed in birds infected with MH2. This virulent strain appears to be particularly oncogenic. It contains besides v-*myc* a second oncogene, v-*mil*. The cooperation of these two oncogenes presumably increases the oncogenic potential of the virus. In vitro, viruses of the MC29 group transform fibroblasts of avian and mammalian origin. Bone marrow cells transformed in vitro resemble the immature myeloid cells observed in tumorigenesis in vivo (Graf and Beug, 1978).

The v-*myc* oncogenes are derived from the cellular chicken c-*myc* gene. It is composed of three exons separated by two intervening sequences, $intron_1$ and $intron_2$. The first exon is untranslatable, only $exon_2$ and $exon_3$ are coding and are transduced into all four viral isolates. The nucleotide sequences of the v-*myc* and chicken c-*myc* are very closely related and differ in MC29 and CMII in only five and seven amino acids, respectively, and in OK10 in only two. v-*myc* of MH2 differs in 27 amino acid substitutions and deletions of four codons. The three chicken c-*myc* exons have complexities of 340, 703, and 980 base pairs, respectively, encoding a protein of 416 amino acids. The structure of the mammalian c-*myc* genes is very similar to that of the chicken c-*myc* locus. The first noncoding exon of both human and mouse c-*myc* contains two active promoters, P_1 and P_2, 150 nucleotides apart (Battey et al., 1983; Cory et al., 1983). $Exon_1$ is untranslatable owing to the presence of multiple termination codons. $Exon_2$ with a complexity of 772 base pairs and $exon_3$ with 900, code for a protein of 439 amino acids. Sequence conservation between v-*myc* and c-*myc* genes is highest in $exon_3$ (Bernard et al., 1983). The noncoding first exons of human and murine c-*myc* genes exhibit about 70% homology in contrast to the first exon of the chicken v-*myc* which is unrelated (Linial and Groudine, 1985). The mammalian c-*myc*–derived mRNAs have complexities of 2.25 and 2.4 kilobases and differ at their 5′ ends, indicating that both promoter sites are used in transcription (Battey et al., 1983).

Recently, Bentley and Groudine (1986a) characterized in human cells two minor *myc*-RNA species of 2.5 and 3.2 kbp. Both are generated by differential splicing of transcripts initiated at a new promoter, P_0, located 0.6

kbp upstream of P_1, and use the same polyadenylation site as the regular c-*myc* RNAs. Unlike P_1 and P_2, P_0 does not have a TATAA box and gives rise to RNAs of 5′ heterogeneity. The 2.5-kbp species exhibits two open reading frames (ORF) coding for a 114 amino acid peptide of unknown function in addition to the c-*myc* protein of 439 amino acids. The 3.2-kbp species has three ORFs coding for two putative extra peptides of 114 and 188 amino acids in addition to the 439–amino acid c-*myc* protein. Synthesis of an extra 188–amino acid peptide from an ORF in human c-*myc* $exon_1$ has also been proposed by Gazin et al. (1984) on the basis of sequencing data, and was recently identified in HeLa cells (Gazin et al., 1986). Existence of this $exon_1$-coded protein raises questions about the evolution of the c-*myc* gene and the divergence of $exon_1$. In contrast to the human $exon_1$, the corresponding murine and chicken exons are clearly noncoding. Whether other parts of the genome take over the role of a missing $exon_1$ coded protein as suggested by Gazin et al. (1986) needs to be demonstrated. In any event, the persistence of a noncoding $exon_1$ at the c-*myc* locus in all species suggests that it may carry some important regulatory elements independent of a coding capacity. $Exon_1$ is likely to play an essential role in regulation of c-*myc* expression by either binding molecules which regulate transcription or by posttranscriptional mechanisms. The activating event crucial for tumorigenicity of c-*myc* involves truncation of $exon_1$, which in the oncogenic viruses is replaced by viral LTRs. In Burkitt's lymphoma (BL) truncation of $exon_1$ is achieved by chromosomal translocations which replace $exon_1$ by immunoglobulin (Ig) gene control elements (Haluska et al., 1983).

The Protein Products

Analyses of *myc* gene products have predominantly been performed with v-*myc*–transformed cells in which expression is about 100-fold higher than in normal cells or human tumor cell lines. In small cell lung cancer cells (SCLC) for instance, the c-*myc* protein level is only about 0.001% of the total cellular protein content in spite of highly amplified c-*myc* DNA sequences (Moelling et al., 1986). Most analyses have been carried out with the MC29-coded *gag-myc* fusion protein $p110^{gag\text{-}myc}$, but no significant difference in function can be detected between this protein and $p90^{gag\text{-}myc}$ of CMII, $p200^{gag\text{-}pol\text{-}myc}$ of OK10, or $p61^{v\text{-}myc}$ of MH2 (for review, see Moelling, 1985). All viral *myc* proteins are phosphoproteins containing phosphoserine and phosphothreonine. Cell fractionation and immunofluorescence analysis have indicated that *myc* is a nuclear protein (Alitalo et al., 1983; Donner et al., 1982; Hann et al., 1983). In dividing cells most of the *myc* protein diffuses out of the nucleus into the cytoplasm (Winquist et al., 1984). Only a small proportion of the protein was detected in chromatin preparations (< 20%) (Bunte et al., 1982). Two forms of c-*myc* protein (p65/p67) have been identified which, however, do not differ in their degree of phosphorylation (Evan and Hancock, 1985; Hann and Eisenmann et al., 1984; Persson and Leder, 1984), suggesting that p65 and p67 may differ in their primary structure. Avian v-*myc* and human c-*myc* proteins show a discrepancy between their predicted molecular mass and their migration behavior on SDS polyacrylamide gels, which may be due to unusual structural features of the protein, such as high proline content and clustering of basic residues in the carboxyterminal domain.

Association of the *myc* protein with the nuclear matrix (Hann et al., 1983) has been shown to be a consequence of experimental conditions (exposure of isolated nuclei to 38 °C). Rather, the *myc* protein belongs to a discrete subset of nuclear proteins that can be extracted at low salt concentrations (Evan and Hancock, 1985). In contrast to *fos* and *myb* proteins, *myc* is not readily released from nuclei by DNase treatment, suggesting different intranuclear molecular interactions (Lorenz and Moelling, unpublished observation). The purified v-*myc* and c-*myc* proteins bind to double-stranded DNA in vitro (Beimling et al., 1985; Donner et al., 1982; Persson and Leder, 1984). Recent evidence indicated a preferential binding of v-*myc* and c-*myc* protein to specific cellular DNA sequences next to the LTR integration site of the MC29 provirus (Moelling et al., 1986). Bacterially expressed c-*myc* protein binds to DNA but does not exhibit any sequence specificity (Watt et al., 1985). Whether this reflects an intrinsic property of *myc* protein, or is due to conformational differences, or to the absence of phosphorylation remains to be investigated. Interestingly, the *myc* proteins of the three nontransforming MC29-deletion mutants exhibit a reduced ability to bind to DNA in vitro (Donner et al., 1983), suggesting a role of nucleic acid interaction in transformation. A subfraction of the viral *myc* protein of about 5% was found to be tightly bound to DNA resisting extraction of 2M NaCl. Molecular cloning of this DNA did not result in a specific DNA fragment (Lorenz and Moelling, unpublished observation).

Recent analyses have pointed out two alternative functions of the *myc* protein. According to Spector et al. (1987), the *myc* protein colocalizes in situ with small nuclear ribonucleoprotein particles. Although this finding may suggest a function for c-*myc* in posttranscriptional regulatory processes, the significance of this colocalization remains to be shown. In an alternative approach, Watt and her collaborators have shown the *myc* protein to be involved in DNA replication (Studzinski et al., 1986). These observations raise the possibility that *myc* protein may have more than one function.

In two recent studies functional regions were mapped in the MC29 v-*myc* and the human c-*myc* coding regions by site-directed mutagenesis

(Heaney et al., 1986, Stone et al., 1987; see Fig. 9). These investigators determined the effects of mutations on the nuclear localization of the protein and its capacity to cooperate with *ras* in the transformation of nonestablished rat fibroblasts. The results indicate that a conserved region in the middle of $exon_2$ (amino acids 105–143) and the half of $exon_3$ (321–439) are essential for transformation and contain at least two sequences required for nuclear localization. The N-terminal of the protein is also required for transformation, but sequences of 10–40 amino acids can be deleted at any position in this region without destroying the transforming potential of the protein. This suggests that the N-terminal does not provide any crucial functions, but is rather required for expression of a stable protein or acquisition of a favorable conformation. Interestingly, transformation of hematopoietic chicken cells (macrophages) depends on an additional small residue of 11 amino acids in the central part (239–249) (see Fig. 9).

Regulation of c-*myc* Expression

Since no significant functional differences in the c-*myc* and v-*myc* coded protein products have been detected so far, even in proteins which differ in

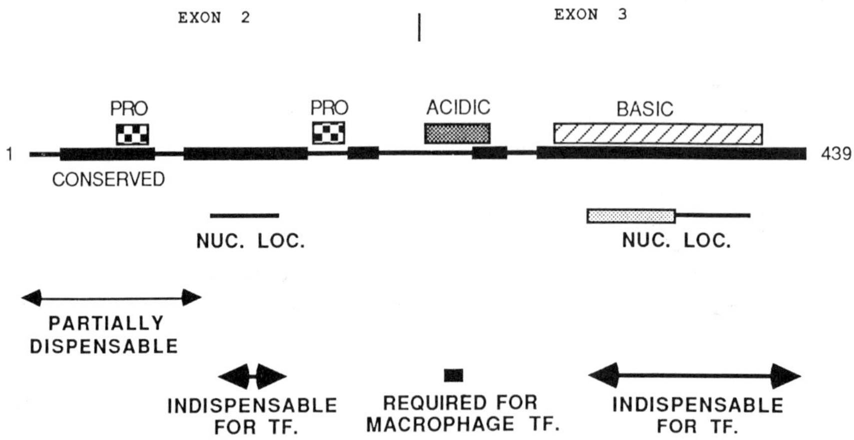

Figure 9 Structure-function analysis of *myc* protein. The top part of the scheme shows the location of prolin-rich stretches in chicken c-*myc*, charged clusters of amino acids, and evolutionarily conserved domains. The position of sequences required for nuclear localization is shown below, the boxed area harboring a major signal sequence. Functionally indispensable regions are shown at the bottom. See text for details. Tf: transformation.

27 amino acids, activation of transforming potential of the c-*myc* proto-oncogene seems to be associated with changes in the mode of its expression. It has been shown that expression of the c-*myc* gene is subject to both transcriptional as well as posttranscriptional regulation (see Fig. 10). Various groups have recently analyzed transcriptional regulation by in vitro elongation of nascent RNA transcripts in isolated nuclei (run-on experiments). The c-*myc* gene can be down-regulated at the transcriptional level by inhibition at P_1 and P_2, which is responsible for allelic exclusion taking place in some plasmacytomas and BLs (Bentley and Groudine, 1986a; Fahrlander et al., 1985). Furthermore, a block in elongation has been observed in differentiated HL60 cells (Bentley and Groudine, 1986b). The density of RNA polymerase II molecules is not constant throughout the entire span of the transcribed gene, suggesting that there is a more or less stable block of elongation. $Exon_1$ appears more heavily loaded with polymerase II than any other region of the coding strand (Bentley et al., 1986b; Nepveu and Marcu, 1986). It is not known whether this higher polymerase density results from a pause in elongation or from premature termination near the end of $exon_1$. Discontinuous transcription appears to be regulated by a secondary structure of the RNA which prevents elongation and also by short-lived proteins, since inhibitors of protein synthesis can partially release this block (for review, see Piechaczyk et al., 1987). A complex block of elongation at the end of $exon_1$ can develop during in vitro differentiation of human promyelocytic HL60 cells into granulocytes

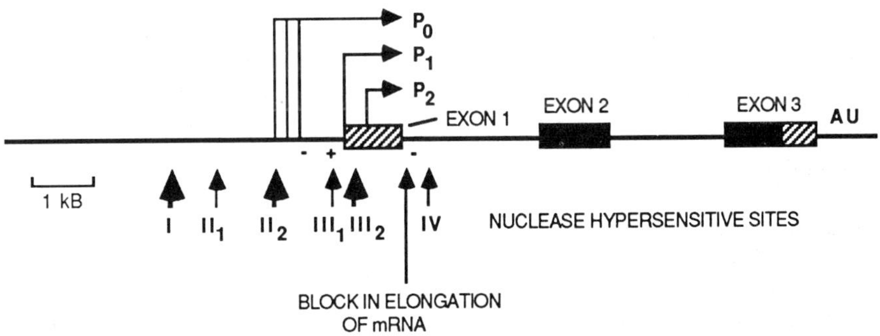

Figure 10 Regulatory regions in the human c-*myc* gene. P_0, P_1, P_2: transcription initiation sites. The heterogeneity of transcripts starting at P_0 is symbolized by a tripled line. DNase I–hypersensitive sites are numbered as described by Siebenlist et al. (1984). AU indicates the region of mRNA instability. (−) and (+) represent positive and negative regulatory elements (Chung et al., 1968).

(Bentley and Groudine, 1986b; Eick and Bornkamm, 1986) and of mouse Friend erythroleukemia cells into red blood cells (Mechti et al., 1986). Block in elongation of transcription can also occur in $intron_1$ in human lymphoid cells treated with butyrate (Blanchard et al., 1985). Transcription has also been observed in the antisense direction. In human cells antisense transcription has been detected only upstream of P_1, but in mouse cells the c-*myc* locus appears to be made up of several antisense transcription units (Nepveu and Marcu, 1986; Mechti et al., 1986). The role of antisense transcription of c-*myc* is so far totally unknown.

The identification of several DNase I–hypersensitive sites in c-*myc* chromatin (see Fig. 10), some of which are dependent on the transcriptional state of the gene (Siebenlist et al., 1984), suggest that c-*myc* is probably controlled by different regulatory factors. Various groups have reached the conclusion that the complex c-*myc* promoter region is regulated via the cooperation of positively and negatively acting factors (for review, see Piechaczyk et al., 1987). Using c-*myc*–CAT hybrid genes and cotransfection of competing DNA fragments from putative control regions, measurement of CAT activity allowed the identification of positive and negative regulatory elements, most of which did not correspond to DNase I–hypersensitive sites (Remmers et al., 1986; Yang et al., 1986).

Expression of the c-*myc* gene is regulated also at the posttranscriptional as well as the posttranslational level. Both its protein and its mRNA are very short lived (15–30 min) (Beimling et al., 1985; Dani et al., 1985; Hann and Eisenmann, 1984). The rate and turnover throughout the various stages of the cell cycle appears to be constant (Hann et al., 1985). Inhibition of protein synthesis in most cell types results in a dramatic stabilization of c-*myc* mRNA and increase of protein level (Dani et al., 1985; Kelly et al., 1983). This suggests that the controlling element is itself a protein involved in mRNA turnover (perhaps a ribonuclease). The finding that the translational efficiency of c-*myc* mRNA is 10-fold higher with transcripts starting at P_2 compared to P_1 transcripts (Darveau et al., 1985) raised the possibility that these two transcripts differ in their stability. However, recent experiments suggested that absence of $exon_1$ leads to a higher stability of the c-*myc* mRNA (Butnick et al., 1985; Rabbitts, 1985).

The various translocations of c-*myc* in BLs and plasmacytomas, mostly affecting $exon_1$, offer the opportunity to test how the 5′ sequence influences RNA stability. However, when the 5′ $exon_1$ was appended to a globin mRNA it did not confer increased instability (Piechaczyk et al., 1986), suggesting that $exon_1$ alone is not responsible for mRNA instability. Furthermore, naturally occurring transcripts of high stability bearing an unaltered $exon_1$ have been described (Eick and Bornkamm, 1986), and indicate that additional sequences must affect mRNA degradation. Chimeric constructs in which the 3 ′ noncoding region of c-*myc* mRNA was appended to otherwise stable transcripts resulted in their destabilization (Piechaczyk et al., 1986). This is in agreement with a recently identified AU-rich region at the 3 ′ end of an unstable mRNA which confers instability to other genes (Shaw and Kamen, 1986). Very similar motifs can be found in various unstable mRNAs, including c-*myc* and c-*fos*.

Comparison of the sequences of unstable protein suggest the existence of specific features which might be responsible for rapid protein degradation. A so-called PEST region, rich in proline, glutamic acid, serine, and threonine, has been identified by Rogers et al. (1986). This region is generally flanked by clusters of positively charged amino acids in 10 unstable proteins, including c-*myc*, c-*fos*, and Ela.

Physiological Role of c-*myc*

It is a widely held notion that the c-*myc* gene product is an intranuclear mediator of the cellular response to growth factors (Armclin et al., 1984; Kaczmarek et al., 1985; Kelly et al., 1983; Rapp et al., 1985). The c-*myc* mRNA level was first reported to increase rapidly following the treatment of different cell types with growth-inducing components (Kelly et al., 1983). Within 1 hr of growth stimulation, the steady-state level of c-*myc* mRNA shows an approximately 20-fold increase followed by a slow decrease, reaching basal levels of expression at about 18 hr. Even though c-*myc* mRNA accumulation is an early event, it is preceded by the even more dramatic induction of c-*fos* (Greenberg and Ziff, 1984; Kelly et al., 1983; Müller et al., 1984) Purified growth factors, such as epidermal growth factor (EGF), fibroblast growth factor (FGF), and platelet-derived growth factor (PDGF), have proven to be as efficient at increasing c-*myc* mRNA levels in quiescent NIH3T3 fibroblasts as 10% fetal calf serum (Müller et al., 1984). The accumulation of c-*myc* mRNA in response to growth factor stimulation seems largely to be due to mRNA accumulation rather than to an increase in the transcription rate (Blanchard et al., 1985).

In contrast to c-*fos*, c-*myc* mRNA is expressed at readily detectable levels at all stages of the cell cycle in chicken fibroblasts as well as in human lymphocytes, leukemia cells, and HeLa cells, suggesting that the c-*myc* product plays a role in normally cycling cells (Hann et al., 1985; Rabbitts et al., 1985; Thompson et al., 1985). The level of expression during the cell cycle is, however, lower than in growth factor–stimulated cells. Other evidence for a role of the c-*myc* product in normal cell proliferation is that its expression is high in growing asynchronous cells and very low in quiescent cells. Serum deprivation of asynchronous cultures for a period as short as 2 hr leads to a dramatic decrease in the level of c-*myc* mRNA, indicating that the constant presence of external growth factors is required to sustain the expression of c-*myc* at high levels (Bravo and Müller, 1986).

Quiescent mouse fibroblasts (3T3) briefly exposed to PDGF or FGF become "competent" to synthesize DNA (Stiles et al., 1979). The addition of platelet-poor plasma lacking PDGF allows these cells to progress through G_1 and enter the S phase (Stiles et al., 1979). The observation that induction of c-*myc* and c-*fos* expression is among the earliest events following growth factor stimulation led to their definition as competence genes. This is in agreement with the observation that c-*myc* protein, either microinjected or expressed from an inducible transfected construct, partially abrogates the PDGF requirement of quiescent mouse fibroblasts for growth (Armelin et al., 1984; Kazmarek et al., 1985). The persistence of competence, however, cannot solely be achieved by these proto-oncogenes, since competence lasts about 16 hr (Bravo and Müller, 1986)—far too long compared to the half-lives of both products, which is about 30–60 min only. Abrogation by *myc* expression of growth factor requirements has also been observed in hematopoietic cells; e.g., after infection of lymphoid cells with a v-*myc* containing retrovirus (Rapp et al., 1985).

Further information of the role of c-*myc* in normal cells was provided by analyses of c-*myc* suppression. c-*myc* is turned off in HL60 cells induced to granulocytic differentiation by dimethylsulfoxide (DMSO) (Bentley and Groudine, 1986b; Westin et al., 1982b), or in teratocarcinoma cells treated with retinoic acid leading to endodermal differentiation (Campisi et al., 1984; Dony et al., 1985). Tumor necrosis factor (TNF) as well as interferon (IF), both of which act as growth inhibitors on HeLa cells, cause an inhibition of c-*myc* transcription in these cells (Yarden and Kimchi, 1986). Similarly, Friend cells which can be induced to differentiation by DMSO treatment exhibit down-regulation of c-*myc* expression. The reverse is also true. Constitutive expression of c-*myc* prevents differentiation (Prochownik and Kukowska, 1986). In essence, these studies indicate that in a variety of cell types c-*myc* is turned off when cells enter a resting state (G_0) a situation which can be created by application of growth inhibitors such as TNF or IF, but also during differentiation, a process which in many cell types involves reduced proliferative activity.

Tumorigenic Potential of c-*myc*

Transformed cells differ from normal cells in that they show elevated and deregulated (constitutive) expression of c-*myc* (Campisi et al., 1984). Activation of c-*myc* in tumor cells is achieved by different molecular mechanisms, including (a) deregulation of c-*myc* expression in virally transformed cells by the presence of the viral transcriptional control elements;

(b) truncation of $exon_1$ and replacement by regulatory elements as a consequence of chromosomal translocations, e.g., with an Ig locus in Burkitt's lymphoma (Haluska et al., 1983); and (c) amplification of the c-*myc* gene in human tumor cells such as small cell cancer of the lung and colon tumors (Erisman et al., 1985; Little et al., 1983; Moelling et al., 1986). The presence of activated c-*myc* genes in human tumors suggested that c-*myc* may play a role in tumor development. To investigate this role, several groups produced transgenic mice expressing MMTV-LTR-*myc* or Ig-*myc* fusion genes (Adams et al., 1985; Steward et al., 1984). These mice developed tumors of monoclonal origin after long latency periods in a variety of tissues, including mammary gland (MMTV-*myc*) and B cells (Ig-*myc*). The monoclonality of the tumor cells and the long time required for tumor growth to occur suggest that elevated c-*myc* expression is insufficient for tumor formation unless additional cooperating functions, e.g., as a result of "spontaneous" proto-oncogene activation, are supplied.

The picture of the role of c-*myc* which has emerged indicates that c-*myc* expression is associated with dividing cells and drops as cells enter the resting state. Constitutive *myc* expression above a certain threshold may promote cell division and inhibit differentiation. c-*myc* expression will therefore increase the proportion of cells that are less mature and have greater proliferative capacity. Any accidental event affecting growth control mechanisms may therefore create a malignant tumor of clonal origin.

THE *erb*A GENE

v-*erb*A-Containing Avian Retroviruses: Introduction

The avian erythroblastosis virus strain ES4 (AEV-ES4) was first isolated in 1933 by Engelbreth-Holm (Rothe-Meyer and Engelbreth-Holm, 1933). Early virus isolates were only weakly oncogenic and caused exclusively erythroleukemia, but repeated passaging in chickens and selection for highly oncogenic variants yielded an acutely oncogenic virus that caused sarcomas and fatal leukemias within 2 weeks after injection. Systematic analysis on the AEV virus became possible in 1976 when Graf and Beug (Graf et al., 1976) could transform chicken embryo fibroblasts and bone marrow cells in vitro.

Early molecular work revealed that the AEV-ES4 genome contains two oncogenes, denoted v-*erb*A and v-*erb*B (Anderson et al., 1980; Hayman et al., 1983; Lai et al., 1980; Privalsky et al., 1983; Sheiness et al., 1981; Vennström et al., 1980; Vennström and Bishop, 1982). The v-*erb*A gene is fused to part of the *gag* gene, and is therefore expressed as a 75-kD *gag*–v-*erb*A hybrid protein ($P75^{gag\text{-}v\text{-}erbA}$; Hayman et al., 1979). The v-*erb*B gene is translated from a subgenomic mRNA and yields a heterogeneous set of membrane-associated glycosylated proteins of 66, 68, and 74 kD in molecular weight (Hayman and Beug, 1984; Hayman et al., 1983; Privalsky and Bishop, 1984; Privalsky et al., 1984). However, initiation of translation for the protein takes place at an AUG located in the retroviral RNA leader sequence, and the resulting protein consequently contains six *gag*-derived amino acids in its N-terminus (M. Jansson and B. Vennström, unpublished data). v-*erb* proteins with identical N-termini were subsequently found in several retroviruses isolated from RAV-1–infected, leukemic chicks, in which part of the c-*erb*B locus was activated by integration of the viral genome (Beug et al., 1986; Fung et al., 1983; Gamett et al., 1986; Miles and Robinson, 1985; Nilsen et al., 1985; Raines et al., 1985; Tracy et al., 1985). Since all these new isolates lack v-*erb*A, it is conceivable that v-*erb*A was aquired by AEV-ES4 during selection for enhanced oncogenicity of a preexisting virus strain containing only v-*erb*B.

The cellular c-*erb*A and c-*erb*B loci are located on distinct chromosomes both in the chicken and human genomes, but were syntenic in the mouse genome (Dayton et al., 1984; Spurr et al., 1984; Symonds et al., 1984a; Zabel et al., 1984). Recently, the functions of both of the cellular *erb* genes have been identified: c-*erb*B encodes the receptor for epidermal growth factor (Downward et al., 1984; Ullrich et al., 1984), whereas the c-*erb*A protein is a nuclear receptor for thyroid hormone (Sap et al., 1986; Weinberger et al., 1986; see below).

Activation of the c-*erb*A Gene: Biochemical Properties of c-*erb*A and v-*erb*A

First clues as to the possible functions of v-*erb*A came from its homology to receptors for steroid hormones (Hollenberg et al., 1985; Krust et al., 1986; Weinberger et al., 1985). The highest amino acid homology (45%) is located in the putative DNA-binding region (Fig. 11), which contains many conserved cysteins and positively charged residues, the spacing of which is compatible with a Zn-finger structure. Identification of the c-*erb*A gene as a nuclear receptor for thyroid hormone became possible by expressing a c-*erb*A cDNA clone in a combined in vitro transcription/translation system using T_7 polymerase and rabbit reticulocyte lysate. Subsequent binding studies using iodinated thyroid hormones (triiodothyronine, T_3; thyroxine, T_4) clearly demonstrated that c-*erb*A binds T_3 and T_4 with affinities identical to those found previously for nuclear thyroid hormone receptors (Sap et al., 1986; Weinberger et al., 1986).

Nucleotide sequence comparison between the viral and cellular *erb*A genes revealed several amino acid differences between the encoded proteins. (a) The 5′ untranslated region of the c-*erb*A gene is unusual in that it contains several short open reading frames flanked by start and stop codons,

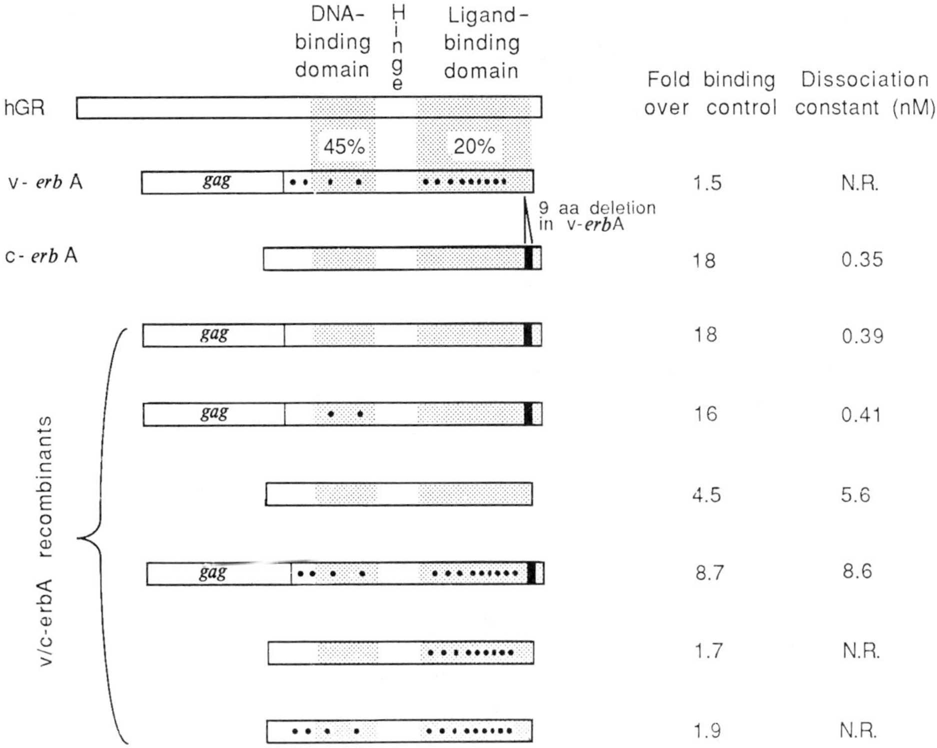

Figure 11 Comparison of the human glucocorticoid receptor to the v-*erb*A protein, of the *erb*A domains of the viral and cellular proteins, and thyroid hormone–binding properties of chimeric v/c-*erb*A proteins. The black dots in v-*erb*A indicate the positions of point mutations. Hormone binding was measured by coretention on nitrocellulose filters of protein-hormone complexes formed at a ligand concentration of 1nM[^{125}I]-T_3, and by Scatchard analysis.

whereas this whole region is removed in v-*erb*A because of its fusion to *gag* sequences. This is probably important for overexpression of the v-*erb*A protein in transformed cells, since the original c-*erb*A cDNA is only expressed at low levels in transfected cells, whereas modified c-*erb*A clones lacking part of the 5′ untranslated sequences are expressed at much higher levels (A. Muñoz and B. Vennström, unpublished data). (b) v-*erb*A contains 13 amino acid substitutions, of which two are located in the putative DNA-binding domain and 11 in other regions (see Fig. 11). (c) the v-*erb*A protein has suffered a nine amino acid internal deletion located three amino acids before the C-terminus. (d) the N-terminus of the c-*erb*A polypeptide is 12 amino acids longer than the *erb*A-specific part of the v-*erb*A protein, since the latter is fused to *gag* at this position. This fusion was probably mediated by a nucleotide sequence homologous to both c-*erb*A and the viral *gag* gene.

The thyroid hormone receptor is known to either positively or negatively regulate the expression of a wide variety of genes, presumably by interaction with their respective promoter regions upon T_3 binding, in a manner similar to those of steroid receptors (for review, see Oppenheimer and Samuels, 1983). Binding studies using v-*erb*A expressed in vitro or in vivo have shown that it has completely lost its ability to bind T_3 and T_4. However, the v-*erb*A protein still binds to DNA on cellulose columns, and elutes at salt concentrations between 0.2 and 0.4 M; i.e. it binds to DNA with an affinity similar to that of thyroid hormone receptor (U. Gehring and H.B., unpublished; McLeod and Baxter, 1976).

To identify the mutations in v-*erb*A that are responsible for its inability to bind hormone, a series of recombinants between the viral and cellular genes has been constructed utilizing restriction sites common to both genes (Fig. 11). Subsequent ligand binding experiments with in vitro synthesized protein has shown that all the proteins having the entire ligand binding domain from v-*erb*A fail to bind hormone. Insertion of the nine amino acid deletion from the C-terminus of v-*erb*A into c-*erb*A considerably diminish but do not completely abolish ligand binding; likewise, reconstitution of the C-terminus of v-*erb*A with that of c-*erb*A increases binding but does not fully restore it to *wt* c-*erb*A levels. Only proteins with the complete ligand binding domain from c-*erb*A bind hormone at high levels. The contribution of the C-terminal deletion versus the point mutations in the *erb*A ligand binding domain to loss of hormone binding has been further elucidated by Scatchard analysis of those chimeric proteins that bind hormone. Both the internal point mutations and the nine amino acid C-terminal deletion alone result in T_3 dissociation constants about 10-fold higher than found for proteins containing the entire c-*erb*A ligand binding domain, indicating that both types of mutations contribute to the loss of T_3 binding in v-*erb*A. In contrast, neither the *gag* region nor the mutations in the DNA-binding region affect the affinity for ligand.

A Family of Related c-*erb*A/Thyroid Hormone Receptor Genes with Distinct Tissue Specifity?

Early work on the identification of human cellular *erb*A genes already suggested the existence of at least two genes with homology to v-*erb*A (Jansson et al., 1983). Recently, additional genes encoding thyroid hormone receptors have been identified and mapped on the human genome. Taken together, the gene most closely homologous to v-*erb*A is located on chromosome 17 (Dayton et al., 1984; Spurr et al., 1984; Zabel et al., 1984), whereas two slightly more distantly related genes reside on chromosome 3 (Weinberger et al., 1986; R. Evans, personal communication). One of the genes on chromosome 3 appears to be preferentially expressed in brain and pituitary tissues, whereas two other genes are expressed at low levels in many types of cells. One additional *erb*A cross-hybridizing sequence has been found on both chromosomes 3 and 17; however, their relatedness to thyroid hormone receptors is as yet unclear (N. K. Spurr, pers. communication; Weinberger et al., 1986). Finally, Dejean et al. (1986) have characterized a gene the transcription of which apparently has been activated by an integrated hepatitis B viral genome in liver tumors. Also, this gene maps to human chromosome 3; however, its amino acid sequence is only about 40% homologous to that of human c-*erb*A, and the encoded protein does not bind thyroid hormones (A. Dejean, personal communication).

v-*erb*A Cooperates with Growth-Promoting Oncogenes in Erythroblast Transformation

The v-*erb*B oncogene as well as a variety of other tyrosine kinase oncogenes (v-*src*, v-*fps*, v-*yes*, v-*sea* and v-*fms*), the serine kinase v-*mil*, and the guanosine diphosphate (GDP)–binding protein v-Ha-*ras* cause the outgrowth of transformed immature erythroid cells from infected bone marrow (Beug et al., 1985a,b; Graf et al., 1976; Kahn et al., 1984; Stanley et al., manuscript in preparation; U. Fuhrmann, and H. Beug, unpublished data), and some of them (v-*erb*B, v-*sea*) cause a mild leukemia in chicks (Beug et al., 1985a; Frykberg et al., 1983; Sealy et al., 1983; Yamamoto et al., 1983). Despite their biochemical diversity, all these oncogenes induce a common transformed phenotype in infected erythroid progenitors: They are induced to self-renew extensively, and are rendered independent of the normal erythroid growth factor erythropoietin. A certain fraction of the transformed erythroblasts, however, undergoes spontaneous differentiation into erythrocytes, again in a hormone-independent manner. Finally, the transformed erythroblasts have rather narrow pH – and ion concentration ranges permitting proliferation in vitro, and cannot be cultivated in most ordinary tissue culture media (Kahn et al., 1986a).

Although the v-*erb*A oncogene has no detectable oncogenic potential of its own in chicks and exhibits no striking effects on fibroblasts or bone marrow cells infected in vitro (Frykberg et al., 1983; Sealy et al., 1983), a number of distinct and measurable effects have been observed upon introduction of v-*erb*A into transformed erythroblasts. (a) v-*erb*A completely blocks spontaneous differentiation of erythroblasts transformed with all growth promoting oncogenes tested so far (Beug et al., 1985b; Frykberg et al., 1983; Kahn et al., 1986a). (b) v-*erb*A enables transformed erythroblasts to grow in normal tissue culture media (Kahn et al., 1986a,b). (c) v-*erb*A restores the erythroblast-transforming potential of transformation-defective v-*erb*B mutants (Damm et al., 1987; Jansson et al., 1987) and enables the non-transforming human EGF-receptor/c-*erb*B gene to transform avian erythroblasts (Khazaie et al., manuscript in preparation). And finally, v-*erb*A causes the sarcoma-inducing oncogene v-*src* to induce rapid fatal erythroleukemia in chicks (Kahn et al., 1986a). In summary, v-*erb*A effectively cooperates with a variety of nonrelated, growth-promoting oncogenes by strongly enhancing their ability to transform erythroid cells in vitro and in vivo.

A Point Mutation in v-*erb*A Affects Its Biological Activity in Erythroblasts

A particularly clear example of how v-*erb*A cooperates with v-*erb*B in erythroblast transformation and how this activity of v-*erb*A could be affected by mutation, comes from the analysis of *td*359 AEV, a transformation-defective mutant of AEV unable to transform erythroblasts, and its revertant (*r*12), obtained after in vivo passage of the *td*359 mutant (Damm et al., 1987). Nucleotide sequence analysis demonstrates that the v-*erb*A protein of *td*359 contains among other substitutions one amino acid change (proline to arginine) located in the short "hinge" region (Fig. 12) at position 144. The v-*erb*A protein of *r*12 has reverted to a proline in this position, and in addition has aquired a 31 amino acid insertion of unknown origin in its *gag* domain. In contrast, the v-*erb*B genes of both the mutant and the revertant carry identical deletions in their 3′-ends: Both of them lack 306 nucleotides which represent most of the region located after the domain of v-*erb*B homologous to tyrosine kinases (Damm et al., 1987, and data not shown).

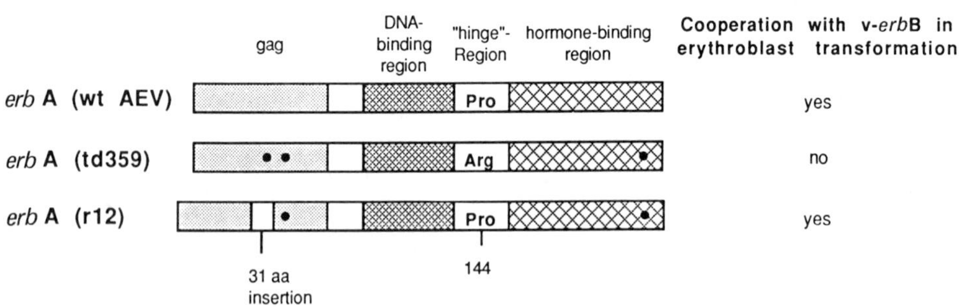

Figure 12 Comparison of v-*erb*A proteins from the *wt*, *td*359, and *r*12 AEVs. Point mutations are indicated by black dots and by the arrow at position 144. The activity of the v-*erb*A proteins was measured in v-*erb*B–transformed erythroblasts.

To analyze the importance of these mutations in v-*erb*A and v-*erb*B for erythroblast transformation, recombinant viruses containing all possible combinations of *wt*, mutant and revertant v-*erb*A and v-*erb*B genes were constructed. Subsequent bone marrow transformation experiments with the resulting viruses has demonstrated that both the *td*359 and the *r*12 v-*erb*B genes are unable to transform erythroblasts when coexpressed with the v-*erb*A gene from *td*359, confirming that the reversion in the *r*12 genome had occurred in its v-*erb*A oncogene (Damm et al., 1987). To unambigously identify the inactivating mutation in the *td*359 v-*erb*A gene, Damm et al. (1987) constructed chimeras between the *td*359 and *r*12 v-*erb*A genes, inserted them into retrovirus constructs with the *td*359 v-*erb*B oncogene, and tested for erythroblast transformation. These studies clearly show that the observed amino acid changes at position 144 are responsible for the inactivation of the *td*359 gene and the respective reactivation of *r*12, suggesting that the hinge region is also important for the structure and function of the v-*erb*A protein.

Mechanism of v-*erb*A Action Involves a Block of Erythrocyte Gene Transcription

Since the thyroid hormone receptor is known to either positively or negatively regulate the expression of a wide variety of genes, presumably by binding to their respective promoter regions, it was thought that v-*erb*A might act through changing the activity of genes involved in erythroid differentiation. To test this directly the observation that v-*erb*A also blocks the temperature-induced differentiation of erythroblasts transformed by temperature-sensitive mutants of the v-*erb*B and v-*sea* oncogenes was exploited, thus allowing study of the effects of v-*erb*A on erythroid differentiation in the absence of a functional, growth-promoting oncogene (Kahn et al., 1986a). Accordingly, recombinant retroviruses containing a *ts erb*B or *ts sea* gene in the presence or absence of a functional v-*erb*A gene were constructed and used for transformation of erythroblasts. After induction of differentiation at 42 °C, the respective cells were analyzed for protein and mRNA expression of a number of erythrocyte-specific genes (Fig. 13A). These studies demonstrated that v-*erb*A selectively arrests expression of two erythrocyte genes, the anion transporter (band 3), which might also serve as a major plasma membrane anchor for the red-cell skeleton (Woods et al., 1986) and δ-aminolevulinic acid synthetase (ALA-S), a key enzyme in hemin synthesis. In contrast, the presence of v-*erb*A does not grossly alter the expression of α- and β-globins or other red-cell skeleton proteins, such as spectrin, β-actin, and band 4.1, or of Na^+K^+ATPase, another protein involved in ion transport (Fig. 13B). To determine if the described effects of

A

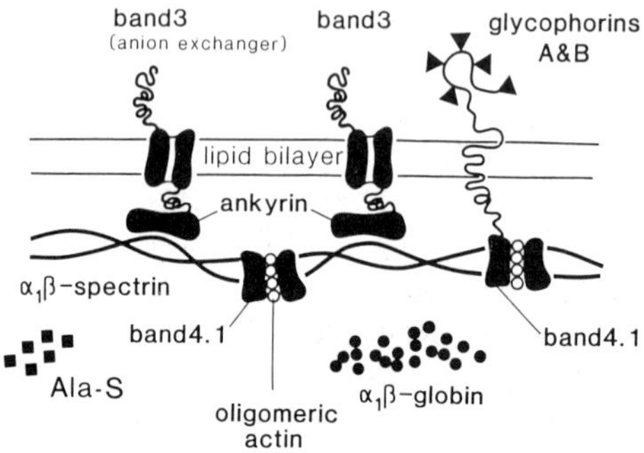

B

Marker	ts *erb*B/*sea*		ts *erb*B/*sea* +*erb*A	
	37 °C	42 °C	37 °C	42 °C
Morphology & differentiation antigens	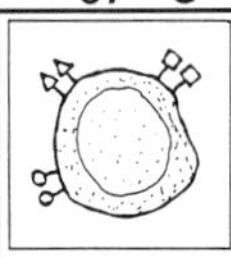	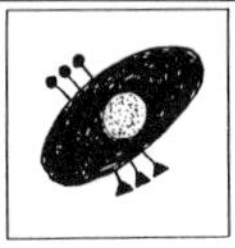	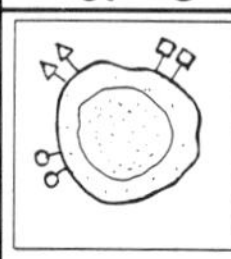	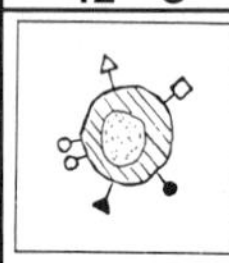
β-globin (a,b)	+	+++	+	++
α-globin (a,b)	+	+++	+	++
Band 3 (a,b)	+	+++	-	-
Band 4.1 (a,b)	++	++	++	++
ALA-S (b)	++	+++	+	+
α/β spectrin (a)	++	++	++	++
β-actin (b)	++	+	++	+
Na+/K+ATPase (b)	++	++	++	++

(a) Protein expression measured by immunoprecipitation
(b) RNA expression measured by Northern blot analysis

Figure 13 A: A scheme depicting subcellular localization and interaction of various erythrocyte-specific proteins. ALA-S, δ aminolevulinic acid synthetase, a key enzyme in hemin biosynthesis. The presence of glycophorins in chick erythrocytes in hypothetical. **B:** Effects of v-*erb*A on the differentiation phenotype of erythrocyte-specific gene expression in *ts* oncogene-transformed erythroblasts. Data are taken from Zenke et al. (manuscript submitted) and Beug et al. (manuscript in preparation). Strength of expression of differentiation antigens (open symbols, erythroblast antigens; closed symbols, erythrocyte antigens) is indicated by one symbol (weak expression in >50% of cells), two symbols (distinct expression in >90% of cells), and three symbols (strong expression in >90% of cells).

v-*erb*A gene expression on anion transporter and ALA-S gene expression occur at the transcriptional or posttranscriptional level, similar cell preparations as used above were subjected to nuclear run-on analysis. The results clearly demonstrate that v-*erb*A causes a marked reduction of the rate of transcription for both genes, suggesting that it acts at the level of transcriptional initiation (Zenke et al., unpublished data).

The v-*erb*A oncogene also arrests anion transporter and ALA-S expression in maturing cells actively transcribing these genes. This was demonstrated by exploiting an earlier observation that temperature-induced *wt-erb*A/*ts-erb*B erythroblasts were blocked in differentiation in normal medium (pH 7.2), but readily differentiated into erythrocytes in a specific, alkaline medium (pH 8.1) (Beug et al., 1982; Beug and Hayman, 1984, and manuscript in preparation). Such cells indeed express high levels of anion transporter protein after temperature induction in alkaline medium, but not at all in normal medium (Fig. 14A). This suggests that some aspect of v-*erb*A function is reversibly blocked by treatment of cells with alkaline medium, thus allowing us to monitor how quickly the oncogene turns off band 3 expression in maturing cells. Consequently, v-*erb*A/*ts* v-*erb*B erythroblasts were induced to differentiate at 42°C in pH 8.1 medium, shifted to pH 7.2 medium for increasing time periods and analyzed for erythrocyte-specific protein and mRNA expression. These studies reveal that v-*erb*A rapidly down-regulates synthesis of anion transporter protein (Fig. 14B) and mRNA (not shown). It also causes a less pronounced and somewhat slower down-regulation of ALA-S mRNA, whereas exerting only minor effects on the other erythrocyte-specific genes tested. Again, the described down-regulation of anion-transporter and ALA-S-mRNA occurs at the level of transcriptional initiation, as shown by nuclear run-on analysis.

Significance of the v-*erb*A–Induced Block of Anion Transporter for Erythroblast Transformation

Taken together, the results described above indicate that erythroblasts transformed by v-*erb*B alone synthesize significant amounts of anion transporter, a process completely blocked by v-*erb*A. It was, therefore, hypothesized that the production of anion transporter could be the cause of the observed stringent pH requirement for growth of the v-*erb*B–transformed cells (Kahn et al., 1986b); i.e., the probably abnormally high activity of band 3 in the immature cells would be toxic to the cells unless this activity was either "balanced" by corresponding pH and ion concentrations in the culture medium, or suppressed by v-*erb*A. To test this, transformed erythroblasts expressing an inactive, mutant *erb*A protein were

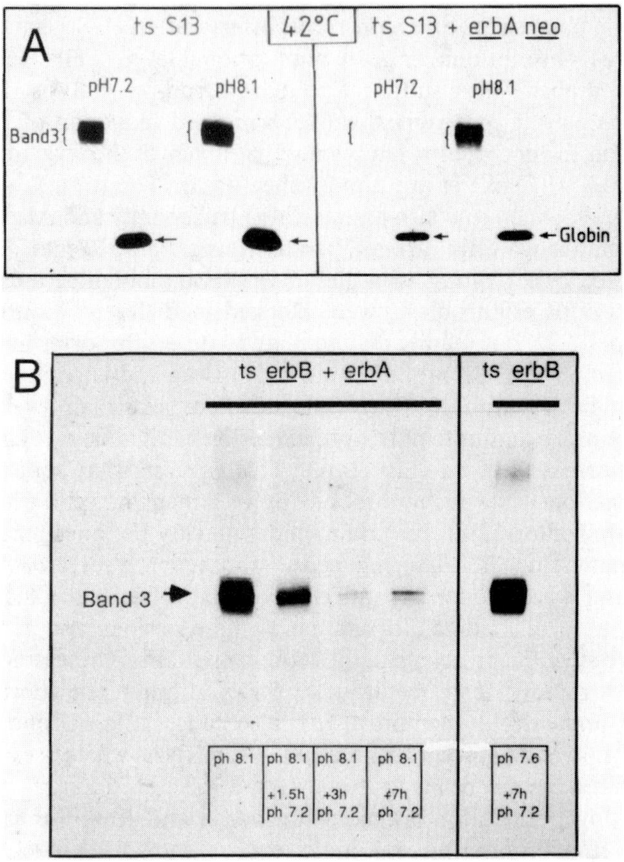

Figure 14 A: Analysis of band 3 expression in *ts* v-*sea*–transformed erythroblasts, containing or not containing v-*erb*A, and grown at 42 °C and pH 7.2 or 8.1. See text for explanations. **B:** Down-regulation of band 3 expression by v-*erb*A upon shift to pH 7.2 medium. Erythroblasts, transformed by *ts* v-*erb*B and v-*erb*A, were grown at pH 8.1 medium for 2 days, which permits synthesis of band 3, and were then shifted to pH 7.2 medium for the times indicated. Extracts from [^{35}S]-methionine–labeled cells were immune precipitated with anti–band 3 antibodies, as indicated in the figure, and analyzed by SDS-PAGE electrophoresis.

incubated with an inhibitor of band 3 activity (DIDS, 4,4′-diisothiocyano-stilbene-2,2′-disulfonate; Falke and Chan, 1986), using a medium that normally does not allow propagation of these cells (H. Beug, unpublished results). In the presence of the drug, the cells incorporate [^{3}H]-thymidine at levels comparable to those of the untreated cells containing v-*erb*A + v-*erb*B. As expected, the cells cease to incorporate [^{3}H]-thymidine and eventually die in the absence of the drug. Likewise, DIDS prevents the extensive vacuolization preceding this medium-induced cell death. The results therefore suggest that the narrow pH requirements for growth of v-*erb*B–transformed erythroblasts are alleviated by v-*erb*A through suppression of synthesis of band 3, a highly active ion transporter apparently toxic to immature erythroid cells when expressed at high levels.

Effects of v-*erb*A in Other Cell Types

Although v-*erb*A-infection of chick embryo fibroblasts does not induce clear-cut phenotypic changes (Frykberg et al., 1983), it enhances the transformed phenotype of fibroblasts infected with a mutant v-*erb*B gene lacking 83 C-terminal amino acids. While fibroblasts containing only this mutant *erb*B protein are partially transformed, exhibiting an enhanced hexose transport rate but essentially normal morphology and actin cable formation, introduction of v-*erb*A induces these cells to assume a transformed phenotype indistinguishable of *wt* AEV–transformed cells (Jansson et al., 1987). In another study, v-*erb*A was found to enhance agar colony formation and in vitro lifespan of infected chick embryo fibroblasts. More importantly, v-*erb*B–transformed fibroblasts superinfected with a v-*erb*A-neo virus cause large, undifferentiated tumors when transplanted onto the chorioallantoic membrane, whereas the same cells without *erb*A formed only small nodules surrounded by large amounts of collagenous matrix (Gandrillon et al., 1987). It is therefore tempting to speculate that v-*erb*A might reduce expression of genes encoding extracellular matrix glues such as collagen or fibronectin, a view that would also explain the above results with mutant *erb*B–infected fibroblasts (Yamamoto et al., 1976).

Functions of v-*erb*A in Leukemic Transformation: Conclusions and Speculations

The v-*erb*A gene encodes a ligand-independent form of the thyroid hormone receptor. The mutations in v-*erb*A responsible for the lack of binding clearly show that the C-terminal half of the molecule represents the domain involved in hormone binding. This region has a similar structure and location as the ligand-binding domains of receptors for steroid hormones, suggesting that these receptors share a common ancestral gene. The fact that both the C-terminal deletion in v-*erb*A and the point mutations are required for abolishing hormone binding suggests that they have accumulated gradually, and that the aquisition of hormone independence has given the virus a selective advantage by increasing the oncogenic activity of v-*erb*B.

The v-*erb*A protein binds to DNA, suggesting that it acts like the thyroid hormone receptor by binding to regulatory elements of specific target genes. Consequently, the v-*erb*A protein might constitutively either up- or down-regulate the expression of its target genes. The nucleotide sequences recognized by v-*erb*A might, however, be distinct from those detected by the c-*erb*A protein, since the viral protein contains two amino acid substitutions in its putative DNA-binding domain. At any rate, if the expression of such genes (or, alternatively, absence thereof) is important for differentiation or growth of erythroblasts, the effects of v-*erb*A on erythroid differentiation could be explained. Experiments designed to test this hypothesis revealed that v-*erb*A specifically blocks transcription of two genes, anion transporter and ALA-S, that may play important roles in red cell differentiation. The down-regulation of band 3 synthesis not only suggests a mechanism by which the oncogene broadens the pH range permissible for erythroblasts growth, but could also have other effects on the erythroblasts. The ion transporter serves as an anchor for the rigid red cell cytoskeleton as well as several enzymes. A lack of proper anchor would naturally disturb the organization of the proteins in the cytoskeletal network, and might subsequently contribute to arresting the cell in an immature stage of differentiation, e.g., by leading to rapid turnover of red cell skeleton proteins (Woods et al., 1986). It is likely, however, that v-*erb*A exerts its effects in erythroblasts pleiotropically, e.g., by affecting the expression of other genes as well. Hemin has been proposed to be a coregulator of erythroid cell differentiation, and the partial block of ALA-S expression caused by v-*erb*A might decrease the synthesis of hemin, thereby contributing to the block of differentiation (Schmidt et al., 1986). Clearly, a more extensive survey of the expression of genes in erythroblasts is required to further clarify this issue.

How do two oncogenes acting in concert, such as the *wt* v-*erb*A and the *td*359 or *r*12 v-*erb*B genes, transform erythroblasts when neither of them by itself is capable to do so? A possible mechanism for the cooperativity between v-*erb*A and v-*erb*B is suggested by analysis of proliferation capacities and state of differentiation of erythroblasts transformed by the *td*359 and *r*12 AEV viruses and their recombinants. On their own, the mutant v-*erb*B genes only induce a weak self-renewal in transformed erythroblasts, which leads to terminal differentiation and thus to an eventual loss of the proliferating cells in the culture. v-*erb*A prevents this cell loss and thus enables the mutant v-*erb*B genes to slowly generate a mass-population of transformed erythroblasts (H. Beug, unpublished observations). The same mechanism might explain, why v-*erb*A confers erythroblast-transforming potential to other mutant-v-*erb*B genes (Janson et al., 1987) and even to the normal human EGF-receptor/c-*erb*B gene (Khazaie et al., manuscript in preparation).

MOLECULAR FUNCTION OF NUCLEAR ONCOPROTEINS: CONCLUSIONS

All available evidence is in agreement with the hypothesis that the nuclear proto-oncogene products play a role in transcriptional or posttranscriptional regulatory mechanisms. The clearest case in this respect is c-*erb*A, which has been shown to encode a thyroid hormone receptor regulating transcription of other genes in response to hormone binding. In contrast, its mutated viral homologue, v-*erb*A, is a constitutively activated trans-regulatory protein, since it regulates the transcription of other genes independent of the binding of a ligand. The first clue as to the function of *erb*A came from its striking homology with steroid hormone receptors, particularly the spacing of cystein residues in the DNA-binding domain (Zn-finger structure), which immediately suggested to search for possible ligands.

In the case of the other nuclear oncoproteins, no extensive homology to nuclear receptors or other known nuclear proteins has been detected so far except for the recently identified avian oncogene *jun*, showing significant homology to the yeast transcriptional activator protein GCN4 (Vogt et al., 1987). The same yeast protein also shows a restricted homology with the conserved center region of *fos* protein, pointing to a possible role for *fos* in the control of gene transcription. This hypothesis is supported by the association of *fos* protein with chromatin, its transactivating effect on the α_1(III) collagen gene and the RSV-LTR and its presence in a protein complex binding to a specific region of the aP2 gene promoter. The latter finding seems to be of particular relevance, since DNA binding of this protein complex depends on the presence of *fos* protein and, on the basis of UV-cross-linking experiments, the *fos* protein may directly interact with the binding site in the aP2 promoter.

Protein-DNA interaction also appears to play a role in *myb* function. *myb*-proteins are associated to some extent with chromatin and bind to DNA in vitro. It has been demonstrated that the DNA-binding domain of *myb* proteins is the most highly conserved region of *myb* proteins, providing a strong argument for the role of DNA binding in *myb* protein function. In addition, it has recently been possible to show that *myb* proteins interact with specific regions on bacteriophage λ DNA, which presumably contains degenerate versions of a binding site(s) for *myb* proteins. The effect of *myb* protein on the promoter activity of other genes, however, remains to be investigated.

Multiple functions have been proposed for the *myc* gene product, another nucleic acid–binding protein. It has been suggested that *myc* protein on the one hand may be directly involved in the DNA replication process because of the inhibitory effect of *myc*-specific antibodies, whereas, on the other hand, its localization with small ribonucleoprotein complexes is suggestive of a function in posttranscriptional control mechanisms. Both these processes would be quite different from those where the other nuclear oncogene products seem to play a role. This is conceivable if one considers the multitude of mechanisms involved in the regulation of gene expression and DNA synthesis. Subversion of any one of these mechanisms may lead to an imbalance in the delicate network of mechanisms regulating differentiation and growth control with the result of advancing the multistage process of neoplastic transformation.

REFERENCES

Adams, J. M., Harris, A. W., Pinkert, C. A., Corcoran, L. M., Alexander, W. S., Cory, S., Palmiter, R. D., and Brinster, R. C. (1985). The c-*myc* oncogene driven by immunoglobulin enhancers induces lymphoid malignancy in transgenic mice. *Nature 318*: 533–538.

Alitalo, K., Ramsay, G., Bishop, J. M., Pfeifer, S. O., Colby, W. W., and Levinson, A. D. (1983). Identification of nuclear proteins encoded by viral and cellular *myc* oncogenes. *Nature 306*: 274–277.

Anderson, S., Hayward, W., Neel, B., and Hanafusa, H. (1980). Avian erythroblastosis virus produces two mRNAs. *J. Virol. 36*: 676–683.

Armelin, H. A., Armelin, M. C. S., Kelly, K., Stewart, T., Leder, P., Cochran, B. H., and Stiles, C. D. (1984). Functional role for c-*myc* in mitogenic response to platelet-derived growth factor. *Nature 310*: 655–660.

Bading, H., Hansen, J., and Moelling, K. (1987). Selective DNA-binding of the human cellular myb isolated by a monoclonal antibody. *Oncogene* (in press).

Battey, J., Moulding, C., Taub, R., Murphy, W., Stewart, T., Potter, H., Lenoir, G., and Leder, P. (1983). Structural consequences of translocation into the IgH locus in Burkitt lymphoma. *Cell 34*: 779–787.

Beimling, P., Benter, T., Sander, T., and Moelling, K. (1985). Isolation and characterization of the human cellular *myc* gene product. *Biochemistry 24*: 6349–6355.

Bender, T. P., and Kuehl, W. M. (1986). Murine *myb* proto-oncogene mRNA: cDNA sequence and evidence for 5′ heterogeneity. *Proc. Natl. Acad. Sci. U.S.A. 83*: 3204–3208.

Bentley, D. L., and Groudine, M. (1986a). Novel promoter upstream of the human c-*myc* gene and regulation of c-*myc* in differentiated HL60 cells. *Mol. Cell. Biol. 6*: 3481–3489.

Bentley, D. L., and Groudine, M. (1986b). A block to elongation is largely responsible for decreased transcription of c-*myc* expression in B-cell lymphomas. *Nature 321*: 702–706.

Bernard, O., Cory, S., Gerondakis, S., Webb, E., and Adams, J. A. (1983). Sequence of the murine and human cellular *myc* oncogenes and two modes of *myc* transcription resulting from chromosome translocation in B-lymphoid tumours. *EMBO J. 2*: 2375–2383.

Beug, H., and Hayman, M. J. (1984). Temperature-sensitive mutants of avian erythroblastosis virus: Surface expression of the *erbB* product correlates with transformation. *Cell 36*: 963–972.

Beug, H., von Kirchbach, A., Döderlein, G., Conscience, J.-F., and Graf, T. (1979). Chicken hematopoietic cells transformed by seven strains of defective avian leukemia viruses display three distinct phenotypes of differentiation. *Cell 18*: 375-390.

Beug, H., Palmieri, S., Freudenstein, C., Zentgraf, H., and Graf, T. (1982). Hormone-dependent terminal differentiation *in vitro* of chicken erythroleukemia cells transformed by *ts* mutants of avian erythroblastosis virus. *Cell 28*: 907–919.

Beug, H., Leutz, A. S., Kahn, P., and Graf, T. (1984). Ts mutants of E26 leukemia virus allow transformed myeloblats, but not erythroblats or fibroblasts, to differentiate at the nonpermissive temperature. *Cell 39*: 579-588.

Beug, H., Hayman, M. J., Graf, T., Benedict, S. H., Wallbank, A. M., and Vogt, P. K. (1985a). S13, a rapidly oncogenic replication-defective avian retrovirus. *Virology 145*: 141–153.

Beug, H., Kahn, P., Döderlein, G., Hayman, M. J., and Graf, T. (1985b). Characterization of hematopoietic cells transformed *in vitro* by AEV-H, an *erb*-B containing avian erythroblastosis virus. In *Modern Trends in Human Leukaemia VI,* Vol. 29 (Neth, Gallo, Greaves, and Janka, eds.). Springer-Verlag, Berlin-Heidelberg, pp. 290–297.

Beug, H., Hayman, M., Raines, M.-B., Kung, H.-J., and Vennström, B. (1986). RAV-1 induced erythroleukemic cells exhibit a weakly transformed phenotypes *in vitro*, and release c-*erb*B containing retroviruses unable to transform fibroblasts. *J. Virol. 57*: 1127–1138.

Bister, K., and Duesberg, P. (1979). Structure and specific sequences of avian erythroblastosis virus RNA: Evidence for multiple classes of transforming genes among avian tumor viruses. *Proc. Natl. Acad. Sci. U.S.A. 76*: 5023–5027.

Bister, K., Nunn, M., Moscovici, C., Perbal, B., Baluda, M. A., and Duesberg, P. H. (1982). Leukemia viruses E26 and avian myeloblastosis virus have related transformation-specific RNA sequences but different genetic structures, gene products and oncogenic properties. *Proc. Natl. Acad. Sci. U.S.A. 79*: 3677–3681.

Blanchard, J. M., Piechaczyk, M., Dani, C., Chambard, J.-C., Franchi, A., and Pouyssegur, J. and Jeanteur, P. (1985). c-*myc* gene is transcribed at high rate in G0-*arrested fibroblasts* and is post-transcriptionally regulated in response to growth factors. *Nature 317*: 443–445.

Boyle, W. J., Lipsick, J. S., Reddy, E. P., and Baluda, M. A. (1983). Identification of the leukemogenic protein of avian myeloblastosis virus and of its normal cellular homologue. *Proc. Natl. Acad. Sci. U.S.A. 80*: 2834–2838.

Boyle, W. J., Lampert, M. A., Lipsick, J. S., and Baluda, M. A. (1984). Avian myeloblastosis virus and E26 virus oncogene products are nuclear proteins. *Proc. Natl. Acad. Sci. U.S.A. 81*: 4265–4269.

Boyle, W. J., Lampert, M. A., Li, A. L., and Baluda, M. A. (1985). Nuclear compartmentalization of the v-*myb* oncogene product. *Mol. Cell. Biol. 5*: 3017–3023.

Bravo, R., and Müller, R. (1986). Involvement of proto-oncogenes in growth control: The induction of c-*fos* and c-*myc* by growth factors. In *Oncogenes and Growth Control* (Kahn, P., and Graf, T., eds.). Springer-Verlag, Berlin-Heidelberg, pp. 198–202.

Bravo, R., Neuberg, M., Burckhardt, J., Almendral, J., Wallich, R., and Müller, R. (1987). Involvement of common and cell type-specific pathways in c-*fos* gene control: Stable induction by cAMP in macrophages. *Cell 48*: 251–260.

Bunte, T., Greiser-Wilke, I., Donner, P., and Moelling, K. (1982). Association of *gag-myc* proteins from avian myelocytomatosis virus wild-type and mutants with chromatin. *EMBO J. 1*: 919–927.

Butnick, N. Z., Miyamoto, C., Chizzonite, R., Cullen, B. R., Ju, G., and Skalka, A. M. (1985). Regulation of the human c-*myc* gene: 5′ Non-coding sequences do not affect translation. *Mol. Cell. Biol. 5*: 3009–3016.

Campisi, J., Gray, H. E., Pardee, A. B., Dean, M., and Soensheim, G. E. (1984). Cell-cycle control of c-*myc* but not c-*ras* expression is lost following chemical transformation. *Cell 36*: 241–247.

Castle, S., and Sheiness, D. (1985). Structural organization of the mouse proto-*myb* gene. *Biochem. Biophys. Res. Commun. 132*: 688–695.

Chung, J., Sinn, E., Reed, R. R., and Leder, P. (1986). Transacting elements modulate expression of the human c-*myc* gene in Burkitt lymphoma cells. *Proc. Natl. Acad. Sci U.S.A. 83*: 7918–7922.

Craig, R. W., and Block, A. (1984). Early decline in c-*myb* oncogene expression in the differentiation of human myeloblastic leukemia (ML-1) cells induced with 12-0-tetradecanoylphorbol-13-acetate. *Cancer Res. 44*: 442–446.

Curran, T., and Morgan, J. I. (1985). Superinduction of the c-*fos* by nerve growth factor in the presence of peripherally active benzodiazepines. *Science 229*: 1265–1268.

Curran, T., Miller, A. D., Zokas, L., and Verma, I. M. (1984). Viral and cellular *fos* proteins: A comparative analysis. *Cell 36*: 259–268.

Curran, T., Van Beveren, C., Ling, N., and Verma, I. M. (1985). Viral and cellular *fos* proteins are complexed with a 39.000 dalton cellular protein. *Mol. Cell. Biol. 5*: 167–172.

Damm, K., Beug, H., Graf, T., and Vennström, B. (1987). Cooperativity between the oncogenes of avian erythroblastosis virus (AEV): A mutant v-*erb*B gene defective in erythroblast transformation can be fully complemented by a highly active v-*erb*A gene. *EMBO J. 6*: 375–382.

Dani, C., Mechti, N., Piechaczyk, M., Lebleu, B., Jeanteur, P., and Blanchard, J. M. (1985). Increased rate of degradation of c-*myc* mRNA in interferon-treated Daudi cells. *Proc. Natl. Acad. Sci. U.S.A. 82*: 4896–4899.

Darby, M. K., Herrera, R. E., Vosberg, H. P., and Nordheim, H. (1986). DNA topoisomerase II cleaves at specific sites in the 5¾flanking region of the c-*fos* proto-oncogene. *EMBO J. 5*: 2257–2265.

Darveau, A., Pelletier, J., and Sonenberg, N. (1985). Differential efficiencies of in vitro translation of mouse c-*myc* transcripts differing in the 5¾untranslated region. *Proc. Natl. Acad. Sci. U.S.A. 82*: 2315–2319.

Dayton, A. I., Selden, J. R., Laws, G., Dorney, D. J., Finan, J., Tripputi, P., Emanuel, B. S., Rovera, G., Nowell, P. C., and Croce, C. M. (1984). A human c-*erb*A oncogene homologue is closely proximal to the chromosome 17 breakpoint in acute promyelocytic leukemia. *Proc. Natl. Acad. Sci. U.S.A. 81*: 4495–4499.

Dejean, A., Bougouleret, L., Grzeschnik, K.-H., and Tiollais, P. (1986). Hepatitis B virus DNA integration in a sequence homologous to v-*erb*A and steroid hormone receptor genes in a hepatocellular carcinoma. *Nature 322*: 70–72.

Deschamps, J., Mejlink, F., and Verma, I. M. (1985). Identification of a transcriptional enhancer element upstream from the proto-oncogene *fos*. *Science 230*: 1265–1268.

Distel, R. J., Ro, H.-S., Rosen, B. S., Groves, D. L., and Spiegelman, B. M. (1987). Nucleoprotein complexes that regulate gene expression in adipocyte differentiation: Direct participation of c-*fos*. *Cell 49*: 835–844.

Donner, P., Greiser-Wilke, I., and Moelling, K. (1982). Nuclear localization and DNA-binding of the transforming gene product of avian myelocytomatosis virus. *Nature 296*: 262–266.

Donner, P., Bunte, T., Greiser-Wilke, I., and Moelling, K. (1983). Decreased DNA-binding ability of purified transformation-specific proteins from deletion mutants of the acute avian leukemia virus MC29. *Proc. Natl. Acad. Sci. U.S.A. 80*: 2861–2865.

Dony, C., and Gruss, P. (1987). Protooncogene c-*fos* expression in growth regions of foetal bone and mesodermal web tissue during murine development. *Nature* (in press).

Dony, C., Kessel, M., and Gruss, P. (1985). Post-transcriptional control of c-*myc* and p53 expression during differentiation of the embryonal carcinoma cell kine F9. *Nature 317*: 636–639.

Downward, J., Yarden, Y., Mayes, E., Scrace, G., Totty, N., Stockwell, P., Ullrich, A., Schlessinger, J., and Waterfield, M. D. (1984). Close similarity of epidermal growth factor receptor and v-*erb*B oncogene protein sequences. *Nature 307*: 521–527.

Eick, D., and Bornkamm, G. (1986). Transcriptional arrest within the first exon is a fast control mechanism in c-*myc* gene expression. *Nucl. Acids Res. 14*: 8331–8346.

El Sabouty, S., Marty, L., and Jeanteur, P. (1984). Extreme instability of *myc* mRNA in normal and transformed human cells. *Proc. Natl. Acad. Sci. U.S.A. 81*: 7046–7050.

Erisman, M. D., Rothberg, P. G., Diehl, R. E., Morse, C. C., Spandorfer, J. M., and Astrin, S. M. (1985). Deregulation of c-*myc* gene expression in human colon carcinoma is not accompanied by amplification or rearrangement of the gene. *Mol. Cell. Biol. 5*: 1969–1976.

Evan, G. I., and Hancock, D. C. (1985). Studies on the interaction of the human c-*myc* protein with cell nuclei: p62$^{c\text{-}myc}$ as a member of a discrete subset of nuclear proteins. *Cell 43*: 253–261.

Evan, G. I., Lewis, G. K., and Bishop, J. M. (1984). Isolation of monoclonal antibodies specific for products of avian oncogene *myb*. *Mol. Cell. Biol. 4*: 2843–2850.

Fahrlander, P. D., Piechaczyk, M., and Marcu, K. B. (1985). Chromatin structure of the murine c-*myc* locus: Implications for the regulation of normal and chromosomally translocated genes. *EMBO J. 4*: 3195–3202.

Falke, J., and Chan, S. (1986). Molecular mechanisms of band 3 inhibitors. 1. Transport site inhibitors. *Biochemistry 25*: 7888–7894.

Finkel, M. P., Biskis, B. O., and Jinkins, P. B. (1966). Virus induction of osteosarcomas in mice. *Science 151*: 698-701.

Finkel, M. P., Reilly, C. A., and Biskis, B. O. (1975). Viral etiology of bone cancer. *Front. Radiat. 10*: 28–39.

Fort, P., Rech, J., Vie, A., Piechaczyk, M., Bonnieu, A., Jeanteur, P., and Blanchard, J.-M. (1987). Regulation of c-*fos* gene expression in hamster fibroblasts: Initiation and elongation of transcription and mRNA degradation. *Nucl. Acids Res.* (in press).

Franza, B. R., Jr., Sambucetti, L. C., Cohen, D. R., and Curran, T. (1987). Analysis of Fos protein complexes and Fos-related antigens by high-resolution two-dimensional gel electrophoresis. *Oncogene 2*: 213–221.

Frykberg, L., Palmieri, S., Beug, H., Graf, T., Hayman, M. J., and Vennstrom, B. (1983). Transforming capacities of avian erythroblastosis virus mutants deleted in the *erb*A or *erb*B oncogenes. *Cell 32*: 227–238.

Fung, Y. K. T., Lewis, W. G., Kung, H. J., and Crittenden, L. B. (1983). Activation of the cellular oncogene c-*erb*B by LTR insertion: Molecular basis for induction of erythroblastosis by avian leukosis virus. *Cell 33*: 357–368.

Gamett, D. C., Tracy, S. E., and Robinson, H. L. (1986). Differences in sequences encoding the carboxyl-terminal domain of the epidermal growth factor receptor correlate with differences in the disease potential of viral *erb*B genes. *Proc. Natl. Acad. Sci. U.S.A. 83*: 6053–6057.

Gandrillon, O., Jurdic, P., Benchaibi, M., Xiao, J.-H., Ghysdael, J., and Samarut, J. (1987). Expression of the v-*erb*A oncogene in chicken embryo fibroblasts stimulates their proliferation *in vitro* and enhances tumor growth *in vivo*. *Cell 49*: 687–697.

Gazin, C., Dupont de Dinechin, S., Hampe, A., Masson, J.-M., Martin, P., Stehelin, D., and Galibert, F. (1984). Nucleotide sequence of the human c-*myc* locus: Provocative open reading frame within the first exon. *EMBO J. 3*: 383–387.

Gazin, C., Rigolet, M., Briand, J. P., Van Regenmortel, M. H., and Galibert, F. (1986). Immunochemical detection of proteins related to the human c-*myc* exon$_1$. *EMBO J. 5*: 2241–2250.

Gerondakis, S., and Bishop, J. M. (1986). Structure of the protein encoded by the chicken proto-oncogene c-*myb*. *Mol. Cell. Biol. 6*: 3677–3684.

Gilman, M. Z., Wilson, R. N., and Weinberg, R. A. (1986). Multiple protein binding sites in the 5′-flanking region regulate c-*fos* expression. *Mol. Cell. Biol. 6*: 4305–4316.

Gonda, T. J., and Bishop, J. M. (1983). Structure and transcription of the cellular homolog (c-*myb*) of the avian myeloblastosis virus transforming gene (v-*myb*). *J. Virol. 46*: 212–220.

Gonda, T. J., and Metcalf, D. (1984). Expression of *myb, myc* and *fos* proto-oncogenes during differentiation of a murine myeloid leukemia. *Nature 310*: 249–251.

Gonda, T. J., Sheiness, D. K., Fanshier, L., Bishop, J. M., Moscovici, C., and Moscovici, M. G. (1981). The genome and the intracellular RNAs of avian myeloblastosis virus. *Cell. 23*: 279–290.

Gonda, T. J., Sheiness, D. K., and Bishop, J. M. (1982). Transcripts from the cellular homologs of retroviral oncogenes: Distribution among chicken tissues. *Mol. Cell. Biol. 2*: 617–624.

Gonda, T. J., Gough, N. M., Dunn, A. R., and de Blaquiere, J. (1985). Nucleotide sequence of cDNA clones of the murine *myb* proto-oncogene. *EMBO J. 4*: 2003–2008.

Graf, T., Royer-Pokora, B., Schubert, G. E., and Beug, H. (1976). Evidence for the multiple oncogenic potential of cloned leukemia virus: *In vitro* and *in vivo* studies with avian erythroblastosis virus. *Virology 71*: 423–433.

Graf, T., and Beug, H. (1978). Avian leukemia viruses: Interaction with their target cells *in vivo* and *in vitro*. *Biochim. Biophys. Acta 516*: 269–299.

Graf, T., Oker-Blom, N., Todorov, T. G., and Beug, H. (1979). Transforming capacities and defectiveness of avian leukemia viruses OK10 and E26. *Virology 99*: 431–436.

Greenberg, M. E., and Ziff, E. B. (1984). Stimulation of mouse 3T3 cells induces transcription of the c-*fos* oncogene. *Nature 311*: 433-438.

Greenberg, M. E., Greene, L. A., and Ziff, E. B. (1985). Nerve growth factor and epidermal growth factor induce rapid transient changes in proto-oncogene transcription in PC12 cells. *J. Cell. Biol. 260*: 14101–14110.

Greenberg, M. E., Ziff, E. B., and Greene, L. A. (1986). Stimulation of neuronal acetylcholine receptors induces rapid gene transcription. *Science 234*: 80–83.

Greenberg, M. E., Siegfried, Z., and Ziff, E. B. (1987). Mutation of the c-*fos* gene dyad symmetry element inhibits serum inducibility of transcription *in vivo* and the nuclear regulatory factor binding *in vitro*. *Mol. Cell. Biol. 7*: 1217–1225.

Haluska, F. G., Tsujimoto, Y., and Croce, C. M. (1983). Mechanisms of chromosome translocation in B- and T-cell neoplasia. *Trends Gen. 3*: 11–16.

Hann, S. R., and Eisenmann, R. N. (1984). Proteins encoded by the human c-*myc* oncogene: Differential expression in neoplastic cells. *Mol. Cell. Biol. 4*: 2486–2497.

Hann, S. R., and Eisenman, R. N. (1985). c-*myc* oncogene protein synthesis is independent of the cell cycle in human and avian cells. *Nature 314*: 366–369.

Hann, S. R., Abrams, H. D., Rohrschneider, L. R., and Eisenman, R. N. (1983). Proteins encoded by v-*myc* and c-*myc* oncogenes: Identification and localization in acute leukemia virus transformants and bursal lymphoma cell lines. *Cell 34*: 789–798.

Hayes, T. E., Kitchen, A. M., and Cochran, B. T. (1987). Inducible binding of a factor to the *fos* regulatory region. *Proc. Natl. Sci U.S.A. 84*: 1272–1276.

Hayman, M. J., and Beug, H. (1984). Identification of a form of the avian erythroblastosis virus *erb*B gene product at the cell surface. *Nature 309*: 460–462.

Hayman, M. J., Royer-Pokora, B., and Graf, T. (1979). Defectiveness of avian erythroblastosis virus: Synthesis of a 75K *gag*-related protein. *Virology 92*: 31–45.

Hayman, M. J., Ramsay, G. M., Savin, K., Kitchener, G., Graf, T., and Beug, H. (1983). Identification and characterization of the avian erythroblastosis virus *erb*B gene product as a membrane glycoprotein. *Cell 32*: 579–588.

Heaney, M. L., Pierce, J., and Parsons, J. T. (1986). Site-directed mutagenesis of the *gag-myc* gene of avian MC29: Biological activity and imtracellular localization of structurally altered proteins. *J. Viol. 60*: 167–176.

Hollenberg, S. M., Weinberger, C., Ong, E. S., Cerelli, G., Oro, A., Lebo, R., Thompson, E. B., Rosenfeld, M. G., and Evans, R. M. (1985). Primary structure and expression of a functional human glucocorticoid receptor cDNA. *Nature 318*: 635–641.

Holt, J. T., Gopüal, T. V., Moulton, A. D., and Nienhuis, A. W. (1986). Inducible production of c-*fos* antisense RNA inhibits 3T3 cell proliferation. *Proc. Natl. Acad. Sci. U.S.A. 83*: 4794–4798.

Jansson, M., Philipson, L., and Vennström, B. (1983). Isolation and characterization of multiple human genes homologous to the oncogenes of avian erythroblastosis virus. *EMBO J. 2*: 561–565.

Jansson, M., Beug, H., Graf, T., Gray, C., and Vennström, B. (1987). The viral *erb*A gene restores weakly transforming activities of mutant *v-erb*B genes in transformation of chicken fibroblasts and erythroblasts. *Oncogene.*

Jenuwein, T., and Müller, R. (1987). Structure-function analysis of *fos* protein: A single amino acid change activates the immortalizing potential of v-*fos*. *Cell 48*: 647–657.

Jenuwein, T., Müller, D., Curran, T., and Müller, R. (1985). Extended life span and tumorigenicity of nonestablished mouse connective tissue cells transformed by the *fos* oncogene of FBR-MuSV. *Cell 4*: 629–637.

Kaczmarek, L., Hyland, J., Watt, R., Rosenberg, M., and Baserga, R. (1985). Microinjected c-*myc* as a competence factor. *Science 228*: 1313–1314.

Kahn, P., Adkins, B., Beug, H., and Graf, T. (1984). *src*- and *fps*-containing avian sarcoma viruses transform chicken erythroid cells. *Proc. Natl. Acad. Sci. U.S.A. 81*: 7122–7126.

Kahn, P., Frykberg, L., Brady, C., Stanley, I. J., Beug, H., Vennström, B., and Graf, T. (1986a). *v-erb*A cooperates with sarcoma oncogenes in leukaemic cell transformation. *Cell 45*: 349–356.

Kahn, P., Frykberg, L., Graf, T., Vennström, B., and Beug, H. (1986b). Cooperativity between v-*erb*A and v-*src*-related oncogenes in erythroid cell transformation. In Proceedings. Hamburg. F. Deinhardt, ed. Springer-Verlag, Berlin-Heidelberg, pp. 41–50.

Katzen, A. L., Kornberg, T. B., and Bishop, J. M. (1985). Isolation of the proto-oncogene c-*myb* from D. melanogaster. *Cell 41*: 449–456.

Kelly, K., Cochran, B. H., Stiles, C. D., and Leder, P. (1983). Cell-specific regulation of the c-*myc* gene by lymphocyte mitogens and platelet-derived growth factor. *Cell 35*: 603–610.

Klempnauer, K.-H., and Sippel, A. E. (1986). Subnuclear localization of proteins encoded by the oncogene v-*myb* and its cellular homolog c-*myb*. *Mol. Cell. Biol. 6*: 62–69.

Klempnauer, K.-H., Gonda, T. J., and Bishop, J. M. (1982). Nucleotide sequence of the retroviral leukemia gene v-*myb* and its cellular progenitor c-*myb*: The architecture of a transduce oncogene. *Cell 31*: 453–463.

Klempnauer, K.-H., Ramsay, G., Bishop, J. M., Moscovici, M. G., Moscovici, C., McGrath, J. P., and Levinson, A. D. (1983). The product of the retroviral transforming gene v-*myb* is a truncated version of the protein encoded by the cellular oncogene c-*myb*. *Cell 33*: 345–355.

Klempnauer, K.-H., Symonds, G., Evan, G. I., and Bishop, J. M. (1984). Subcellular localization of proteins encoded by oncogenes of avian myeloblastosis virus and avian leukemia virus E26 and by the chicken c-*myb* gene. *Cell 37*: 537–547.

Klempnauer, K.-H., Bonifer, C., and Sippel, A. E. (1986). Identification and characterization of the protein encoded by the human c-*myb* proto-oncogene. *EMBO J. 5*: 1903–1911.

Kruijer, W., Cooper, J. A., Hunter, T., and Verma, I. M. (1984). Platelet-derived growth factor induces rapid but transient expression of the c-*fos* gene and protein. *Nature 312*: 711–716.

Kruijer, W., Schubert, D., and Verma, I. M. (1985). Induction of the proto-oncogene *fos* by nerve growth factor. *Proc. Natl. Acad. Sci. U.S.A. 82*: 7330–7334.

Krust, A., Green, S., Argos, P., Kumar, V., Walter, P., Bornert, J.-M., and Chambon, P. (1986). The chicken oestrogen receptor sequence: Homology with v-*erb*A and the human oestrogen and glucocorticoid receptors. *EMBO J. 5*: 891–897.

Lai, M., Hu, S., and Vogt, P. (1979). Avian erythroblastosis virus: Transformation-specific sequences form a contigous segment of 3.25 kb located in the middle of the 6 kb genome. *Virology 97*: 366–377.

Lai, M. M. C., Neil, J. C., and Vogt, P. K. (1980). Cell-free translation of avian erythroblastosis virus RNA yields two specific and distinct proteins with molecular weights of 75.000 and 40.000 Dalton. *Virology 100*: 475–483.

Lavu, S., and Reddy, E. P. (1986). Structural organization and nucleotide sequence of the mouse c-*myb* oncogene: Activation in ABPL tumors is due to viral integration in an intron which results in the deletion of 5′ coding sequences. *Nucl. Acids Res. 14*: 5309–5320.

Leprince, D., Gegonne, A., Coll, J., de Taisne, C., Schneeberger, A., Lagrou, C., and Stehelin, D. (1983). A putative second cell-derived oncogene of the avian leukemia retrovirus E26. *Nature 306*: 395–397.

Linial, M., and Groudine, M. (1985). Transcription of three c-*myc* exons is enhanced in chicken bursal lymphoma cell lines. *Proc. Natl. Acad. Sci. U.S.A. 82*: 53–57.

Little, C. D., Lau, M. M., Carney, D. N., Gazdar, A. F., and Minna, J. D. (1983). Amplification and expression of the c-*myc* oncogene in human lung cancer cell lines. *Nature 306*: 194–196.

Majello, B., Kenyon, L. C., and Dalla-Favera, R. (1986). Human c-*myb* protooncogene: Nucleotide sequence of cDNA and organization of the genomic locus. *Proc. Natl. Acad. Sci. USA 83*: 9636–9640.

McLeod, K., and Baxter, J. (1976). Chromatin receptors for thyroid hormones. *J. Biol. Chem. 251*: 7380–7387.

Mechti, N., Piechaczyk, M., Blanchard, J.-M., Marty, L., Bonnieu, A., Jeanteur, P., and Lebleu, B. (1986). Transcriptional and post-transcriptional regulation of c-*myc* expression during the differentiation of murine erythroleukemia Friend cells. *Nucl. Acids Res. 14*: 9653–9666.

Meijlink, F., Curran, T., Miller, D. A., and Verma, I. M. (1985). Removal of a 67-base-pair sequence in the noncoding region of protooncogene *fos* converts it to a transforming gene. *Proc. Natl. Acad. Sci. U.S.A. 82*: 4987–4991.

Miles, B. D., and Robinson, H. L. (1985). High-frequency transduction of c-*erbB* in avian leukosis virus-induced erythroblastosis. *J. Virol. 54*: 295–303.

Moelling, K. (1985). Fusion proteins in retroviral transformation. In *Advances in Cancer Research*, Vol. 43. Weinhouse, S., and Klein, G., eds. Academic Press, New York, pp. 205–239.

Moelling, K., Pfaff, E., Beug, H., Beimling, P., Bunte, T., Schaller, H. E., and Graf, T. (1985). DNA-Binding activity is associated with purified *myb* proteins from AMV and E26 viruses and is temperature-sensitive for E26 ts mutants. *Cell 40*: 983–990.

Moelling, K., Lorenz, U., Beimling, P., Heimann, B., Thomas, G., Bading, H., and Sander, T. (1986). Biochemical properties of oncogene-coded proteins. In *Cell Cycle and Oncogenes*. Gallwitz, D., and Tanner, W., eds. Springer-Verlag, Berlin-Heidelberg, pp. 105–113.

Moelling, K., Heimann, B., Beimling, P., Bepler, G., Köppler, H., Havemann, K., and Balzer, T. (1987). Analysis of oncogene proteins in human cell cancer tumor lines. In *Contributions to Oncology*, Vol. 24. Munk, K., and Hofschneider, P. H., eds. Karger, Basel, pp. 76–86.

Moran, E., and Mathews, M. B. (1987). Multiple functional domains in the adenovirus E1A gene. *Cell 48*: 177–178.

Morgan, J. I., and Curran, T. (1986). Role of ion influx in the control of c-*fos* expression. *Nature 322*: 552–555.

Moscovici, M. G., and Moscovici, C. (1983). Isolation and characterization of a temperature sensitive mutant of avian myeloblastosis virus. *Proc. Natl. Acad. Sci. U.S.A. 80*: 1421–1425.

Moscovici, C., Gazzolo, L., and Moscovici, M. G. (1975). Focus assay and defectiveness of avian myeloblastosis virus. *Virology 68*: 173–181.

Moscovici, C., Samarut, J., Gazzolo, L., and Moscovici, M. G. (1981). Myeloid and erythroid neoplastic responses to avian defective leukemia viruses in chickens and in quail. *Virology 118*: 765–768.

Moscovici, M. G., Jurdic, P., Samarut, J., Gazzolo, L., Mura, C. V., and Moscovici, C. (1983). Characterization of the hematopoietic target cells for the avian leukemia virus E26. *Virology 129*: 65–78.

Müller, R. (1986). Cellular and viral *fos* genes: Structure, regulation of expression and biological properties of their encoded products. *Biochem. Biophys. Acta 823*: 207–225.

Müller, R., Bravo, R., Burckhardt, J., and Curran, T. (1984). Induction of c-*fos* gene and protein by growth factors precedes activation of c-*myc*. *Nature 312*: 716–720.

Müller, R., Müller, D., Verrier, B., Bravo, R., and Herbst, H. (1986). Evidence that expression of c-*fos* protein in anion cells is regulated by external signals. *EMBO J. 5*: 311–316.

Müller, R., Bravo, R., Müller, D., Kurz, C., and Renz, M. (1987). Different modifications in *fos* and its associates protein p39: Modulation of DNA binding by phosphorylation. *Oncogene Res.* (submitted).

Nepveu, A., and Marcu, K. B. (1986). Intragenic pausing and anti-sense transcription within the murine c-*myc* locus. *EMBO J. 5*: 2859–2865.

Nilsen, T. W., Maroney, P. A., Goodwin, R. G., Rottman, F. M., Crittenden, L. B., Raines, M. A., and Kung, H. (1985). c-*erb*B activation in ALV-induced erythroblastosis: Novel RNA processing and promoter insertion result in expression of an amino-truncated EGF receptor. *Cell 41*: 719–726.

Nishikura, K., and Murray, J. M. (1987). Antisene RNA of proto-oncogene c-*fos* blocks renewed growth of quiescent 3T3 cells. *Mol. Cell. Biol. 7*: 639–649.

Nover, L. (1984). Inducers of heat shock protein synthesis. In *Heat Shock Response of Eukaryotic cells*. Nover, L., ed. Springer-Verlag, Heidelberg.

Nunn, M. F., Seeburg, P. H., Moscovici, C., and Duesberg, P. H. (1983). Tripartite structure of the avian erythroblastosis virus E26 transforming gene. *Nature 306*: 391–395.

Oppenheimer, H., and Samuels, H. H. (eds.) (1983). *Molecular Basis of Thyroid Hormone Action*. Academic Press, New York.

Persson, H., and Leder, P. (1984). Nuclear localization and DNA binding properties of protein expressed by human c-*myc* oncogene. *Science 225*: 718–721.

Piechaczyk, M., Bonnieu, A., Eick, D., Remmers, E., Yang, J.-Q., Marcu, K., Jeanteur, P., and Blanchard, J.-M. (1986). Altered c-*myc* RNA metabolism in Burkitt's lymphomas and mouse plasmacytomas. *Curr. Top. Microbiol. Immunol. 132*: 331–338.

Piechaczyk, M., Blanchard, J.-M., and Jeanteur, P. (1987). c-*myc* gene regulation still holds its secret. *Trends Gen. et. 3*: 47–51.

Privalsky, M. L., and Bishop, J. M. (1984). Subcellular localization of the v-*erb*B protein, the product of a transforming gene of avian erythroblastosis virus. *Virology 135*: 356–368.

Privalsky, M. L., Sealy, L., Bishop, J. M., McGrath, J. P., and Levinson, A. D. (1983). The product of the avian erythroblastosis virus *erb*B locus is a glycoprotein. *Cell 32*: 1257–1267.

Privalsky, M. L., Ralston, R., and Bishop, J. M. (1984). The membrane glycoprotein encoded by the retroviral oncogene v-*erb*B is structurally related to tyrosine-specific protein kinases. *Proc. Natl. Acad. Sci. U.S.A. 81*: 704–707.

Prochownik, E. V., and Kukowska, J. (1986). Deregulated expression of c-*myc* by murine erythroleukemia cells prevents differentiation. *Nature 322*: 848–850.

Prywes, R., and Roeder, R. (1986). Inducible binding of a factor to the c-*fos* enhancer. *Cell 47*: 777–784.

Rabbitts, T. H. (1985). The c-*myc* proto-oncogene: Involvement in chromosomal abnormalities. *Trends Genet.* 327–331.

Rabbitts, P. H., Watson, J. V., Lamond, A., Forster, A., Stinson, M. A., Evan, G., Fischer, W., Atherthon, E., Sheppard, R., and Rabbitts, T. H. (1985). Metabolism of c-*myc* gene products: c-*myc* mRNA and protein expression in the cell cycle. *EMBO J. 4*: 2009–2015.

Radke, K., Beug, H., Kornfeld, S., and Graf, T. (1982). Transformation of both erythroid and myeloid cells by E26, an avian leukemia virus that contains the *myb* gene. *Cell 31*: 643–653.

Rahmsdorf, H. J., Schönthal, A., Angel, P., Rüther, U., and Herrlich, P. (1987). Posttranscriptional regulation of c-*fos* mRNA expression. *Nucl. Acids Res. 15*: 1643–?.

Raines, M. A., Lewis, W. G., Crittenden, L. B., and Kung, H. (1985). *c-erbB* activation in avian leukosis virus-induced erythroblastosis: Clustered integration sites and the arrangement of provirus in the c-*erb*B alleles. *Proc. Natl. Acad. Sci. U.S.A. 82*: 2287–2291.

Rapp, U. R., Cleveland, J. L., Brightman, K., Scott, A., and Ihle, J. N. (1985). Abrogation of IL-3 and IL-2 dependence by recombinant murine retroviruses expressing v-*myc* oncogenes. *Nature 317*: 434–438.

Reich, N. C., Oren, M., and Levine, A. J. (1983). Two distinct mechanisms regulate the levels of a cellular tumor antigen, p53. *Mol. Cell. Biol. 3*: 2143–2150.

Remmers, E. F., Yang, J.-Q., and Marcu, K. B. (1986). A negative transcriptional control element located upstream of the murine c-*myc* gene. *EMBO J. 5*: 899–904.

Renz, M., Verrier, B., Kurz, C., and Müller, R. (1987). Chromatin association and DNA-binding properties of the c-*fos* proto-oncogene product. *Nucleic Acids Res. 15*: 277–292.

Rogers, S., Wells, R., and Rechsteiner, M. (1986). Amino acid sequences common to rapidly degraded proteins: The PEST hypothesis. *Science 234*: 364–368.

Rosson, D., and Reddy, E. P. (1986). Aberrant splicing events that are induced by proviral integration: Implications for *myb* oncogene activation. *Nature 319*: 604–606.

Rothe-Meyer, A., and Engelbreth-Holm, J. (1933). Experimentelle Studien über die Beziehungen zwischen Hühnerleukose und Sarkom an der Hand eines Stammmes von übertragbaren Leukose-Sarkom-Kombinationen. *Acta Pathol. Microbiol. Scand. 10*: 380–427.

Roussel, M., Saule, S., Lagrou, C., Rommens, C., Beug, H., Graf, T., and Stehelin, D. (1979a). Nucleotide sequence of chicken c-*myb* complementary DNA and implications for *myb* oncogene activation. *Nature 281*: 452–455.

Roussel, M., Saule, S., Rommens, L., Beug, H., Graf, T., and Stehelin, D. (1979b). Three types of viral oncogenes of cellular origin specific for haematopoetic cell transformation. *Nature 281*: 452–455.

Rüther, U., Garber, C., Komitowski, D., Müller, R., and Wagner, E. (1987). Deregulated c-*fos* expression interferes with normal bone development in transgenic mice. *Nature 325*: 412–416.

Sambucetti, L., and Curran, T. (1986). The *fos* protein complex is associated with DNA in isolated nuclei and binds to DNA cellulose. *Science 234*: 1417–1419.

Sap, J., Muñoz, A., Damm, K., Ghysdael, J., Leutz, A., Beug, H., and Vennström, B. (1986). The c-*erb*A protein is a high affinity receptor for thyroid hormone. *Nature 324*: 635–640.

Sassone-Corsi, P., and Borelli, E. (1987). Promoter *trans*-activation of c-*fos* and c-*myc*, but not Ha-*ras*, by the adenovirus E1A products. *Proc. Natl. Acad. Sci. U.S.A.* (in press).

Sassone-Corsi, P., and Verma, I. M. (1987). Modulation of c-*fos* gene transcription by negative and positive cellular factors. *Nature 326*: 507–510.

Schmidt, J. A., Marshall, J., Hayman, M. J., Pouka, P., and Beug, H. (1986). Control of erythroid differentiation: Possible role of the transferrin cycle. *Cell 46*: 41–51.

Sealy, L., Privalsky, M. L., Moscovici, G., Moscovici, C., and Bishop, J. M. (1983). Site-specific mutagenesis of avian erythroblastosis virus: *erb*B is required for oncogenicity. *Virology 130*: 155–178.

Setoyama, C., Frunzio, R., Liau, G., Mudryj, M., and de Crombrugghe, B. (1986a). Transcriptional activation encoded by the v-*fos* gene. *Proc. Natl. Acad. Sci. U.S.A. 83*: 3213–3217.

Setoyama, C., Hatamochi, A., Peterkofsky, B., Prather, W., and de Crombrugghe, B. (1986b). v-*fos* stimulates expression of the a_1(III) collagen gene in NIH3T3 cells. *Biochem. Biophys. Res. Commun. 136*: 1042–1048.

Shaw, G., and Kamen, R. (1986). A conserved AU sequence from the third untranslated region of GM-CSF mRNA mediates selective mRNA degradation. *Cell 46*: 659–667.

Sheiness, D., and Gardinier, M. (1984). Expression of a proto-oncogene (proto-*myb*) in hematopoietic tissues of mice. *Mol. Cell. Biol. 4*: 1206–1212.

Sheiness, D., Vennström, B. and Bishop, J. M. (1981). Virus-specific RNAs in cells infected by avian myelocytomatosis virus and avian erythroblastosis virus: Modes of oncogene expression. *Cell 23*: 291–300.

Shen-Ong, G. L., Morse, H. C., Potter, M., and Mushinski, J. F. (1986). Two modes of c-*myb* action in virus-induced mouse myeloid tumors. *Mol. Cell. Biol. 6*: 380–392.

Siebenlist, U., Henninghausen, I., Battey, J., and Leder, P. (1984). Chromatin structure and protein binding in the putative regulatory regions of the c-*myc* gene in Burkitt lymphoma. *Cell 37*: 381–391.

Slamon, D. J., Boone, T. C., Murdock, D. C., Keith, D. E., Press, M. F., Larson, R. A., and Souza, L. M. (1986). Studies of the human c-*myb* gene and its product in human acute leukemias. *Science 233*: 347–351.

Souza, L. M., Strommer, J. N., Hillyard, R. L., Komaromy, M. C., and Baluda, M. A. (1980). Cellular sequences are present in the presumptive avian myeloblastosis virus genome. *Proc. Natl. Acad. Sci. U.S.A. 77*: 5177–5181.

Spector, D. L., Watt, R. A., and Sullivan, N. F. (1987). The v- and c-*myc* oncogene poteins colocalize *in situ* with small nuclear ribonucleoprotein particles. *Oncogene 1*: 5–12.

Spindler, K. R., and Berk, A. J. (1984). Rapid intracellular turnover of adenovirus 5 early region 1A proteins. *J. Virol. 52*: 706–710.

Spurr, N. K., Solomon, E., Jansson, M., Sheer, D., Goodfellow, P. N., Bodmer, W. F., and Vennström, B. (1984). Chromosomal localisation of the human homologues to the oncogenes *erb*A and B. *EMBO J. 3*: 159–163.

Stewart, T. A., Pattengale, P. K., and Leder, P. (1984). Spontaneous mammary adenocarcinoma in transgenic mice that carry and express MTV/*myc* fusion genes. *Cell 38*: 627–637.

Stone, J., de Lange, T., Ramsay, G., Jakobovits, E., Bishop, J. M., Varmus, H., and Lee, W. (1987). Definition of regions in human c-*myc* that are involved in transformation and nuclear localization. *Mol. Cell. Biol. 7*: 1697–1709.

Stuart, T. A., Bellvé, A. R., and Leder, P. (1984). Transcription and promoter usage of the *myc* gene in normal somatic and spermatogenic cells. *Science 226*: 707–710.

Studzinsky, G. P., Brelvi, Z. S., Feldman, S. C., and Watt, R. A. (1986). Participation of c-*myc* protein in DNA synthesis of mammalian cells. *Science 234*: 467–470.

Symonds, G., Klempnauer, K.-H., Evan, G. I., and Bishop, J. M. (1984a). Induced differentiation of avian myeloblastosis virus-transformed myeloblasts: Phenotypic alteration of the viral oncogene. *Mol. Cell. Biol. 4*: 2587–2593.

Symonds, G., Stubblefield, E., Guyaux, M., and Bishop, J. M. (1984b). Cellular oncogenes (c-*erb*A and c-*erb*B) located on different chicken chromosomes can be transduced into the same retroviral genome. *Mol. Cell. Biol. 4*: 1627–1630.

Thompson, C. B., Challoner, P. B., Neiman, P. E., and Groudine, M. (1985). Levels of c-*myc* oncogene mRNA are invariant throughout the cell cycle. *Nature 314*: 363–366.

Thompson, C. B., Challoner, P. B., Neiman, P. E., and Groudine, M. (1986). Expression of the c-*myb* proto-oncogene during cellular proliferation. *Nature 319*: 374–380.

Tracy, S. E., Woda, B. A., and Robinson, H. L. (1985). Induction of angiosarcoma by a c-*erb*B transducing virus. *J. Virol. 54*: 304–310.

Treisman, R. (1985). Transient accumulation of c-*fos* RNA following serum-stimulation requires a conserved 5′ element and c-*fos* 3′ sequences. *Cell 42*: 889–902.

Treisman, R. (1986). Identification of a protein-binding site that mediates transcriptional response of the c-*fos* gene to serum factors. *Cell 46*: 567–574.

Ullrich, A., Coussens, L., Hayflick, J. S., Dull, T. J., Gray, A., Tam, A. W., Lee, J., Yarden, Y., Libermann, T. A., Schlessinger, J., Downward, J., Mayes, E. L. V., Whittle, N., Waterfield, M. D., and Seeburg, P. H. (1984). Human epidermal growth factor receptor cDNA sequence and aberrant expression of the amplified gene in A431 epidermoid carcinoma cells. *Nature 309*: 418–425.

Van Beveren, C., van Straaten, F., Curran, T., Müller, R., and Verma, I. M. (1983). Analysis of FBJ-MuSV provirus and c-*fos* (mouse) gene reveals that viral and cellular *fos* gene products have different carboxy termini. *Cell 32*: 1241–1255.

van Straaten, F., Müller, R., Curran, T., Van Beveren, C., and Verma, I. M. (1983). Complete nucleotide sequence of a human c-*onc* gene: Deduced amino acid sequence of the human c-*fos* protein. *Proc. Natl. Acad. Sci. U.S.A. 80*:3183–3187.

Vennström, B., and Bishop, J. M. (1982). Isolation and characterization of chicken DNA homologous to the two putative oncogenes of avian erythroblastosis virus. *Cell 28*: 135–143.

Vennström, B., Fanshier, L., Moscovici, C., and Bishop, J. M. (1980). Molecular cloning of the avian erythroblastosis virus genome and recovery of oncogenic virus by transfection of chicken cells. *J. Virol. 36*: 575–585.

Vogt, P. K., Bos, T. J., and Doolittle, R. F. (1987). Homology between the DNA-binding domain of the GCN4 regulatory protein of yeast and the carboxyl-terminal region of a protein coded for by the oncogene *jun*. *Proc. Natl. Acad. Sci. U.S.A. 84*: 3316–3319.

Watson, R. J., Dyson, P. J., and McMahon, J. (1987). Multiple c-*myb* transcript cap sites are variously utilized in cells of mouse haematopoietic origin. *EMBO J. 6*: 1643–1651.

Watt, R. A., Shatzman, A. R., and Rosenberg, M. (1985). Expression and characterization of the human c-*myc* DNA-binding protein. *Mol. Cell. Biol. 5*: 448–456.

Weinberger, C., Hollenberg, S. M., Rosenfeld, M. G., and Evans, R. M. (1985). Domain structure of human glucocorticoid receptor and its relationship to the v-*erb*A oncogene product. *Nature 318*: 670–672.

Weinberger, C., Thompson, C., Ong, E., Gruol, D., and Evans, R. (1986). The c-*erb*A gene encodes a thyroid hormone receptor. *Nature 324*: 641–646.

Weinstein, Y., Ihle, J. N., Lavu, S., and Reddy, E. P. (1986). Truncation of the c-*myb* gene by a retroviral integration in an interleukin 3-dependent myeloid leukemia cell line. *Proc. Natl. Acad. Sci. U.S.A. 83*: 5010–5014.

Westin, E. H., Gallo, R. C., Arya, S. K., Souza, L. M., Baluda, M. A., Aaronson, S. A., and Wong-Staal, F. (1982a). Differential expression of the *amv* gene in human haematopoietic cells. *Proc. Natl. Acad. Sci. U.S.A. 79*: 2194–2198.

Westin, E. H., Wong-Staal, F., Gelmann, E. P., Dalla-Favera, R., Papas, T. S., Lautenberger, J. A., Eva, A., Reddy, E. P., Tronick, S. R., Aaronson, S. A., and Gallo, R. C. (1982b). Expression of cellular homologues of retroviral *onc* genes in human hematopoietic cells. *Proc. Natl. Acad. Sci. U.S.A. 79*: 2490–2494.

Winqvist, R., Saksela, K., and Alitalo, K. (1984). The *myc* proteins are not associated with chromatin in mitotic cells. *EMBO J. 3*: 2947–2950.

Woods, C. M., Boyer, B., Vogt, P. K., and Lazarides, E. (1986). Control of erythroid differentiation: Asynchronous expression of the anion transporter and the peripheral components of the membrane skeleton in AEV- and S13-transformed cells. *J. Cell. Biol. 103*: 1789–1798.

Yamamoto, K. M., Yamada, S. S., and Pastan, I. (1976). Cell surface protein partially restores morphology, adhesiveness and contact inhibition of movement to transformed fibroblasts. *Proc. Natl. Acad. Sci. U.S.A. 73*: 1217–1221.

Yamamoto, T., Hihara, H., Nishida, T., Kawai, S., and Toyoshima, K. (1983). A new avian erythroblastosis virus, AEV-H, carries an *erb*B gene responsable for the induction of both erythroblastosis and sarcomas. *Cell 34*: 225–232.

Yang, J. -Q., Remmers, E. F., and Marcu, B. (1986). The first exon of the c-*myc* proto-oncogene contains a novel positive control element. *EMBO J.5*: 3553–3562.

Yarden, A., and Kimchi, A. (1986). Tumor necrosis factor reduces c-*myc* expression and cooperates with interferon-l in HeLa cells. *Science 234*: 1413–1417.

Zabel, B. U., Fournier, R. E., Lalley, P. A., Naylor, S. L., and Sakaguchi, A. Y. (1984). Cellular homologs of the avian erythroblastosis virus *erb*A and *erb*B genes are synthenic in mouse but asyntenic in man. *Proc. Natl. Acad. Sci. U.S.A. 81*: 4874–4878.

TWO

Insertional Activation of Proto-Oncogenes Previously Identified as Viral Oncogenes

Bruce E. Clurman and William S. Hayward
Sloan-Kettering Institute for Cancer Research
New York, New York

INTRODUCTION

The ribonucleic acid (RNA) tumor viruses can be classified into two groups. The acute, or rapidly transforming retroviruses, induce neoplastic disease within weeks after infection of the host, and transform appropriate target cells in tissue culture. In contrast, the nonacute, or slowly transforming retroviruses, induce neoplasms with a much longer latent period, and are usually unable to morphologically transform cells in vitro. It has become clear that the differences in the pathogenic properties of these two classes are attributable to the presence of oncogenes in the genomes of the acute retroviruses. Approximately 25 viral oncogenes (v-*onc* genes) have now been identified.

The finding that a homolog of the v-*src* gene of Rous sarcoma virus was present in the normal cell (Stehelin et al., 1976) provided the first evidence for the existence of cellular genes with oncogenic potential. Cellular homologs of all of the known retroviral oncogenes have now been identified. These genes have been termed cellular oncogenes (c-*onc* genes), or proto-oncogenes. Inherent in the latter term is the important concept that in their normal cellular configurations proto-oncogenes are not oncogenic—they require some type of modification to activate their oncogenic potential. It is generally believed that genes that function to control cellular growth or differentiation would be likely candidates for oncogenic activation. The identification of some proto-oncogene products as growth factors or growth factor receptors has given credence to this idea. Alterations in these genes can thus result in a disruption of normal cellular control processes, resulting in the abnormal growth patterns characteristic of neoplastic transformation.

While the discovery of viral oncogenes and their cellular progenitors provided an explanation for the oncogenic properties of the acute retroviruses, the nonacute retroviruses, which lack oncogenes yet efficiently induce neoplasms, remained an enigma. A model to explain the oncogenicity of these viruses evolved from the discovery of host proto-oncogenes, and from certain features of the retroviral life cycle. As an obligatory step in their life cycle, retroviruses integrate into the host cell chromosomes. The integrated viral genome, called a provirus, thus becomes a stable component of the host genome. Integration can occur at many different sites in the host genome, possibly at random, although factors other than deoxyribonucleic acid (DNA) sequence may influence the relative availability of different regions. Thus as a rare event, viral insertions might occur within the vicinity of a proto-oncogene in such a way that the oncogenic potential of the gene is activated.

As originally formulated, this model proposed that the provirus, integrated upstream of the coding sequences of the proto-oncogene, would provide an active promoter (located within the viral long terminal repeat [LTR]), from which transcription of the adjacent host gene would initiate (Neel et al., 1981; Payne et al., 1981) (see Fig. 1). According to this model (the promoter insertion model), the inappropriate expression of the proto-oncogene, under control of the proviral regulatory sequences, would result in disruption of normal cellular growth controls, leading to neoplastic transformation of the target cell.

The demonstration that the c-*myc* gene is insertionally activated in avian leukosis virus (ALV)-induced bursal lymphomas (Hayward et al., 1981) provided a solid basis for the notion that host proto-oncogenes could be oncogenically activated by direct mutational events. In the case of the ALV-induced lymphomas, insertional activation of c-*myc* occurs precisely as predicted by the promoter insertion model (see following section). However, subsequent studies of both retroviral and nonviral neoplasms have revealed other mechanisms for mutationally activating proto-oncogenes. In general, these fall into two classes: regulatory and structural (i.e., changes in the coding region resulting in synthesis of an altered gene

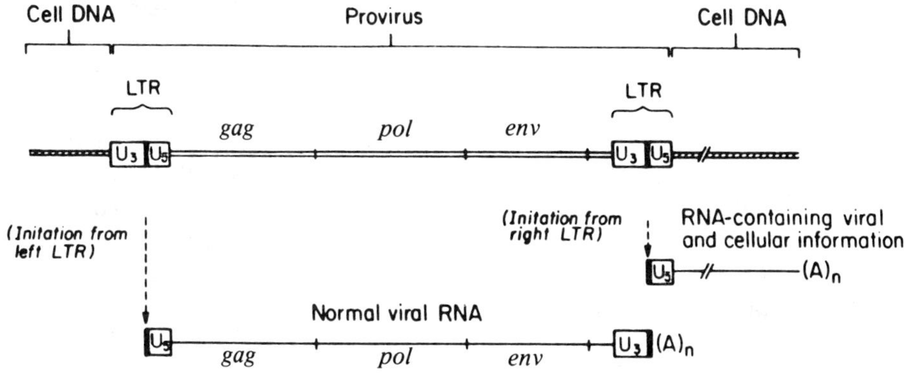

Figure 1 Structure and transcription of an integrated retroviral genome (provirus). Viral genes required for replication are *gag* (structural proteins), *pol* (reverse transcriptase and integrase), and *env* (envelope glycoprotein). Various *cis*-acting sequences, including the promoter, enhancer, and poly(A) addition signals, are encoded in the 5′ (left) and 3′ long terminal repeats (LTRs). Transcription of viral RNA normally initiates within the 5′ LTR, and poly(A) addition occurs in the 3′ LTR. The promoter in the 3′ LTR is normally used inefficiently, if at all (Herman and Coffin, 1986). However, in some neoplasms induced by nonacute retroviruses (e.g., ALV-induced B-cell lymphomas), proto-oncogene activation results from transcription initiating within the 3′ LTR, and continuing into adjacent host proto-oncogene sequences, as predicted by the promoter insertion model. Efficient utilization of the 3′ promoter may require deletion of critical regions within the provirus (see text). In some other systems, insertional activation involves 5′ LTR-initiated transcription, which proceeds past the 3′ poly(A) addition signal at low frequency, and into the adjacent proto-oncogene. Abnormal splicing events result in a closer juxtaposition of viral and proto-oncogene sequences in the chimeric RNA. (Adapted from Neel et al., 1981; used with permission.)

product). Both types of alterations can be introduced by retroviral insertions. Many different strategies for achieving these alterations have been found in the various host-virus systems studied. This chapter will focus on the insertional activation of only those genes that were previously identified as viral oncogenes. Other cellular targets for insertional activation will be discussed in Chapter 3.

MECHANISMS OF INSERTIONAL ACTIVATION IN DIFFERENT VIRUS-HOST SYSTEMS

c-*myc*

The first demonstration of insertional activation was in ALV-induced bursal lymphomas, in which the activated gene was identified as c-*myc* (see below).

The *myc* gene was originally identified as a viral oncogene present in four independent isolates of avian acute retroviruses, MC29, MH2, OK10, and CMII (Roussel et al., 1979). The v-*myc* genes of each of the acute viruses carry the complete coding region of c-*myc*, but the transduced genes have sustained at least one (CMII), and as many as 27 (MH2) missense mutations (Alitalo et al., 1983; Hayflick et al., 1985; Kan et al., 1984; Reddy et al., 1983; Walther et al., 1986; Watson et al., 1983). The v-*myc* genes of MH2 and OK10 are expressed as independent proteins, whereas in CMII and MC29 they are expressed as *gag-myc* fusion proteins. MH2 also carries a second oncogene, v-*mil*.

ALV-Induced B-Cell Lymphomas

Avian leukosis viruses induce a variety of neoplasms, including B-cell lymphomas, nephroblastomas, firbosarcomas, carcinomas, and erythroblastosis (Beard, 1963; Purchase et al., 1977; Weiss et al., 1982). The pathogenic spectrum of these viruses is strongly dependent on such factors as time of infection, route of infection, viral strain, and host strain. The neoplasm most commonly observed is a B-cell lymphoma (classically termed lymphoid leukosis), which arises in the bursa of Fabricius and later metastasizes to other organs such as liver, kidney, and spleen. This disease is generally characterized by extensive bursal involvement and development of discrete bursal nodules (Cooper et al., 1968; Neiman et al., 1980).

The first presumptive evidence for insertional activation was based on three predictions of the promoter insertion model: (a) tumors should be clonal, arising from a single initially infected cell that had sustained an appropriate integration event; (b) proviruses should be integrated within a common chromosomal region in independently derived tumors; and (c) novel chimeric messenger RNAs (mRNAs), encoding both viral (U_5) and cellular information should be expressed in tumor cells (see Fig. 1). All three of these predictions were met in the ALV-induced B-cell lymphomas (Neel et al., 1981; Payne et al., 1981). A fourth prediction, that the provirus should be integrated adjacent to a host gene with oncogenic potential, was met when the adjacent host DNA was identified as the c-*myc* gene (Hayward et al., 1981; Neel et al., 1982), and the cell-derived sequences on the tumor-specific U_5-positive RNA transcripts were shown to be from the c-*myc* gene. The U_5-*myc* transcripts are generally somewhat smaller (about 2.3 kb) than the normal c-*myc* mRNA (2.4 kb), and are expressed at levels 30- to 100-fold higher than in normal tissues.

More than 100 integrated *myc*-associated proviruses in bursal lymphomas, induced by various strains of ALV, have now been mapped (Fung et al., 1981, 1982; Goodenow and Hayward, 1987; Neel et al., 1981, 1982; Payne et al., 1981, 1982; Robinson and Gagnon, 1986; Rovigatti et al., 1982; Shih et al., 1984). Approximately 70% are located in the first intron, and the majority of these are within a 300-bp region just upstream of $exon_2$, the first coding exon (see Fig. 2A). Most of the remaining integrations are within or upstream of the first exon. Approximately 95% are in the same transcriptional orientation as c-*myc*. Payne et al. (1982), however, identified some important exceptions to this pattern. Several examples of integrations upstream but in the opposite orientation were found, and one

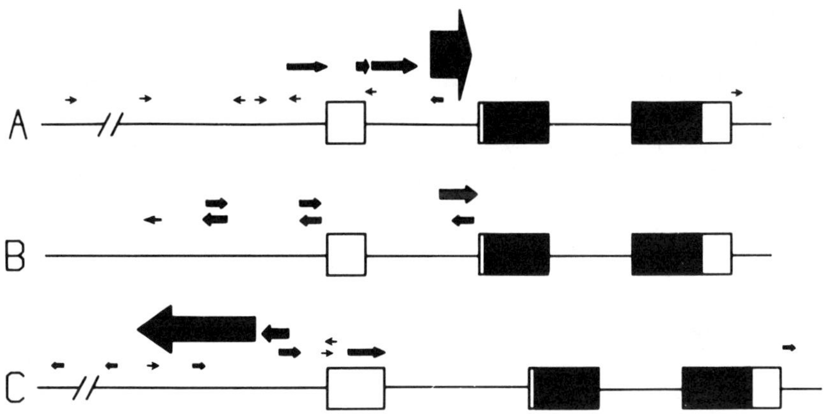

Figure 2 Orientation and distribution of integrations within c-*myc* loci insertionally activated by ALV, REV, and MuLV. Integration sites and transcriptional orientation of the proviruses are indicated by arrows. The width of each arrow reflects the relative number of integrations within the indicated region. (The smallest arrow in each case represents a single integration event.) The three exons of c-*myc*, oriented 5′ to 3′ (left to right), are represented by boxes. Open boxes: noncoding regions; closed boxes: coding regions. A. ALV-induced B-cell lymphomas in chickens. B. REV-induced T-cell lymphomas in chickens. C. MuLV-induced T-cell lymphomas in mice. Data were compiled from the following sources: A. Goodenow and Hayward, 1987; Linial et al., 1985; Robinson and Gagnon, 1986; Payne et al., 1982; Shih et al., 1984 (approximately 100 independent integrations are represented). B. Isfort et al., 1987 (14 integrations). C. Li et al., 1984; Reicin et al., 1986; Selten et al., 1984 (approximately 70 integrations).

integration was found to map downstream of c-*myc*. These exceptions provided the first evidence that the viral enhancer could influence transcription from a cellular promoter, thus obviating the requirement for LTR-initiated transcription of the activated proto-oncogene. Although relatively rare in ALV-induced lymphomas, this orientation predominates in many other systems that were characterized later (see below, and Chapter 3).

Several examples of "unusual" transcription patterns have been reported in cell lines derived from ALV-induced lymphomas (Linial and Groudine, 1985). Integrations within certain regions appear to activate cryptic promoters in the first intron, and one cell line with an integration in $intron_1$ and in the same transcriptional orientation contained transcripts initiated on the normal c-*myc* promoter. Whether these patterns represent changes that are selected for during in vitro passage, or reflect the patterns in the original tumors, has not been determined. All studies to date on RNA recovered directly from tumors have revealed LTR-initiated transcripts (Goodenow and Hayward, 1987; Hayward et al., 1981; Neel et al., 1981; Payne et al., 1982).

Another unexpected characteristic of the ALV integrations near c-*myc*, observed early on (Fung et al., 1981; Neel et al., 1981; Payne et al., 1981), was the existence of deletions in a high proportion of the integrated proviruses. Based on the loss of a SacI site near the 5′ end of the provirus, it was originally suggested that the 5′ LTR was deleted in these *myc*-associated proviruses (Rovigatti et al., 1982). This led to the suggestion that deletion of the 5′ promoter, and the resulting block of 5′-initiated transcription, would facilitate utilization of the 3′ promoter (Cullen et al., 1984; Hayward et al., 1982; Neel et al., 1981). The 3′ promoter of nondefective ALV is used only minimally, if at all, in a randomly infected cell population (Herman and Coffin, 1986). Cullen et al. (1984) tested this model (transcriptional interference model) by linking a marker gene downstream of a complete provirus, and to a provirus in which the 5′ end had been removed, and transfecting these constructs into tissue culture cells. Removal of the 5′ LTR resulted in a five- to 10-fold increase in expression of the downstream marker gene.

More complete analyses of the *myc*-associated proviruses (Goodenow and Hayward, 1987; Robinson and Gagnon, 1986) have shown that although most carried deletions near the 5′ end of the provirus, the 5′ LTR was generally intact. Deletions were present in all of 25 randomly selected proviruses analyzed by Goodenow and Hayward (1987). In about 85% of these, the proviral deletion included a region just downstream of the viral 5′ LTR—a region that has been implicated in both *cis*- and *trans*-acting regulatory functions (Arrigo et al., 1987; Broome and Gilbert, 1985; Herman and Coffin, 1986). In three cases, however, deletions were within the 3′ half of the provirus. Interestingly, no 5′-initiated transcripts were detectable from these proviruses, even when the 5′ LTR was structurally intact, suggesting that the internal deletions disrupt some important regulatory regions (Goodenow and Hayward, 1987). Thus the transcriptional interference model is still tenable, although it may not be the complete answer. A deletion has also been found in one provirus that was inserted in the opposite transcriptional orientation from c-*myc* (Payne et al., 1982), a configuration in which transcriptional initiation from the 3′ LTR would presumably be unnecessary. Several other explanations for the deletions, not mutually exclusive, have also been proposed (Goodenow and Hayward, 1987; Hayward et al., 1982; Swift et al., 1987): A block in the expression of viral genes—in particular the *env* gene, whose product is localized on the surface of the infected cell—might allow the infected cell to escape detection by the host immune system. The absence of *env* expression would also allow superinfection of the infected cell. (Superinfection by retroviruses of the same subgroup is normally blocked by "interference," which is thought to be mediated by saturation of viral binding sites on the cell surface by the envelope glycoprotein synthesized in the infected cell [Weiss et al., 1982].) This would allow subsequent integrations in cells with an activated c-*myc* gene, raising the possibility of further proto-oncogene activations that might complement the activated c-*myc* gene. Consistent with this interpretation, recent studies, using a protocol that involves sequential infection with ALVs of two different subgroups, have resulted in identification of a new oncogene (termed *bic*), which is insertionally activated in approximately 50% of the metastatic lymphomas induced with the two virus protocol (Clurman and Hayward, manuscript in preparation). Most of these tumors also contained *myc* activations, suggesting that *myc* and *bic* might provide complementary functions required for induction of a fully malignant state.

Insertions near c-*myc* are found in the vast majority of B-cell lymphomas induced by ALV (85–100% in different studies). However, a new class of rapidly appearing B-cell lymphomas, induced by a recombinant ALV, is not associated with c-*myc* activation, but rather with integrations into c-*myb* (see below). Only one example of insertional activation of c-*myc* in a nonlymphoid tumor has been reported. This tumor, diagnosed as an adenocarcinoma of the omentum, was induced by ring-necked pheasant virus (RPV), and contained a provirus integrated upstream of $exon_1$, and in the same transcriptional orientation (Simon et al., 1984).

Reticuloendotheliosis Virus-Induced Lymphomas

The reticuloendotheliosis viruses (REVs), which were originally isolated from various types of poultry (chicken, turkey, and duck), have little homology with the chicken ALVs, and appear to be more closely related to the murine leukemia viruses (Wilhelmsen et al., 1984). However, like ALV, they induce primarily bursal lymphomas in chickens (Witter and Crittenden, 1979). These lymphomas are characterized, in over 70% of cases, by integrations within the c-*myc* locus (Noori-Daloii et al., 1981; Swift et al., 1985). The mechanism involved is indistinguisable from that in the ALV-induced B-cell lymphomas. The distribution of integrations is similar to that for ALV-induced lymphomas (Fig. 2A), with the vast majority (90%) located within the first intron. Transcription initiates within the 3′ LTR. The *myc*-associated proviruses also contain deletions, as in the ALV system (Swift et al., 1985, 1987).

REV also induces a low incidence of T-cell lymphomas in most chicken lines, and in some lines, which are resistant to B-cell lymphoma, induces only T-cell lymphomas (Witter et al., 1986). These tumors are characterized by integrations within c-*myc* (14/14 tumors), but the distribution and orientation patterns are strikingly different from those in either the ALV- or REV-induced B-cell lymphomas (Isfort et al., 1987). Six of the 14 tumors had integrations within the first intron, just upstream of $exon_2$, but eight integrations were upstream of $exon_1$. Furthermore, half of the proviruses were in the opposite transcriptional orientation from c-*myc* (see Fig. 2B).

Transcription initiates within the 3′ LTR of proviruses integrated in the first intron and in the same transcriptional orientation; however, in tumors that carry proviruses upstream of $exon_1$, in either orientation, transcription initiates from a cryptic c-*myc* promoter within $intron_1$ (Isfort et al., 1987). Thus REV appears to exert an enhancer-like activity in these cases. It is not clear why the enhancer should activate transcription from the cryptic promoter, since the normal c-*myc* promoter(s) are closer to the viral enhancer. One possibility is that the upstream integrations disrupt control sequences required for transcription from the normal promoters. The levels of *myc* mRNA in these tumors are elevated (four- to 18-fold over levels in normal thymus), but not to the same extent as that in either ALV-or REV-induced B-cell lymphomas. The lower level of expression may be more favorable for T-cell lymphomagenesis, thus resulting in a selection for proviruses that are not integrated in the promoter insertion orientation (Isfort et al., 1987).

MuLV-Induced T-Cell Lymphomas

T-cell and occasionally B-cell lymphomas can be induced in mice by exogenous murine leukemia virus (MuLV), or in "high-incidence" mouse strains by germ-line transmission of MuLV or transmission through the mother's milk (Weiss et al., 1982). Tumor induction is usually accompanied by the generation of mink cell focus-forming (MCF) viruses, which are recombinants between exogenous ecotropic viruses, and endogenous viral sequences related to the xenotropic MuLVs (Chattopadhyay et al., 1982; Cloyd et al., 1980; Elder et al., 1977; Hartley et al., 1977; Ruscetti et al., 1979, 1981). MCF viruses are characterized by the acquisition of *env*-LTR sequences from the endogenous source (for a review see Famulari, 1983; Holland et al., 1985). The precise role of these sequences is unknown, although they may facilitate infection of, or expression in, appropriate target cells, or allow superinfection of cells previously infected with the primary virus (possibly allowing multihit insertional activations to occur). A more direct role for the MCF envelope glycoprotein in the oncogenic process has also been proposed (Famulari et al., 1983; Weiss et al., 1982).

Initial efforts to demonstrate insertional activation in MuLV-induced tumors were hampered by the high background of endogenous proviruses in mice (as many as 50–100 copies per cell), which made identification of novel tumor-specific junction fragments with viral probes virtually impossible. Several laboratories have overcome this difficulty by using rats rather than mice as the host because of the absence of MuLV-related endogenous proviruses in the rat (Steffen, 1984; Tsichlis et al., 1983). Another approach was to molecularly tag the exogenous virus with nonviral (prokaryotic) sequences inserted into the LTR (Li et al., 1984). In some cases, direct analysis for rearrangement of known proto-oncogenes has been used in the initial screening, thus bypassing the need to identify unique virus-cell junction fragments.

The first proto-oncogene to be implicated in MuLV-induced T-cell leukemias and lymphomas was c-*myc* (Cuypers et al., 1984; Li et al., 1984; Selten et al., 1984; Steffen, 1984). The incidence of c-*myc* involvement varies considerably from one system to another, and is lower (0–60%) than in the avian systems. Approximately 90% of c-*myc* integrations in MuLV systems are upstream of the first exon, and in the opposite transcriptional orientation (Cuypers et al., 1984; Li et al., 1984; O'Donnell et al., 1985; Reicin et al., 1986; Selten et al., 1984) (see Fig. 2C). Approximately 10% are within $exon_1$, in either orientation. Two examples of integrations downstream of c-*myc* and in the same transcriptional orientation have been reported. No integrations have been found within the first intron—the major target in ALV- and REV-induced B-cell lymphomas. Thus enhancer insertion appears to be the preferred mechanism of c-*myc* activation in these systems.

The observation that the majority of integrations occur about 0.5–1.5 kb upstream of the first c-*myc* promoter raises the possibility that disruption of putative control sequences located in this region plays an important role in the activation process (Reicin et al., 1986). The levels of c-*myc* mRNA in MuLV-induced tumors are not elevated substantially over those in normal lymphoid cells, suggesting that deregulation, rather than overexpression, may be the important factor. Reicin et al. (1986) also observed a change in utilization of the two normal c-*myc* promoters, P_1 and P_2. An increased P_1/P_2 utilization ratio was seen in all tumors that carried c-*myc*–associated proviruses. Interestingly, this ratio was also increased in many lymphomas that did not display c-*myc* integrations, suggesting that integrations may have occurred outside the region analyzed by restriction analysis, perhaps acting by some long-distance *cis*-acting mechanism. In this respect, it is perhaps relevant that several common integration sites that have not been demonstrated to be functional genes are closely linked to the c-*myc* locus in mice (P. Tsichlis, personal communication). Alternatively, c-*myc* expression might be altered by integrations into unlinked loci involved in *trans*-acting regulation of the c-*myc* gene.

Cuypers et al. (1984) and Selten et al. (1984) have analyzed c-*myc* activations in a variety of murine systems, and report a correlation between tumor latency and incidence of c-*myc* involvement. They define three groups with latencies of 3–6, 6–12, and 12–16 months. Activation of c-*myc* was found in approximately 40% of 66 tumors from group 1 (which included BALB/c or C57BL mice infected with moloney MuLV (Mo-MuLV) as newborns, and AKR mice infected with MCF247), whereas no c-*myc* activations were found in 16 tumors from the 12-16 month group (C57BL or BALB/c infected as newborns with MCF1130, and C57BL infected with milk-transmitted C57-MLV). Selten et al. (1984) also analyzed the *myc*-associated proviruses in the Mo-MuLV-infected BALB/c mice (group 1) to test for involvement of MCF recombinant viruses. Approximately 50% of the c-*myc* activations in these tumors resulted from integrations of MCF viruses, as determined by the presence of MCF-specific restriction sites in the integrated proviruses.

Many other common integration sites have been identified by proviral tagging in the MuLV-induced lymphomas (see Chapter 3). Activation of c-*myc* is often accompanied by integrations within one of these additional sites, which may represent proto-oncogenes that cooperate with c-*myc* to induce the fully malignant state (Cuypers et al., 1984). An analysis of early stage tumors by O'Donnell et al. (1985) indicated that c-*myc* activation may be either an early or late event in tumor progression.

Induction of Feline Leukemia Virus (FeLV)-Induced T-Cell Lymphomas

One of the most common causes of death in domestic cats is T-cell lymphoma. These tumors are often, but not always, associated with evidence of FeLV infection (Hardy, 1982). In an analysis of 16 field-isolated or experimentally induced virus-positive T-cell lymphomas and cell lines, three showed evidence of proviral insertions adjacent to c-*myc* (Neil et al., 1984). Two of these were upstream of $exon_2$, and one appeared to be downstream.

Somewhat surprising was the observation of Neil et al. (1984) that five of the 16 tumors that did not have insertional activations of c-*myc* contained *myc*-transducing retroviruses. Two other groups also identified *myc*-transducing viruses in a high percentage of T-cell lymphomas, but found no evidence for insertional activation of c-*myc* in any tumors (Levy et al., 1984; Mullins et al., 1984). The detection of *myc*-transducing viruses at such high frequency suggests that transduction is the predominant mechanism of c-*myc* activation in the FeLV system. It is possible that the structure of FeLV is particularly favorable for generating a transducing virus (Stewart et al., 1986).

Common Features of c-*myc* Activation

Although the molecular details of insertional activation of c-*myc* differ in the various systems described above, the basic strategy is the same; namely, a disruption or alteration of the normal cellular control of c-*myc* expression. Of more than 200 integrations analyzed in many different systems no integrations were found to disrupt the coding region of c-*myc*. Thus there must be a very strong selection for maintaining the integrity of the normal c-*myc* protein. This contrasts with the situation seen with c-*erb*B and c-*myb*, where insertional activation is invariably associated with truncation of the gene product (see below). Furthermore, with one possible exception, fusion of the c-*myc* gene product with viral sequences has not been observed. (The exception is the RP9 cell line, derived from an ALV-induced lymphoma, in which the protein appears to be translated by initiation at the *gag* AUG on a spliced mRNA, yielding a protein that has 14 additional amino acids at its N-terminus. [Linial and Groudine, 1985; C.-K. Shih and W. S. Hayward, unpublished].)

Likewise, point mutations within the coding region do not appear to be essential for activation of c-*myc*, at least in the ALV system where three activated c-*myc* genes have been cloned and sequenced. In the first reported case (Westaway et al., 1984), three base changes were found in a short region that was sequenced near the 5′ end of the coding region. One of these was shown to be a somatic mutation (by demonstrating the loss of a SacI site present in the normal c-*myc* locus in the same animal), and one was a missense mutation. However, two other ALV-activated c-*myc* genes, sequenced more recently, contained no missense mutations (M. Hahn and W. S. Hayward, 1988). Similarly, in human Burkitt's lymphomas examples of both mutated (Murphy et al., 1986; Rabbitts et al., 1983), and nonmutated

(Battey et al., 1983; Wiman et al., 1984) c-*myc* coding regions have been reported. Thus although missense mutations are sometimes found, they are clearly not essential for the oncogenic activation of c-*myc*.

In contrast, the v-*myc* genes of MC29, MH2, CMII, and OK10 all contain missense mutations, and in two cases (MC29 and CMII) are expressed as *gag-myc* fusion proteins. These mutations may help to "fine tune" the oncogenic properties of the v-*myc* gene, or extend the range of target tissues in which it can induce transformation (Enrietto et al., 1983a,b).

c-*erb*B

The *erb*B gene was first identified in avian erythroblastosis virus (AEV), which contains two transduced cellular genes, v-*erb*A and v-*erb*B (Privalsky and Bishop, 1982; Vennstrom and Bishop, 1982; for a review, see Graf and Stehelin, 1982). The isolation of acute retroviruses containing only v-*erb*B, and studies with AEV deletion mutants indicate that the v-*erb*B gene is the primary transforming gene of AEV, and that v-*erb*A augments the transforming activitites of v-*erb*B, particulary in erythroid cells (Beug et al., 1985; Graf and Beug, 1983; Frykberg et al., 1983; Miles and Robinson, 1985; Nishida et al., 1984; Sealy et al., 1983). The v-*erb*B protein is a 61-kD membrane-associated glycoprotein (Hayman and Beug, 1984; Privalsky and Bishop, 1984; Privalsky et al., 1983). Nucleotide sequencing has demonstrated that v-*erb*B is a truncated version of the receptor for epidermal growth factor (EGF) (Downward et al., 1984; Ullrich et al., 1984; Yamamoto et al., 1983). The EGF receptor, encoded by the c-*erb*B gene, consists of three domains, an extracellular ligand binding domain, a transmembrane region, and an intracellular tyrosine kinase domain. The v-*erb*B truncation removes most of the extracellular ligand-binding domain while leaving the remainder of the receptor except for 32 C-terminal amino acids intact; v-*erb*B is thus truncated at both termini relative to c-*erb*B. Activation of the viral gene is thought to result from deregulation of the tyrosine kinase activity.

Insertional Activation of c-*erb*B by ALV

Infection of line 15_1 chickens with ALV results in a high incidence of erythroblastosis (Fung et al., 1983; Robinson et al., 1985). H.-J. Kung and collaborators have shown that ALV-induced erythroblastosis is associated with proviral insertions within the c-*erb*B locus (Fung et al., 1983; Raines et al., 1985). Ninety percent of the integrations are within a 1500-bp region of DNA 5′ to the first v-*erb*B homologous exon (vE_1) of c-*erb*B. These integrations separate the c-*erb*B–specific exons from the v-*erb*B homologous portion of the gene; most are clustered within a few hundred bases immediately upstream of vE_1. The proviruses are in the same transcriptional orientation as c-*erb*B, and most appear to be structurally intact.

All of the tumors contained high levels of tumor-specific c-*erb*B–related mRNAs (Fung et al., 1983; Goodwin et al., 1986; Nilsen et al., 1985). Northern analysis demonstrated two predominant mRNA species of 7.0 and 3.6 kb. Both transcripts were found in all of the tumors examined regardless of their precise site of proviral integration. S1-nuclease analysis of tumor cell RNAs, and sequence analysis of tumor-derived cDNA clones revealed that these transcripts result from a complex series of RNA-processing events (Nilson et al., 1985; Goodwin et al., 1986). Both the 7.0- and 3.6-kb mRNAs initiate within the viral 5′-LTR. The splice donor sequence in the viral *gag* gene is joined to the splice acceptor sequence just upstream of *env* in a manner analogous to that used in the generation of the normal subgenomic *env* mRNA. A cryptic splice donor signal within *env* is then fused to the splice acceptor sequence of vE_1. This splicing pattern is found in both the 7.0- and 3.6-kb mRNAs. The transcripts differ only in their 3′-untranslated regions. The 3.6-kb mRNA contains 900 bp of 3′-untranslated sequences, whereas the larger transcript has 4.3 kb of 3′-untranslated information. A functional role for the variable amount of 3′-untranslated information has not yet been determined.

This complex RNA processing results in chimeric viral c-*erb*B mRNAs containing 575 bp of viral information, 1917 bp of c-*erb*B coding sequence, and variable 3′ untranslated regions. Despite the splicing complexity, all of the sequences have been joined in the same translational reading frame. The protein encoded by the activated c-*erb*B transcript consists of six *gag*-derived amino acids, 53 *env*-derived amino acids, and 639 c-*erb*B residues. The activated c-*erb*B gene is thus 5′ truncated at exactly the same point as the v-*erb*B gene. The tumor-specific transcripts, however, do contain the C-terminal 32 amino acids that are deleted in AEV.

Sequence analysis of tumor cDNAs revealed a third c-*erb*B mRNA (Goodwin et al., 1986). This transcript is 5.2 kb and contains only *gag* and c-*erb*B sequences. The *gag* splice donor is joined directly to vE_1. Since it is not detected by Northern analysis, the 5.2-kb transcript appears to be a very minor component of the activated c-*erb*B mRNAs.

Acute transforming viruses containing transduced c-*erb*B sequences have been found in many cases of ALV-induced erythroblastosis (Beug et al., 1986;

Gamett et al., 1986; Miles and Robinson, 1985). Beug et al. (1986) found that about 15% (2/14) of the ALV-induced tumors they examined released acute viruses, whereas 50% (10/20) of the tumors characterized by Miles and Robinson (1985) shed *erb*B-containing viruses. It is likely that the remaining 10% of the tumors studied by Kung's group (Fung, et al., 1983; Raines et al., 1985) that displayed unusual c-*erb*B rearrangements also contained transduced c-*erb*B sequences. The reason for the discrepancy between the observed transduction frequencies is unclear.

The high frequency of c-*erb*B transduction in ALV-induced erythroblastosis is most likely due to the structure of the c-*erb*B–associated proviruses. The integration sites, orientation, and sequence content of these insertions probably result in production of packageable virally initiated *erb*B transcripts that could be intermediates in the formation of transducing viruses (Miles and Robinson, 1985). The *erb*B-containing viruses released from these tumors have restricted transforming abilities relative to AEV. Recent studies have revealed C-terminal deletions in some of these transduced genes (Gamett et al., 1986).

Determinants of c-*erb*B Activation

ALV activation of c-*erb*B provided the first example of abnormal splicing events and *gag*/c-*onc* fusion during insertional activation of a proto-oncogene. Many factors undoubtedly contribute to the complex mechanism of c-*erb*B activation. Unlike ALV activation of c-*myc*, truncation of the gene product appears to be a fundamental component of c-*erb*B activation. The finding that the cluster of c-*erb*B–associated proviruses all result in the same 5′ truncation, and that this is exactly the same deletion found in v-*erb*B, argues strongly for an important role for truncation. It is interesting to note that although the v-*erb*B genes are 3′ truncated, the virally promoted c-*erb*B mRNAs contain the entire 3′ c-*erb*B coding sequence. Thus 3′ truncation may not be an essential feature of c-*erb*B activation. C-terminal deletion may, however, serve to modulate the transforming properties of activated c-*erb*B alleles.

The 5′ truncation of c-*erb*B removes the normal translation initiation signal. In the chimeric mRNAs, an AUG is provided by the viral leader region. The requirement for a functional translational initiation signal may explain the exclusive use of the 5′ viral LTR in the activated c-*erb*B mRNAs. Initiation within the 3′ LTR, as in the case of c-*myc* activation by ALV, would result in virally promoted chimeric mRNAs without a functional AUG.

Another consequence of 5′ truncation of c-*erb*B is deletion of the signal sequence normally used in positioning the EGF receptor within the plasma membrane. The *env* sequences found in the chimeric transcripts encode most of the *env* signal sequence (Nilsen et al., 1985). Plasma membrane association may be required for the activities of both c-*erb*B and v-*erb*B, and selection for *env/erb*B fusion may reflect this requirement for cell surface localization. However, the finding of chimeric c-*erb*B mRNAs containing only *gag* and c-*erb*B sequences (although this mRNA is a minor component and may not be functionally significant), and the observation that v-*erb*B does not contain the c-*erb*B signal sequence yet is found at the plasma membrane (Hayman and Beug, 1984; Privalsky and Bishop, 1984) obscure the contribution of the *env* information to the transforming properties of the virally promoted c-*erb*B mRNAs.

c-*myb*

The avian defective leukemia viruses AMV and E26 contain the oncogene v-*myb* (Boyle et al., 1983; Duesberg et al., 1980; Gonda et al., 1981; Klempnauer et al., 1983; Nunn et al., 1983). In a viral context, v-*myb* rapidly induces myeloid leukemias in infected chickens and transforms myeloid precursor cells in tissue culture (Beug et al., 1979; Boettiger and Durban, 1984; Gazzolo et al., 1979; for reviews see Graf and Beug, 1978, and Moscovici, 1975). Nucleotide sequencing of c-*myb* cDNAs has shown that when compared with c-*myb*, v-*myb* alleles are truncated at both their 5′ and 3′ termini (Bender and Keuhl, 1986; Gerondakis and Bishop, 1986; Klempnauer et al., 1982; Nunn et al., 1983; Rosson and Reddy, 1986). While the precise extent of these structural alterations remains unknown (due mostly to some uncertainty about the structure of the 5′ end of chicken c-*myb*), transduction of c-*myb* by AMV and E26 resulted in N-terminal truncations of at least 71 and 80 amino acids, respectively. At their C-termini, AMV and E26 truncate 199 and 278 amino acids, respectively. It is thought that both N- and C-termini deletions contribute to the transforming activity of v-*myb*. In addition to these deletions, both v-*myb* genes have sustained missense mutations (Gerondakis and Bishop, 1986; Rosson and Reddy, 1986).

Proviral Insertions Within the 5′ Region of c-*myb* in Murine Myeloid Tumors

Abelson murine leukemia virus induces hemopoietic tumors in pristane-primed BALB/c mice (Mushinski et al., 1983; Reddy et al., 1975). These tumors include plasmacytomas, and tumors composed of cells that morphologically appear to be plamacytoid lymphosarcomas (called ABPL tumors). While the latter tumors were originally thought to be B-cell derived, more recent evidence indicates that ABPL tumors actually consist of early myeloid cells (Shen-Ong et al., 1986).

Shen-Ong et al. (1984, 1986) examined a series of six ABPL tumors. Surprisingly, most of the tumors lacked the replication-defective transforming component of the Abelson complex (Mushinski et al., 1983; Shen-Ong et al., 1984). All of the tumors, however, contained insertions of the Mo-MuLV helper virus within the c-*myb* locus. Each of the *myb*-associated proviruses was found within the 1.5 kb of cellular DNA 5′ to the first v-*myb* homologous exon (vE_1), and all were in the same transcriptional orientation as the c-*myb* gene (see Fig. 3B). Most of these proviruses had sustained deletions within their *gag, pol,* or *env* genes.

Proviral insertions within c-*myb* in ABPL tumors are associated with abnormal *myb* transcripts (Mushinski et al., 1983; Shen-Ong et al., 1986) that are both overproduced and increased in size compared with c-*myb* mRNA in normal tissues. Whereas the normal thymus c-*myb* mRNA is approximately 3.8 kb, the ABPL tumors express predominant species of 4, 5, and 7 kb. Northern blot and S1 nuclease analysis showed that the majority of the aberrant ABPL *myb* transcripts initiate within the 5′ Mo-MuLV LTR. A cryptic splice donor sequence in the viral *gag* region is joined to the natural splice acceptor immediately upstream of vE_1, creating a chimeric mRNA containing approximately 1500 bp of viral information fused to the c-*myb* sequences. This transcript is thought to correspond to the 5-kb mRNA, although this designation awaits further characterization of the 5′ end of these messages. Although most of the *myb*-associated proviruses are internally deleted, all have retained the cryptic *gag* splice donor.

Recently, Gonda et al. (1987) have described insertional activation of c-*myb* in two murine monocytic leukemia cell lines. Like the ABPL tumors, both WEHI-265 and WEHI-274 contain deleted Mo-MuLV proviruses within the 5′ region of, and in the same transcriptional orientation as, c-*myb*. These tumors express abundant 5′ LTR–initiated, *myb*-related mRNAs of 5.3 and 3.9 kb. These mRNA species probably correspond to the 4- and 5-kb ABPL mRNAs of Shen-Ong et al. (1986). The 5-kb transcript initiates within the 5′ LTR and continues through *gag* until reaching the cryptic splice donor used in the ABPL transcripts. The cryptic splice donor is then joined to a normal c-*myb* acceptor, as in ABPL tumors. However, whereas in WEHI-265 the vE_1 splice acceptor is used, in the WEHI-274 mRNA the cryptic *gag* donor is joined to the c-*myb* exon immediately 5′ to vE_1. The virally promoted *myb* mRNAs in WEHI-274 thus contain additional upstream c-*myb* sequences. The smaller 3.9-kb transcript appears to be derived from the 5.3-kb mRNAs

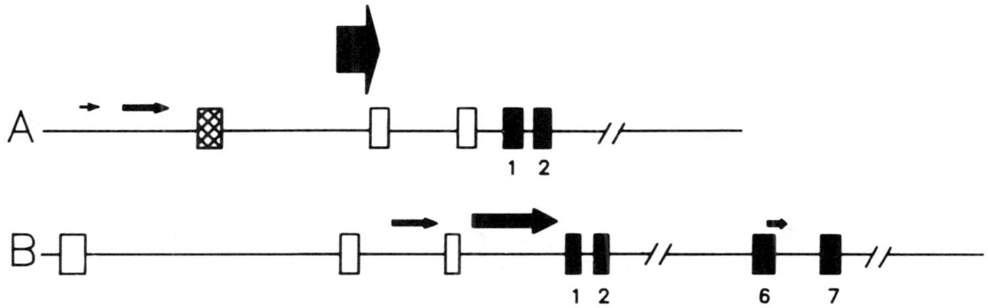

Figure 3 Orientation and distribution of integrations within c-*myb* loci insertionally activated by EU-8 and MuLV. The c-*myb* exons, oriented 5′ to 3′ (left to right), are represented by boxes. (Only relevant portions of the c-*myb* loci are shown.) Closed boxes: v-*myb*–homologous exons (numbered); open boxes: c-*myb*–specific exons; hatched box: chicken c-*myb*–specific exon that has not been precisely localized. Other symbols are as described in the legend to Fig. 2. A. EU-8 virus-induced lymphomas in chickens. B. MuLV-induced murine myelooid tumors and cell lines. Data were complied from the following sources: A. S. L. Hahn et al., unpublished observations; Kanter et al., 1987 (25 integrations). B. Gonda et al., 1987; Weinstein et al., 1986, 1987; Shen-Ong et al., 1986 (10 integrations).

by an additonal splice from the normal *gag* splice donor to a cryptic splice acceptor within *gag*, 230 bp upstream of the cryptic *gag* splice donor. The two transcripts thus differ only in the amount of *gag* sequences present.

All of the activated c-*myb* alleles with 5′ insertions in murine myeloid tumors overexpress aberrant *myb* mRNAs. It remains unclear, however, precisely how the structure of the c-*myb* protein encoded by the activated genes is altered. Sequencing of cDNAs has shown that the fusion of *gag* and *myb* has placed the two genes in different translational reading frames (Gonda et al., 1987; Rosson et al., 1987; Shen-Ong et al., 1986). While the natural *gag* AUG is the closest to the 5′ end of the chimeric mRNAs, a frameshift supression mechanism must be invoked if it is to initiate the activated *myb* protein. Although several possible start sites exist within the *gag* region found in the chimeric transcripts, the AUG 86 bp upstream of the *gag* cryptic splice donor is currently the favored translational initiation codon (Gonda et al., 1987; Shen-Ong et al., 1986). In the 5-kb mRNA, utilization of this AUG might be very inefficient, since it is about 1500 bp from the 5′ end of the mRNA and might require reinitiation to be functional (because of the presence of several upstream AUGs). The 4-kb transcript, however, deletes most of *gag*, including the *gag* AUG while retaining this possible start site, and thus may be responsible for synthesizing the transforming protein (Gonda et al., 1987).

Proviral Integrations Altering the 3′ Region of c-*myb* in Murine Myeloid Tumors

Two groups have examined cell lines derived from virally induced murine myeloid leukemias for c-*myb* rearrangements (Shen-Ong et al., 1986; Weinstein et al., 1986). The cell line NFS-60 was found to contain a 3′ c-*myb* rearrangement. This rearrangement resulted from the insertion of a Cas-Br MuLV provirus into the sixth v-*myb* homologous exon (vE_6). The provirus is structurally intact and in the same transcriptional orientation as c-*myb*.

Northern analysis of NFS-60 revealed a highly expressed, novel 2.3-kb c-*myb* mRNA. Sequence analysis of the *myb*-proviral junction showed that the deletion of two nucleotides from the LTR U_3 region (a normal consequence of the retroviral integration process), resulted in the formation of a translational termination codon within vE_6, and the loss of 240 amino acids from the C-terminus of the c-*myb* protein. This truncation is intermediate to those in the transduced c-*myb* gene of AMV and E26.

Another example of 3′-c-*myb* truncation by viral insertion is the murine myeloid cell line VFLJ2 (Weinstein et al., 1987). This line was derived from in vitro infection of murine fetal liver cells with the recombinant virus J2 (which contains c-*myc* and c-*raf*) and the Leuk-1 strain of Mo-MuLV as the helper virus. Remarkably this line contains a Mo-MuLV insertion within c-*myb* at the same nucleotide as in the NFS-60 integration. Thus, like Cas-Br–MuLV, the Leuk-1 provirus introduces a termination codon into vE_6 and the activated c-*myb* mRNA expressed in VFLJ2 is identical to that observed in NFS-60.

Recent evidenced has suggested that integrations 5′ of vE_1 can result in 3′ c-*myb* splicing aberrations in addition to 5′ truncation of the c-*myb* gene. Rosson et al. (1987) have sequenced a *myb* cDNA from ABPL2 and have found intron sequences within the cDNA. The inclusion of these sequences resulted from the use of cryptic splice donor and acceptor sequences present in the intron just downstream of vE_6, adding 353 bases to the *myb* mRNA. However, Shen-Ong (1987) has recently demonstrated the presence of a similarly-spliced *myb* RNA in normal tissues, thus raising doubt as to the significance of the alternative 3′ splicing pattern in oncogenesis.

Insertional Activation of the Chicken c-*myb* Gene by EU-8 Virus

EU-8 virus is a replication competent avian leukosis virus that contains the subgroup A *env* gene of UR2AV inserted into the ring-necked pheasant virus (RPV) genome in place of the RPV subgroup F *env* gene (Simon et al., 1987). When injected i.v. into 10-day-old chicken embryos, EU-8 rapidly induces a high incidence of lymphoma (Kanter et al., 1988; Simon et al., 1987). EU-8 disease can be distinguished from typical ALV-induced lymphoid leukosis (see above) by its very short latency (4-8 weeks). In this respect, it resembles those induced by the acute avian leukemia viruses. Unlike the acute viruses, however, EU-8 does not carry an oncogene and induces tumors that are clonal in origin. EU-8 virus therefore appears to be intermediate in latency to the traditional classes of acute and nonacute avian retroviruses. These tumors differ from classic lymphoid leukosis in that they present with widespread metastasis in the absence of distinct bursal nodules. EU-8–induced lymphomas are clearly B-cell derived, however, as shown by the detection of rearranged immunoglobulin genes and expression of both immunoglobulin mRNA and protein (Kanter et al., 1988).

Examination of a series of EU-8-induced tumors (Kanter et al., 1988) demonstrated that 100% (25/25) of these tumors contained EU-8 proviruses within the c-*myb* locus. This is in contrast to the longer latency lymphomas induced by other ALVs, in which c-*myc* is insertionally activated (see above). The activation of c-*myc* and c-*myb* appear to be mutually exclusive events. The majority of the c-*myb*-associated proviruses are structurally intact and in the same transcriptional orientation as c-*myb*. Approximately 70% of the integrations are clustered within a 700-bp region approximately 3 kb 5′ to vE_1. The remainder occur further upstream in a 2.5-kb region approximately 6 kb 5′ of vE_1 (see Fig. 3A).

All of the EU-8 tumors express elevated levels of altered c-*myb* mRNA. Most of the tumors express a 4.0- to 4.1-kb tumor-specific *myb* mRNA, which initiates within the 5′ LTR and contains upstream c-*myb*-specific sequences in addition to the v-*myb* homologous information. These transcripts presumably arise from a common splicing event from a donor sequence within the virus to a c-*myb* acceptor sequence. The signals used to generate these transcripts, however, have not yet been identified. Since the integrations result in loss of 5′-sequences from c-*myb*, additional information, derived from either the virus or the c-*myb* locus, must be included to account for the increased size of these transcripts.

There is currently some uncertainty regarding the organization of the 5′ end of the chicken c-*myb* gene (Gerondakis and Bishop, 1986; Rosson and Reddy, 1986). The extent of c-*myb* truncation in the tumor-specific *myb* transcripts is thus unknown. Clearly, since the most proximal integrations leave c-*myb* sequences upstream of vE_1 intact, the extent of 5′ truncation in EU-8–induced tumors is less than that observed either in retroviral transduction of c-*myb*, or in insertional activation of c-*myb* in the murine myeloid leukemias. The localization of upstream EU-8 integration sites also raises the possibility that some of the EU-8 tumors might express virally initiated *myb* mRNAs that contain the complete c-*myb* coding sequence.

Whereas EU-8 induces *myb*-associated neoplasms at an exceptionally high frequency, some other ALVs are also able to insertionally activate c-*myb* (B. E. Clurman and W. S. Hayward, manuscript in preparation; E. Humphries, personal communication). Preliminary analysis of five rapidly appearing lymphomas induced by other ALVs suggests that the integrations within c-*myb* resemble those found with EU-8. The determinants underlying the high efficiency of c-*myb* activation in EU-8–induced lymphomas are currently unknown.

Mechanisms of c-*myb* Activation

When compared with c-*myb*, the v-*myb* genes of AMV and E26 have undergone four alterations that might contribute to their tumorigenicity: (a) 5′ truncation, (b) 3′ truncation, (c) missense mutations, and (d) transcriptional deregulation as a result of linkage to constitutively active viral transcription elements. Because all of these differences occur simultaneously, it is difficult to assess the relative role each plays in the activation of c-*myb*. The observation that AMV and E26 differ in their transforming properties (Moscovici et al., 1983; Radke et al., 1982) may reflect, in part, the differences in their *myb* genes, although E26 also carries an additional oncogene, v-*ets*.

Insertional activation of the c-*myb* gene has been observed in several systems. The distribution of these integrations is summarized in Fig. 3. In general, viral insertions within the c-*myb* gene tend to mimic the structural changes found in v-*myb* alleles. The 5′ truncations of c-*myb* in murine myeloid tumors closely resemble those found in v-*myb* genes. Initiation of the tumor-specific *myb* transcripts within the viral LTR results in high levels of constitutively expressed 5′-truncated *myb* mRNAs. The combination of an LTR linked to a 5′-deleted c-*myb* gene, as found in the murine myeloid tumors, approximates the structure of AMV. In some cases, viral insertations within c-*myb* in murine myeloid tumors also result in 3′ truncations. The 3′ truncations found in NFS-60 and VFLJ2 fall between the AMV and E26 3′ deletions.

The integration of EU-8 virus into the chicken c-*myb* gene provides the first example of an association between insertional activation of c-*myb* and lymphomagenesis. While the structure of the 5′ end of the viral-*myb* junctions is still under study, these tumors clearly have less extensive 5′ deletions of c-*myb* than their murine myeloid counterparts. Like the murine tumors, however, initiation within the viral LTR results in high-level constitutive production of the chimeric *myb* transcripts. The relative contribution of structural and transcriptional alterations of c-*myb* in these tumors awaits further investigation.

c-*mos*

Activation of c-*mos* in Mineral Oil–Induced Murine Plasmacytomas

Two examples of c-*mos* rearrangements have been found in murine plasmacytomas (Cohen et al., 1983; Gattoni-Celli et al., 1983; Rachevi et al.,

1982). Both rearrangements resulted from the insertion of an intracisternal A particle (IAP) (for review see Stoye and Coffin, 1985) within the 5′ region of c-*mos*, but in opposite transcriptional orientations. Whereas expression of normal c-*mos* mRNA in most mouse tissues is too low to be detected by Northern analysis (Probst and Vande Woude, 1985), c-*mos*-related mRNA was detectable in the tumors. Interestingly, the head-to-head orientation (opposite transcriptional orientation to c-*mos*) resulted in higher levels of *mos* mRNA than did the insertion in the same transcriptional orientation.

Intracisternal A particle insertion may activate the transforming activity of c-*mos* in several ways. Transcriptional activation, either by enhancer or promoter/enhancer insertion, appears to have resulted in overexpression of *mos*. An additional consequence of the integration events may be the removal of a negative regulatory element that has been identified in the c-*mos* upstream region (Wood et al., 1984). Intracisternal A particle insertion might therefore result in both the removal of cellular negative transcriptional control elements and the insertion of LTR-like elements. The finding that the transforming activity of c-*mos* can be activated by an LTR placed upstream of the coding sequences (Blair et al., 1981) provides strong support for a transcriptional activation model in IAP c-*mos* insertions.

c-Ha-*ras*

The *ras* family of oncogenes has been implicated in a broad range of human tumors as well as in experimentally induced tumors in mice (see Chapt. 8). In most cases, activation involves a missense mutation at sites corresponding to codons 12, 59, or 61 of c-Ha-*ras*. Thus, *ras* would not appear to be a likely candidate for insertional activation. However, two isolated examples of insertional activation have been reported, one in an ALV-induced nephroblastoma and one in an MuLV-induced lymphoma.

The avian nephroblastoma carrying the activated *ras* gene was induced by MAV, an ALV strain that induces a high incidence of nephroblastoma (Watts and Smith, 1980). The insertion of a provirus near c-Ha-*ras* in this tumor could not be demonstrated directly, but its existence was inferred from the presence of a chimeric message encoding both viral (U_5) and host c-Ha-*ras* sequences (Westaway et al., 1986). The U_5-*ras* linkage was found in a number of independent complementary DNA (cDNA) clones from the same tumor, and was thus unlikely to represent a cloning artifact. Expression of c-Ha-*ras* was elevated 25-fold in this tumor compared to normal kidney tissues. Sequencing of the cDNA clones revealed no missense mutations within the coding region of the gene.

The failure to identify an integrated provirus adjacent to c-Ha-*ras* in this tumor suggests that integration had occurred a long distance upstream of the gene, beyond the region accessible to restriction analysis. No evidence for c-Ha-*ras* rearrangements was found in any of a large number of other MAV-induced nephroblastomas, or in nephroblastomas induced by other ALV strains.

Recently, insertional activation of c-Ha-*ras* was found in an MuLV-induced leukemia cell line, which was originally composed of early stem cells, but later differentiated into more mature T cells (P. Ihle, personal communication). The *ras* gene rearrangement was also present in the original tumor, and thus was not related to the further differentiation of the cell line. The provirus was integrated just upstream of the first coding exon of c-Ha-*ras*, and in the same transcriptional orientation. As in the MAV case, no missense mutations were found within the coding region of the first three exons of the rearranged gene, including the critical sequences at positions 12 and 59/61. (The fourth coding exon from these cells has not yet been cloned and sequenced.) The level of c-Ha-*ras* expression, as measured by p21 levels, was high in these cells, whereas p21 was undetectable in other MuLV-induced leukemic cell lines. Sequence analysis of the cloned locus revealed a rather complex rearrangement of upstream sequences, involving two proviruses, and possibly a translocation mediated by proviruses integrated at different sites in the host genome.

Activation of the c-Ha-*ras* genes in the two cases described above appears to be the result of overexpression or deregulation rather than point mutation. This is not, however, without precedent. Chang et al. (1982) observed transformation of NIH3T3 cells following transfection with a c-Ha-*ras* gene linked to an MuLV LTR, but not with c-Ha-*ras* alone, although the efficiency of transformation was much lower than that with an LTR-v-*ras* construct. However, cells can be transformed by normal c-Ha-*ras* if multiple copies of the transfected DNA are introduced, suggesting a requirement for substantial overexpression of the c-*ras* gene (Pulciani et al., 1985). Examples of *ras* gene amplification have been reported in several different human tumors (George et al., 1985; Schwab et al., 1983). Although the possibility cannot be ruled out that one or more of the amplified genes carried a point mutation, it seems likely that overexpression of c-*ras* is also the relevant mechanism in these tumors.

c-*fms*

Activation of c-*fms* in Friend MuLV–Induced Myeloid Leukemias

Friend MuLV (F-MuLV) induces a variety of neoplasms in mice, including T- and B-cell leukemias, erythroleukemias, and myeloid leukemias (Wendling et al., 1983). Three common integration sites, designated *fim*-1, *fim*-2, and *fim*-3, have been identified in F-MuLV–induced myeloid leukemias (Bordereaux et al., 1987; Sola et al., 1986). The *fim*-2 locus was involved in 20% of the F-MuLV–induced myeloid tumors and transformed myeloid cell lines.

By sequencing the cloned locus, Gisselbrecht et al. (1987) recently identified *fim*-2 as the upstream portion of the c-*fms* proto-oncogene. Expression of c-*fms* mRNA was substantially elevated in the myeloid tumors. Integrations mapped upstream of the first c-*fms* exon, and in the opposite transcriptional orientation. The c-*fms* RNA was similar in size to that in the normal cell, suggesting that the transcripts initiate at the normal promoter, and encode an unaltered c-*fms* protein.

The v-*fms* gene, first identified in the McDonough strain of FeSV (SM-FeSV) (Frankel et al., 1979), has been shown to be derived from the cellular CSF-1 receptor gene (Sherr et al., 1985). The viral gene product is truncated at its C-terminus, and displays constitutive kinase activity that is not influenced by the presence or absence of CSF-1 (Sacca et al., 1986). The data of Gisselbrecht et al. (1987), however, raise the possibility that insertional activation of c-*fms* by F-MuLV does not involve truncation, and that overexpression or deregulation is sufficient to activate its oncogenic potential. However, a much more complete characterization of c-*fms* proteins and cDNAs from tumor cells will be required to substantiate this possibility.

CONCLUSIONS

Insertional Activation versus Transduction of Proto-Oncogenes

Approximately two dozen viral oncogenes have been identified in acute retroviruses, yet only a handful of these has been implicated in oncogenesis by insertional activation of the corresponding proto-oncogenes. This unequal representation may reflect in part a bias in the types of tumors analyzed (mostly lymphomas and leukemias), or the catalog of genes that are most commonly utilized in screening for activated proto-oncogenes. However, to a large extent it probably reflects the limitations imposed by the types of mutations that can be induced by proviral integrations, and by the particular structural and functional features of each proto-oncogene that can be altered to activate the oncogenic potential of the gene.

Integrations can cause changes in both the regulation of a proto-oncogene, and the structure of its gene product. Many different strategies exist for altering gene expression, including introduction of viral enhancers or promoter/enhancer units, disruption or circumvention of various control regions within the resident gene, or (possibly) changes in mRNA structure that alter its stability. The repertoire of possible changes in the structure of the gene product, however, are more limited. Truncations (either 5′ or 3′) can result from integration within the coding region, and several examples of fusion between viral and host genes as a result of unusual splicing events have been found.

These same types of changes are found in many transduced oncogenes. However, the viral oncogenes almost invariably also contain missense point mutations, which cannot be induced by proviral insertion. Although many of the point mutations may be benign, others have been shown to be important in activating the oncogenic potential of the gene, as in the case of *src* (Hanafusa. 1986) and *ras* (Tabin et al., 1982; Reddy et al., 1982). If a particular proto-oncogene can only be activated in this way, it would be an unlikely candidate for insertional activation.

Somatic mutations occur at low frequency in resident cellular genes, but the opportunity for such mutations to occur is greatly enhanced in a gene that is transduced by a retrovirus. The viral genome can undergo an enormous number of replications in a very short period of time because of the spread of virus to neighboring cells. A single viral genome may be amplified some 10^8-fold in a matter of days, a period during which a cellular gene might be amplified eight-fold as a consequence of cell division. Thus the target size for potential mutations is vastly increased, and the number of replication events, a major source of mutations, is similarly increased. In addition, the viral reverse transcriptase appears to be highly error prone (Mizutani and Temin, 1976), increasing the probability of introducing point mutations at each round of replication. Thus in an infected animal, retroviral transduction of a proto-oncogene can rapidly generate a large population of genetic variants from which an oncogenic mutant can be selected. Selection, of course, is in the form of tumor growth following infection of cells with an oncogenic mutant.

Insertional Activation by Altering Proto-Oncogene Expression

A major factor in most insertional activations is disruption of the normal controls that govern the expression of the target proto-oncogene. In some cases, deregulation or overexpression alone appears to be sufficient, whereas in others the regulatory changes are accompanied by alterations in the gene product. Deregulation appears to occur primarily at the transcription level, with transcription of the proto-oncogene initiating on either a viral or host promoter. Five different patterns of promoter usage have been recognized: initiation from (a) the viral 3′ LTR, (b) the viral 5′ LTR, or (c) the normal cellular promoter; (d) altered utilization of alternative normal cellular promoters; and (e) activation of cryptic cellular promoters.

The first two of these provide a proviral promoter/enhancer complex, which displaces the normally used cellular promoter, and can occur only when the virus is integrated upstream of the proto-oncogene coding sequences and in the same transcriptional orientation. The other three patterns occur primarily when the provirus is upstream in the opposite orientation, or downstream in the same orientation, although a few exceptions have been reported (e.g., in REV-induced T-cell lymphomas, and in some cell lines derived from ALV-induced B-cell lymphomas).

The c-*myc* gene appears to be an example of a gene that can be oncogenically activated by disrupting its expression without altering the structure of its gene product. The fact that insertional activations have involved c-*myc* more frequently than any other proto-oncogene may be a reflection of this. Although the known v-*myc* genes are mutationally altered, these changes are probably not essential for oncogenesis. However, some of the mutations appear to alter the pathogenic properties or extend the target range of the transducing virus. This may explain the broader spectrum of neoplasms induced by v-*myc* viruses (myeloid leukemias, B-cell lymphomas, carcinomas, and fibrosarcomas) compared to that in which insertional activation of c-*myc* has been observed (almost exclusively T- or B-cell neoplasms).

Presumably, the major factor in transcriptional activation is the placement of proto-oncogene expression under the control of the viral enhancer or promoter/enhancer. However, the integration event may play an additional role in some cases, by disrupting or displacing normal regulatory sequences. In MuLV-induced lymphomas, for example, the major cluster of integration sites falls within a region of c-*myc* thought to regulate initiation of transcription (Chung et al., 1986; Remmers et al., 1986; Siebenlist et al., 1984). The normal c-*myc* gene is also regulated at the level of RNA chain elongation (Bentley and Groudine, 1986; Nepveu and Marcu, 1986), with a block in elongation occurring near the 3′ end of $exon_1$ in the repressed state. Initiation within the first intron, either from a proviral LTR as in most ALV-induced B-cell lymphomas, or from a cryptic cellular promoter as in some REV-induced T-cell lymphomas, would allow a bypass of the elongation block.

Hann et al. (1988) have recently proposed another model that may be relevant to many of the examples of insertional activation. They have identified a *myc* protein that is somewhat larger than $p60^{myc}$ (which initiates from the AUG in $exon_2$) and is usually less abundant. Sequencing of the N-terminus of the larger protein has shown that it initiates at a rare initiation codon near the 3′ end of $exon_1$. The ratio of the two *myc* proteins is altered in many tumor cells, although not always in the same direction. The authors have raised the interesting possibility that a change in this ratio is important in oncogenesis. This model would be relevant to the examples discussed above in which the first exon is absent from the tumor RNA as a result of initiations within the first intron, or in less common cases (such as in the RP9 cell line) where the first exon is removed by splicing. It is less clear how upstream integrations would alter this ratio, although changes in promoter usage might result in altered ratios if the two mRNAs differ in their translational efficiencies from the first and second exon sites. There is as yet no direct evidence that the ratio of the two *myc* proteins plays a role in oncogenesis. If the model is valid, however, a single integration event within the first intron might simultaneously alter *myc* expression in four different ways: place c-*myc* under transcriptional control of the viral LTR sequences, displace upstream transcriptional control sequences, bypass the transcription elongation block, and abolish synthesis of the larger c-*myc* protein that initiates in $exon_1$. Further studies will be required to evaluate the relative contribution of each of these factors.

Activation of Proto-Oncogenes by Altering the Structure of the Gene Product

The potential for proto-oncogene activation by qualitative changes is probably inherent in the proteins themselves. For example, deletion of a regulatory domain might lead to activation if the regulatory and functional domains of the target protein can be physically dissociated without abolishing the essential biological activity of the protein. Certain groups of proteins, such as growth factor receptors, seem to be particularly amenable to these sorts of changes. Other oncoproteins, such as c-*myc*, may contain several functional domains, but disruption of any particular domain might not be sufficient to lead to oncogenic activation, or might result in complete abrogation of protein function.

Two viral oncogenes have been identified as truncated versions of cellular genes encoding known growth factor receptors: the EGF receptor (c-*erb*B) and the CSF-1 receptor (c-*fms*). Several other oncogenes encode proteins with structures similar to known receptors, but their ligands have not yet been identified. These include v-*kit*, v-*ros*, and *neu* (Besmer et al., 1986; Neckameyer and Wang, 1984; Schector et al., 1984). The proto-oncogenes from which these oncogenes were derived encode proteins that share the structural features of an extracellular ligand-binding domain, a transmembrane domain, and an intracellular domain possesing tyrosine kinase activity. The plethora of tyrosine kinases suggests that the function and control of each one must be highly specialized and tightly regulated. The extracellular and intracellular domains each participate in this regulation—both are potential targets for insertional activation.

The most extensively studied example of oncogenic activation of a growth factor receptor gene is c-*erb*B. The known viral insertions within c-*erb*B all result in the same N-terminal truncation, which is identical to the truncation in the AEV v-*erb*B gene product. This truncation removes most of the extracellular EGF-binding domain, and appears to result in a deregulation of the enzymatic activity of the intracellular kinase domain of the protein. The invariant association of this truncation with activated *erb*B genes suggests that it is a critical step in the activation process. The C-terminus of the EGF receptor also appears to be a target for activation, but its role is less clear. Although v-*erb*B is 3′ truncated, the chimeric transcripts resulting from ALV insertions are not. Furthermore, both 3′ truncated and 3′ nontruncated c-*erb* genes are found in transducing viruses shed by ALV-induced erythroid tumors. (All are 5′ truncated.) However, viruses carrying genes with intact 3′ ends are more restricted in their transforming abilities, indicating that alterations in the C-terminus of the protein significantly influence the oncogenic properties of the protein.

While structural alteration is the hallmark of c-*erb*B activation, it is important to keep in mind that transcriptional deregulation of c-*erb*B also occurs as the chimeric transcripts are placed under the control of the viral LTR. The functional significance of the overexpression of the activated receptor is unknown, but an increase in receptor expression could certainly contribute to the transforming ability of the insertionally activated gene. Transcriptional activation of a growth factor receptor may be particularly important in cell lineages in which the receptor is not normally expressed.

Truncation is also an invariant feature of c-*myb* insertional activation. Although the c-*myb* gene does not encode a tyrosine kinase growth factor receptor, the structural alterations found in activated c-*myb* alleles are remarkably similar to those observed in activated c-*erb*B genes. Both 5′ and 3′ truncations seem to participate in c-*myb* activation. While the majority of the oncogenically activated c-*myb* genes are 5′ truncated, some contain 3′ truncations. In two cases (NFS-60 and VFLJ2), 3′ deletion appears to be the only structural change within the activated gene. Like *erb*B, both c-*myb* termini appear to contain oncogenic determinants. Since the function of c-*myb* is unknown, it is difficult to speculate as to how truncation results in oncogenic activation of the protein.

Provirus Structure, Integration Site, and Orientation

The nonrandom distribution and distinct patterns of proviral integrations in each system probably reflect, to a large extent, the selective factors imposed by unique structural and functional features of both the virus and the proto-oncogene involved. For example, there are clearly limits to the amount of truncation that can be tolerated and still retain functional activity. There are also restrictions as to the minimal amount of deletion that will result in oncogenic activation. These considerations should delineate a region within each gene that is amenable to insertional activation. This seems to be the case of both c-*erb*B and c-*myb*, both of which exhibit clustered integration sites.

The selection between 5′ and 3′ LTR usage for transcription initiation may be strongly influenced by gene-specific factors. In cases where truncation is important, transcription from the 5′ LTR allows utilization of the *gag* AUG to replace initiation codons lost by truncation, and can also provide viral coding sequences—usually as a result of abnormal splicing patterns—that may contribute to the altered properties of the activated gene product. The 3′ LTR of most retroviruses cannot provide a usable initiation codon. This might be an advantage, however, for a gene such as c-*myc* that retains its own initiation codon. Furthermore, the known examples of 3′ LTR utilization—primarily the ALV- and REV-induced bursal lymphomas—appear to express the activated gene at higher levels than those in which the 5′ LTR is used, or in which "enhancer" insertion is involved. The higher level of expression from the 3′ LTR might be an advantage in some proto-oncogene/target cell combinations.

Utilization of the 3′ LTR is invariably associated with internal deletions in the provirus, which may play an essential role in "activating" the 3′ viral promoter. When the 5′ LTR is used, transcription must read through the poly(A) addition signal in the 3′ LTR of the integrated provirus and into the adjacent cellular gene. A low level of readthrough appears to occur normally in the avian retrovirus system (Herman and Coffin, 1986). If this level of readthrough allows sufficient expression of the activated proto-oncogene, no additional change in the provirus would be required. Indeed, the steady-state levels of ALV-activated c-*erb*B and c-*myb* RNAs are significantly lower than the levels of the normal ALV mRNA in these tumors (Kanter et al., 1988; Nilsen et al., 1985). Deletion of the 3′ LTR would presumably allow higher levels of 5′ LTR-mediated expression, but only one example of this is known: the upstream provirus activating c-*myc* in the RP9 avian lymphoma cell line (Linial and Groudine, 1985). Levels of activated c-*myc* expression are high in this cell line (Hayward et al., 1981).

Another determinant of integration patterns may be chromatin structure. Although there appears to be no sequence specificity for integration sites in the host genome, several lines of evidence suggest that integrations occur preferentially within regions of "open" chromatin structure, as defined by deoxyribonuclease (DNAse) sensitivity (Rohdewohld et al., 1987; Robinson and Gagnon, 1986; Schubach and Groudine, 1984).

Thus insertional activation of a particular proto-oncogene might be extremely rare in a cell in which the gene is not normally transcriptionally active (and therefore in a "closed" conformation)—quite likely a cell that would respond most profoundly to its abnormal expression. This limitation is circumvented by acute retroviruses, which can introduce into the appropriate target cell an oncogene that is already under control of the viral LTR, and often mutationally altered in other ways that contribute to its oncogenic properties.

The most puzzling contrast in integration patterns is between the T-and B-cell lymphomas induced by REV. Since the same virus and the same proto-oncogene (chicken c-*myc*) are involved in both cases, the source of the differences in integration patterns must reside elsewhere. It is possible that the chromatin structures of the c-*myc* genes in the two target cells differ, or that optimal levels of c-*myc* expression required to transform the two cell types are different, thus favoring different modes of activation (Swift et al., 1987). Alternatively, polymorphic differences may be present within the c-*myc* genes of the high- and low-susceptibility chicken strains, altering the accessibility or responsiveness of different portions of the c-*myc* locus.

The range of integration sites that can result in proto-oncogene activation is clearly determined by the interaction of many factors. The selection factors and the determinants of integration site availability are probably different for each combination of host, virus strain, target cell, and proto-oncogene. It is perhaps overly simplistic to think that, in any system studied thus far, all of these contributory factors have been identified.

It is apparent that insertional activation of proto-oncogenes is an important mechanism of oncogenesis. In this chapter, we have discussed only those proto-oncogenes that were originally identified as viral oncogenes in acute retroviruses. While the number of proto-oncogenes that can be insertionally activated is obviously finite, many cellular genes, in addition to the known v-*onc* homologs, are potential targets for insertional activation. Many of these have already been identified as common sites of integration in tumors induced by nonacute retroviruses (see Chap. 3), and many others will certainly follow.

ACKNOWLEDGMENTS

We would like to thank our colleagues, cited in the text, for permission to quote unpublished data. We would also like to thank Eveyon Maldonado for assistance in preparing the manuscript. Work in our laboratory was supported by NIH grants CA-43250 and CA-16599. B. E. C. is a Rudin Fellow in the Medical Scientist Training Program of the Sloan-Kettering Institute and Cornell University Medical College. This chapter is dedicated to the memory of Stanley P. Clurman.

REFERENCES

Alitalo, K., Bishop, J. M., Smith, D. H., Chen, E. Y., Colby, W. W., and Levinson, A. D. (1983). Nucleotide sequence of the v-*myc* oncogene of avian retrovirus MC29. *Proc. Natl. Acad. Sci.* U.S.A. *80*: 100–104.

Arrigo, S., Yun, M., and Beemon, K. (1987). cis-Acting elements within the *gag* genes of avian retroviruses. *Mol. Cell. Biol. 7*: 388–397.

Battey, J., Moulding, C., Taub, R., Murphy, W., Stewart, T., Potter, H., Lenoir, G., and Leder, P. (1983). The human c-*myc* oncogene: Structural consequences of translocation into the IgH locus in Burkitt lymphoma. *Cell 34*: 779–787.

Beard, J. W. (1963). Viral tumors of chickens with particular references to the leukosis complex. *Ann. N.Y. Acad. Sci. 108*: 1057–1085.

Bender, T. P., and Kuehl, W. M. (1986). Structural and expression of c-*myb* proto-oncogene mRNA in murine B cells. *Curr. Topics Microbiol. Immunol. 132*: 153–158.

Bentley, D. L., and Groudine, M. (1986). A block to elongation is largely responsible for decreased transcription of c-*myc* in differentiated HL60 cells. *Nature 321*: 702–706.

Besmer, P., Murphy, J. E., George, P. C., Qiu, F., Bergold, P. J., Lederman, L., Snyder, H. W., Jr., Brodeur, D., Zuckerman, E. E., and Hardy, W. D. (1986). A new acute transforming feline retrovirus and relationship of its oncogene v-*kit* with the protein kinase gene family. *Nature 320*: 415–421.

Beug, H., von Kirchbach, A., Doderlein, G., Conscience, J. F., and Graf, T. (1979). Chicken hemopoietic cells transformed by seven strains of defective avian leukemia viruses display three distinct phenotypes of differentiation. *Cell 18*: 375–390.

Beug, H., Hayman, M. J., Raines, M. B., Kung, H. J., and Vennstrom, B. (1986). Rous-associated virus 1-induced erythroleukemic cells exhibit a weakly transformed phenotype in vitro and release c-*erb*B-containing retroviruses unable to transform fibroblasts. *J. Virol. 57*: 1127–1138.

Beug, H., Kahn, P., Doderlein, G., Hayman, M., and Graf, T. (1985). Characterization of hemopoietic cells transformed in vitro by AEV-H, an *erb*-containing avian erythroblastosis virus. In *Modern Trends in Human Leukemia VI,* Vol. 29. (R. Neth, M. Greaves, and R. Gallow, eds.) Springer-Verlag, Berlin, p. 290–297.

Blair, D. G., Oskarsson, M. K., Wood, T. G., McClements, W. L., Fischinger, P. J., and Vande Woude, G. F. (1981). Activation of the transformation potential of a normal cell sequence: A molecular model for oncogenesis. *Science 212*: 941–943.

Boettiger, D., and Durban, E. M. (1984). Target cells for avian myeloblastosis virus in embryonic yolk sac and relationship of cell differentiation to cell transformation. *J. Virol. 49*: 841–847.

Bordereaux, D., Fichelson, S., Sola, B., Tambourin, P. E., and Gisselbrecht, S. (1987). Frequent involvement of the *fim*-3 region in F-MuLV-induced mouse myeloblastic leukemias. *J. Virol. 61*: 4043-4045.

Boyle, W. J., Lipsick, J. S., Reddy, E. P., and Baluda, M. A. (1983). Identification of the leukemogenic protein of avian myeloblastosis virus and of its normal cellular homologue, *Proc. Natl. Acad. Sci. U.S.A. 80*: 2834–2838.

Broome, S., and Gilbert, W. (1985). Rous sarcoma virus encodes a transcriptional activator. *Cell 40*: 537–546.

Chang, E. H., Furth, M. E., Scolnick, E. M., and Lowy, D. R. (1982). Tumorigenic transformation of mammalian cells induced by a normal human gene homologous to the oncogene of Harvey murine sarcoma virus. *Nature 297*: 479–483.

Chattopadhyay, S. K., Cloyd, M. W., Linemeyer, D. L., Lander, R., Rands, E., and Lowy, D. R. (1982). Cellular origin and role of mink cell focus-forming viruses in murine thymic lymphomas. *Nature 295*: 25–31.

Chung, J., Sinn, E., Reed, R. R., and Leder, P. (1986). trans-Acting elements modulate expression of the human c-*myc* gene in Burkitt lymphoma cells. *Proc. Natl. Acad. Sci. U.S.A. 83*: 7918–7922.

Cloyd, M. W., Hartley, J. W., and Rowe, W. P. (1980). Lymphomagenicity of recombinant mink cell focus-inducing murine leukemia viruses. *J. Exp. Med. 151*: 542-552.

Coffin, J. M. (1982). Structure of the retroviral genome. In *RNA Tumor Viruses.* (R. Weiss, N. Teich, H. Varmus, and J. Coffin, eds.) Cold Spring Harbor Laboratory, Cold Spring Harbor, New York p. 261–368.

Cohen, J. B., Unger, T., Rechavi, G., Canaani, E., and Givol, D. (1983). Rearrangement of the oncogene c-*mos* in mouse myeloma NSI and hybridomas. *Nature 306*: 797–799.

Cooper, M. D., Payne, L. E., Dent, P. B., Burmester, B. P., and Good, R. A. (1968). Pathogenesis of avian lymphoid leukosis. I. Histogenesis. *J. Natl. Cancer Inst. 41*: 374–389.

Cullen, B. R., Lomedico, P. T., and Ju, G. (1984). Transcriptional interference in avian retroviruses—Implications for the promoter insertion model of leukaemogenesis. *Nature 307*: 241–245.

Cuypers, H. T., Selten, G., Quint, W., Zijlstra, M., Maandag, E. R., Boelens, W., van Wezenbeek, P., Melief, C., and Berns, A. (1984). Murine leukemia virus-induced T-cell lymphomagenesis: Integration of proviruses in a distant chromosomal region. *Cell 37*: 141–150.

Downward, J., Yarden, Y., Mayes, E., Scrace, G., Totty, N., Stockwell, P., Ullrich, A., Schlessinger, J., and Waterfield, M. (1984). Close similarity of epidermal growth factor receptor and v-*erb*B oncogene protein sequences. *Nature 307*: 521–527.

Duesberg, P. H., Bister, K., and Moscovici, C. (1980). Genetic structure of avian myeloblastosis virus released from transformed myeloblasts as a defective virus particle. *Proc. Natl. Acad. Sci. U.S.A. 77*: 5120–5124.

Elder, J. H., Gautsch, J. W., Jensen, F. C., Lerner, R. A., Hartley, J. W., and Rowe, W. P. (1977). Biochemical evidence that MCF murine leukemia viruses are envelope (*env*) gene recombinants. *Proc. Natl. Acad. Sci. U.S.A. 74*: 4676–4680.

Enrietto, P. J., Hayman, M. J., Ramsay, G. M., Wyke, J. A., and Payne, L. N. (1983a). Altered pathogenicity of avian myelocytomatosis (MC29) viruses with mutations in the v-*myc* gene. *Virology 124*: 164–172.

Enrietto, P. J., Payne, L. N., and Hayman, M. J. (1983b). A recovered avian myelocytomatosis virus which induces lymphomas in chickens: Pathogenic properties and their molecular basis. *Cell 35*: 369–379.

Famulari, N. G. (1983). Murine leukemia viruses with recombinant *env* genes: A discussion of their role in leukemogenesis. *Curr. Topics Microbiol. Immunol. 103*: 75–108.

Frankel, A. E., Gilbert, J. H. Porzig, K. T., Scolnick, E. M., and Aaronson, S. A. (1979). Nature and distribution of feline sarcoma virus nucleotide sequences. *J. Virol. 30*: 821–827.

Frykberg, L., Palmieri, S., Beug, H., Graf, T., Hayman, M., and Vennstrom, B. (1983). Transforming capacities of avian erythroblastosis virus mutants deleted in the *erb*A or *erb*B oncogenes. *Cell 33*: 357–368.

Fung, Y.-K. T., Fadly, A. M., Crittenden, L. B., and Kung, H.-J. (1981). On the mechanism of retrovirus-induced avian lymphoid leukosis: Deletion and integration of the provirus. *Proc. Natl. Acad. Sci. U.S.A. 78*: 3418–3422.

Fung, Y.-K. T., Crittenden, L. B., and Kung, H.-J. (1982). Orientation and position of avian leukosis virus DNA relative to the cellular oncogene c-*myc* in B-lymphoma tumors of highly susceptible $15I_5X7_2$ chickens. *J. Virol. 44*: 742–746.

Fung, Y.-K. T., Lewis, W. G., Crittenden, L. B., and Kung, H.-J. (1983). Activation of the cellular oncogene c-*erb*B by LTR insertion: Molecular basis for induction of erythroblastosis of avian leukosis virus. *Cell 33*: 357–368.

Gamett, D. G., Tracey, S. E., and Robinson, H. L. (1986). Differences in the sequences encoding the carboxyl-terminal domain of the epidermal growth factor receptor correlated with differences in the disease potential of viral *erb*B genes. *Proc. Natl. Acad. Sci. U.S.A. 83*: 6053–6057.

Gattoni-Celli, S., Hsiao, W.-L., and Weinstein, I. B. (1983). Rearranged c-*mos* locus in a MOPC-21 murine myeloma cell line and its persistence in hybridomas. *Nature 306*: 795–796.

Gazzolo, L. C., Moscovici, C., Moscovici, M. G., and Samurat, J. (1979). Response of hemopoietic cells to avian leukemia viruses: Effects on the differentiation of the target cells. *Cell 16*: 627–638.

George, D. L., Scott, A. F., Trusko, S., Glick, B., Ford, E., and Dorney, D. J. (1985). Structure and expression of amplified c-Ki-*ras* gene sequences in Y1 mouse adrenal tumor cells. *EMBO J. 4*: 1199–1203.

Gerondakis, S., and Bishop, J. M. (1986). Structure of the protein encoded by the chicken proto-oncogene c-*myb*. *Mol. Cell. Biol. 6*: 3677–3684.

Gisselbrecht, S., Fichelson, S., Sola, B., Bodereaux, D., Hampe, A., Andre, C., Galibert, F., and Tambourin, P. (1987). Frequent c-*fms* activation by proviral insertion in mouse myeloblastic leukemia. *Nature 329*: 259–261.

Gonda, T., Sheiness, D. L., Fanshier, L., Bishop, J. M., Moscovici, C., and Moscovici, M. G. (1981). The genome and the intracellular RNAs of avian myeloblastosis virus. *Cell 23*: 279–290.

Gonda, T. J., Cory, S., Sobieszczuk, P., Holtzman, D., and Adams, J. (1987). Generation of altered transcripts by retroviral insertion in the c-*myb* gene in two murine monocytic leukemas. *J. Virol. 61*: 2754–2763.

Goodenow, M. M., and Hayward, W. S. (1987). 5′ Long terminal repeats of *myc*-associated proviruses appear structurally intact but are functionally impared in tumors induced by avian leukosis viruses. *J. Virol. 61*: 2489–2498.

Goodwin, R. G., Rottman, F. M., Callaghan, T., Kung, H. J., Maroney, P. A., and Nilsen, T. W. (1986). c-*erb*B activation in avian leukosis virus induced erythroblastosis: Multiple epidermal growth factor receptor mRNAs are generated by alternative RNA processing. *Mol. Cell. Biol. 6*: 3128–3133.

Graf, T., and Beug, H. (1978). Avian leukemia viruses: Interaction with their target cells in vivo and *in vitro*. *Biochim. Biophys, Acta 516*: 269–299.

Graf, T., and Beug, H. (1983). Role of the v-*erb*A and v-*erb*B oncogenes of avian erythroblastosis virus in erythroid cell transformation. *Cell 34*: 7–9.

Graf, T., and Stehelin, D. (1982). Avian leukemia viruses: Oncogenes and genome structure. *Biochim. Biophys. Acta 651*: 245–271.

Hahn, M., and Hayward, W. S. (1988). Absence of missense mutations in activated c-*myc* genes in avian leukosis virus-induced B-cell lymphomas. *Mol. Cell. Biol.* (in press).

Hanafusa, H. (1986). Activation of the c-*src* gene. In *Oncogenes and Growth Control.* (P. Kahn and T. Graf, eds.) Springer-Verlag, Berlin, pp. 100–105.

Hann, S. R., King, M. W., Bentley, D. L., Anderson, C. W., and Eisenman, R. N. (1988). A non-AUG translational initiation in c-*myc* exon 1 generates an N-Terminally distinct protein whose synthesis is disrupted in Burkitt's lymphomas. *Cell 52*: 185–195.

Hardy, W. (1982). Pathogenesis of feline leukemia and sarcoma viruses. In *RNA Tumor Viruses.* (R. Weiss, N. Teich, H. Varmus, and J. Coffin, eds.) Cold Spring Harbor Laboratory, Cold Spring Harbor, New York, pp. 923–938.

Hartley, J. W., Wolford, N. K., Old, L. J., and Rowe, W. P. (1977). A new class of murine leukemia virus associated with development of spontaneous lymphomas. *Proc. Natl. Acad. Sci. U.S.A. 74*: 789–792.

Hayflick, J., Seeburg, P. H., Ohlsson, R., Pfeiffer-Ohlsson, S., Watson, D., Papas, T., and Duesberg, P. H. (1985). Nucleotide sequence of two overlapping *myc*-related genes in avian carcinoma virus OK10 and their relation to the *myc* genes of other viruses and the cell. *Proc. Natl. Acad. Sci. U.S.A. 82*: 2718–2722.

Hayman, M., and Beug, H. (1984). Identification of a form of the avian erythroblastosis virus *erb*B gene product at the cell surface. *Nature 309*: 460–462.

Hayward, W. S., Neel, B. G., and Astrin, S. M. (1981). Activation of a cellular *onc* gene by promoter insertion in ALV-induced lymphoid leukosis. *Nature 209*: 475–480.

Hayward, W. S., Neel, B. G., and Astrin, S. M. (1982). Avian leukosis viruses: Activation of cellular "oncogenes." In *Advances in Viral Oncology 1*. (G. Klein, ed.) Raven Press, New York, pp. 207–233.

Herman, S. A., and Coffin, J. M. (1986). Differential transcription from the long terminal repeats of integrated avian leukosis virus DNA. *J. Virol. 60*: 497–505.

Holland, C. A., Hartley, J. W., Rowe, W. P., and Hopkins, N. (1985). At least four viral genes contribute to the leukemogenicity of murine retrovirus MCF 247 in AKR Mice. *J. Virol. 53*: 158–165.

Isfort, R., Witter, R. L., and Kung, H. J. (1987). c-*myc* activation in an unusual retrovirus-induced avian T-lymphoma resembling Marek's disease: Proviral insertion 5′ of exon one enhances the expression of an intron promoter. Oncogene Research *2*: 81–94.

Kan, N. C., Flordellis, C. S., Mark, G. E., Duesberg, P. H., and Papas, T. S. (1984). Nucleotide sequence of avian carcinoma virus MH2: Two potential *onc* genes, one related to avian virus MC29 and the other related to murine sarcoma virus 3611. *Proc. Natl. Acad. Sci. U.S.A. 81*: 3000–3004.

Kanter, M. R., Smith, R. E., and Hayward, W. S. (1988) Rapid induction of B-cell lymphomas: Insertional activation of c-*myb* by ALV. *J. Virol. 62*: 1423–1432.

Klempnauer, K.-H., Gonda, T. J., and Bishop, J. M. (1982). Nucleotide sequence of the retroviral leukemia gene v-*myb* and its cellular progenitor c-*myb*: The architecture of a transduced oncogene. *Cell 31*: 453–463.

Klempnauer, K.-H., Ramsay, G., Bishop, J. M., Moscovici, M. G., Moscovici, C., McGrath, J. P., and Levinson, A. D. (1983). The product of the retroviral transforming gene v-*myb* is a truncated version of the protein encoded by the cellular oncogene c-*myb*. *Cell 33*: 345–355.

Levy, L. S., Gardner, M. B., and Casey, J. W. (1984). Isolation of a feline leukemia provirus containing the oncogene *myc* from a feline lymphosarcoma. *Nature 308*: 853–856.

Li, Y., Holland, C. A., Hartley, J. W., and Hopkins, N. (1984). Viral integration near c-*myc* in 10–20% of MCF 247-induced AKR lymphomas. *Proc. Natl. Acad. Sci. U.S.A. 81*: 6808–6811.

Linial, M., and Groudine, M. (1985). Transcription of three c-*myc* exons is enhanced in chicken bursal lymphoma cell lines. *Proc. Natl. Acad. Sci. U.S.A. 2*: 53–57.

Miles, B. D., and Robinson, H. L. (1985). High-frequency transduction of c-*erb*B in avian leukosis virus-induced erythroblastosis. *J. Virol. 54*: 295–303.

Mizutani, S., and Temin, H. (1976). Incorporation of noncomplementary nucleotides at high frequences by ribadeoxyvirus DNA polymerases and *Escherichia coli* DNA polymerase I. *Biochemistry 15*: 1510–1516.

Moscovici, C. (1975). Leukemic transformation with avian myeloblastosis virus: Present status. *Curr. Topics Microbiol. Immunol. 171*: 79–101.

Moscovici, M. G., Jurdic, P., Samarut, J., Gazzolo, L., Mura, C. V., and Moscovici, C. (1983). Characteristics of the hemopoietic target cells for the avian leukemia virus E26. *Virology 129*: 65–78.

Mullins, J. I., Brody, D. S., Binari, R. C., Jr., and Cotter, S. M. (1984). Viral transduction of c-*myc* gene in naturally occuring feline leukemias, 1984. *Nature 308*: 856–858.

Murphy, W., Sarid, J. J., Taub, R., Vasicek, T., Battey, J., Lenoir, G., and Leder, P. (1986). A translocated human c-*myc* oncogene is altered in a conserved coding sequence. *Proc. Natl. Acad. Sci. U.S.A. 83*: 2939–2943.

Mushinski, J. F., Potter, M., Bauer, S. R., and Reddy, E. P. (1983). DNA rearrangement and altered RNA expression of the c-*myb* oncogene in mouse plasmacytoid lymphosarcomas. *Science 220*: 795–798.

Neckameyer, W. S., and Wang, L.-H. (1984). Molecular cloning and characterization of avian sarcoma virus UR2 and comparison of its transforming sequences with those of other avian sarcoma viruses. *J. Virol. 50*: 914–921.

Neel, B. G., Hayward, W. S., Robinson, W. L., Fang, J., and Astrin, S. M. (1981). Avian leukosis virus-induced tumors have common proviral integration sites and synthesize discrete new RNAs: oncogenesis by promoter insertion. *Cell 23*: 323–334.

Neel, B. G., Gasic, G. P., Rogler, C. E., Skalka, A. M., Ju, G., Hishinuma, F., Papas, T., Astrin, S. M., and Hayward, W. S. (1982). Molecular analysis of the c-*myc* locus in normal tissue and in avian leukosis virus-induced lymphomas. *J. Virol. 44*: 158–166.

Neil, J. C., Hughes, D., McFarlane, D., Wilkie, N., Onions, D. E., Lees, G., and Jarret, O. (1984). Transduction and rearrangement of the *myc* gene by feline leukemia virus in naturally occurring T-cell leukemias. *Nature 308*: 814–820.

Neiman, P. E., Jordan, L., Weiss, R. A., and Payne, L. N. (1980). Malignant lymphoma of the bursa of Frabricius and analysis of early transformation. In *Viruses in Naturally Occurring Cancers. Cold Spring Harbor Symposia on Quantitative Biology,* Vol. 7, Book A. (M. Essex, G. Todaro, and H. Zurhausen, eds.) Cold Spring Harbor Laboratory, Cold Spring Harbor, New York pp. 519–528.

Nepveu, A., and Marcu, K. B. (1986). Intragenic pausing and anti-sense transscription within the murine c-*myc* locus. *EMBO J. 5*: 2859–2865.

Nilsen, T. W., Maroney, P. A., Goodwin, R. G., Rottman, F. M., Crittenden, L. B., Raines, M. A., and Kung, H. (1985). c-*erb*B activation in ALV-induced erythroblastosis: Novel RNA processing and promoter insertion result in expression of an amino-truncated EGF receptor. *Cell 41*: 719–726.

Nishida, T., Sakamoto, S. Yamamoto, T., Hayman, M., Kawai, S., and Toyoshima, K. (1984). Comparison of genome structures among 3 different strains of avian erythroblastosis viruses. *Gann 75*: 325–333.

Noori-Daloii, M. R., Swift, R. A., Kung, H. J., Crittenden, L. B., and Witter, R. L. (1981). Specific integration of REV proviruses in avian bursal lymphomas. *Nature 294*: 574–576.

Nunn, M., Weiher, H., Bullock, P., and Duesberg, P. (1983). Avian erythroblastosis virus E26: Nucleotide sequence of the tripartite oncogene and of the LTR, and analysis of the cellular prototype of the viral *ets* sequence. *Virology 139*: 330–339.

O'Donnell, P. V., Fleissner, E., Lonial, H., Koehne, C. F., and Reicin, A. (1985). Early clonality and high-frequency proviral integration into the c-*myc* locus in AKR leukemias. *J. Virol. 55*: 500–503.

Payne, G. S., Courtneidge, S. A., Crittenden, L. B., Fadley, A. M., Bishop, J. M., and Varmus, H. E. (1981). Analysis of avian leukosis virus DNA and RNA in bursal tumors: Viral gene expression is not required for maintenance of the tumor state. *Cell 23*: 311–322.

Payne, G. S., Bishop, J. M., and Varmus, H. E. (1982). Multiple arrangements of viral DNA and an activated host oncogene in bursal lymphomas. *Nature 295*: 209–214.

Privalsky, M. L., and Bishop, J. M. (1982). Proteins specified by avian erythroblastosis virus: Coding region localization and identification of a previously undetected *erb*B polypeptide. *Proc. Natl. Acad. Sci. U.S.A. 79*: 3958–3962.

Privalsky, M. L., and Bishop, J. M. (1984). Subcellular localization of the v-*erb*B protein, the product of a transforming gene of avian erythroblastosis virus. *Virology 135*: 365–368.

Probst, F., and Vande Woude, G. F. (1985). c-*mos* proto-oncogene transcripts are expressed in mouse tissues. *Nature 315*: 515–518.

Pulciani, S., Santos, E., Long, L. K., Sorrentino, V., and Barbacid, M. (1985). *ras* gene amplification and malignant transformation. *Mol. Cell. Biol. 5*: 2836–2841.

Purchase, H. G., Okazaki, W., Vogt, P. K., Hanafusa, H., Burmester, B. R., and Crittenden, L. B. (1977). Oncogenicity of avian leukosis viruses of different subgroups and of mutants of sarcoma viruses. *Infect. Immun. 15*: 423–428.

Rabbitts, T. H., Hamlyn, P. H., and Baer, R. (1983). Altered nucleotide sequences of a translocated c-*myc* gene in Burkitt lymphoma. *Nature 306*: 760–765.

Rachevi, G., Givol, D., and Canaani, E. (1982). Activation of a cellular gene by DNA rearrangement: Possible involvement of an IS-like element. *Nature 300*: 607–611.

Radke, K., Beug, H., Kornfeld, S., and Graf, T. (1982). Transformation of both erythroid and myeloid cells by E26, an avian leukemia virus that contains the *myb* gene. *Cell 31*: 643–653.

Raines, M. A., Lewis, W. G., Crittenden, L. B., and Kung, H.-J. (1985). c-*erb*B activation in avian leukosis virus-induced erythroblastosis: Clustered integration sites and the arrangement of provirus in the c-*erb*B alleles. *Proc. Natl. Acad. Sci. U.S.A. 82*: 2287–2291.

Reddy, E., Potter, M., Singer, P. A., and Sklar, M. D. (1975). Synthesis, surface deposition, and secretion of immunoglobulins by Abelson virus-transformed lymphosarcoma cell lines. *Cell 6*: 149–159.

Reddy, E. P., Reynolds, R. K., Santos, E., and Barbacid, M. (1982). A point mutation is responsible for the acquisition of transforming properties by the T24 human bladder carcinoma oncogene. *Nature 300*: 149–152.

Reddy, E. P., Reynolds, R. K., Watson, D. K., Schultz, R. A., Lautenberger, J., and Papas, T. S. (1983). Nucleotide sequence analysis of the proviral genome of avian myelocytomatosis virus (MC29). *Proc. Natl. Acad. Sci. U.S.A. 80*: 2500–2504.

Reicin, A., Yang, J.-Q., Marcu, K. B., Fleissner, E., Koehne, C. F., and O'Donnell, P. V. (1986). Deregulation of the c-*myc* oncogene in virus-induced thymic lymphomas of AKR/J mice. *Mol. Cell. Biol. 6*: 4088–4092.

Remmers, E. F., Yang, J. Q., and Marcu, K. B. (1986). A negative transcriptional control element located upstream of the murine c-*myc* gene. *EMBO J. 5*: 899–904.

Robinson, H. L., and Gagnon, G. C. (1986). Patterns of proviral insertion and deletion in avian leukosis virus-induced lymphomas. *J. Virol. 57*: 28–36.

Robinson, H. L., Miles, B. D., Catalano, D. E., Briles, W. E., and Crittenden, L. B. (1985). Susceptibility to *erb*B-induced erythroblastosis is a dominant trait in line 15_1 chickens. *J. Virol. 55*: 617–622.

Rohdewohld, H., Weiher, H., Jaenisch, R., and Breindl, M. (1987). Retrovirus integration and chromatin structure: Moloney murine leukemia proviral integration sites map near DNase I-hypersensitive sites. *J. Virol. 61*: 336–343.

Rosson, D., and Reddy, E. P. (1986). Nucleotide sequence of chicken c-*myb* complementary DNA and implications for *myb* oncogene activation. *Nature 319*: 604–606.

Rosson, D., Dugan, D., and Reddy, E. P. (1987). Aberrant splicing events that are induced by proviral integration: Implications for *myb* oncogene activation. *Proc. Natl. Acad. Sci. U.S.A. 84*: 3171–3175.

Roussel, M., Saule, S., Lagrou, C., Rommens, C., Beug, H., Graf, T., and Stehelin, D. (1979). Three new types of viral oncogene of cellular origin specific for hematopoietic cell transformation. *Nature 281*: 452–455.

Rovigatti, U. G., Rogler, C. E., Neel, B. G., Hayward, and Astrin, S. M. (1982). Expression of endogenous oncogenes in tumor cells. In *Tumor Cell Heterogeneity: Origins and Implications.* (A. H. Owens, Jr., D. S. Coffey, and S. B. Baylin, eds.) Academic Press, New York. pp. 319–330.

Ruscetti, S. K., Linemeyer, D., Field, J., Troxler, D., and Scolnick, E. M. (1979). Characterization of protein found in cells infected with the spleen focus-forming virus that shares immunological cross-reactivity with the gp70 in mink cell focus-inducing virus particles. *J. Virol. 30*: 787–798.

Ruscetti, S., Davis, L., Field, I., and Oliff, A. (1981). Friend murine leukemia virus-induced leukemia is associated with the formation of mink cell focus-inducing viruses and is blocked in mice expressing endogenous mink cell focus-inducing xenotropic viral envelope genes. *J. Exp. Med. 154*: 907–920.

Sacca, R., Stanley, E. R., Sherr, C. J., and Rettenmier, C. W. (1986). Specific binding of the mononuclear phagocyte colony-stimulating factor CSF-1 to the product of the v-*fms* oncogene. *Proc. Natl. Acad. Sci., U.S.A. 83*: 3331–3335.

Schector, A. L., Stern, D. F., Vaidyanathan, L., Decker, S. J., Drebin, M. I., and Weinberg, R. A. (1984). The *neu* oncogene: An *erb*B-related gene encoding a 185,000-M_r tumor antigen. *Nature 312*: 513–516.

Schwab, M., Alitalo, K., Varmus, H. E., Bishop, J. M., and George, D. (1983). A cellular oncogene (c-K-*ras*) is amplified, over-expressed, and located within karyotypic abnormalities in mouse adrenocortical tumor cells. *Nature 303*: 497–501.

Sealy, L., Privalsky, M., Moscovici, G., Moscovici, C., and Bishop, J. M. (1983). Site-specific mutagenesis of avian erythroblastosis virus—*erb* is required for oncogenicity. *Virology 130*: 155–178.

Selten, G., Cuypers, H. T., Zijlstra, M., Melief, C., and Berns, A. (1984). Involvement of c-*myc* in MuLV-induced T cell lymphomas in mice: Frequency and mechanisms of activation. *EMBO J. 3*: 3215–3222.

Shaw, J., Hayman, M. J., and Enrietto, P. J. (1985). Analysis of a deleted MC29 provirus: *gag* sequences are not required for fibroblast transformation. *J. Virol 56*: 943–950.

Shen-Ong, G. L. C., Potter, M., Mushinski, J. F., Lavu, S., and Reddy, E. P. (1984). Activation of the c-*myb* locus by viral insertional mutagenesis in plasmacytoid lymphosarcomas. *Science 226*: 1077–1080.

Shen-Ong, G. L. C., Morse, H. C., III, Potter, M., and Mushinski, J. F. (1986). Two modes of c-*myb* activation in virus-induced mouse myeloid tumors. *Mol. Cell. Biol. 6*: 380–392.

Shen-Ong, G. L. (1987). Alternative internal splicing in c-*myb* RNAs occurs commonly in normal and tumor cells. *EMBO J. 13*: 4035–4039.

Sherr, C. J., Rettenmier, C. W., Sacca, R., Roussel, M. F., Look, A. T., and Stanley, E. R. (1985). The c-*fms* proto-oncogene product is related to the receptor for the mononuclear phagocyte growth factor, CSF-1. *Cell 41*: 665–676.

Shih, C.-K., Linial, M., Goodenow, M. M., and Hayward, W. S. (1984). Nucleotide sequence 5′ of the chicken c-*myc* coding region: Localization of a non-coding exon that is absent from *myc* transcripts in most avian leukemia virus-induced lymphomas. *Proc. Natl. Acad. Sci. U.S.A. 81*: 4697–4701.

Siebenlist, U., Hennighausen, L., Battey, J., and Leder, P. (1984). Chromatin structure and protein binding in the putative regulatory region of the c-*myc* gene in Burkitt lymphoma. *Cell 37*: 381–391.

Simon, M. C., Smith, R. E., and Hayward, W. S. (1984). Mechanisms of oncogenesis by subgroup F avian leukosis virus. *J. Virol. 52*: 1–8.

Simon, M. C., Neckameyer, W. S., Hayward, W. S., and Smith, R. E. (1987). Genetic determinants of neoplastic diseases induced by a subgroup F avian leukosis virus. *J. Virol. 61*: 1203–1212.

Sola, B., Fichelson, S., Bordereaux, D., Tambourin, P. E., and Gisselbrecht, S. (1986). *fim*-1 and *fim*-2: Two new integration regions of Friend murine leukemia virus in myeloblastic leukemias. *J. Virol. 60*: 718–725.

Steffen, D. (1984). Proviruses are adjacent to c-*myc* in some murine leukemia virus-induced lymphomas. *Proc. Natl. Acad. Sci. U.S.A. 81*: 2097–2101.

Stehelin, D., Varmus, H. E., Bishop, J. M., and Vogt, P. K. (1976). DNA related to the transforming gene of avian sarcoma viruses is present in normal avian DNA. *Nature 260*: 170–

Stewart, M. A., Forrest, D., McFarlane, R., Onions, D., Wilkie, N., and Neil, J. C. (1986). Conservation of the c-*myc* coding sequence in transduced feline v-*myc* genes. *Virology 154*: 121–134.

Stoye, J., and Coffin, J. (1985). Endogenous retroviruses. In *RNA Tumor Viruses 2/Supplements and Appendixes.* (R. Weiss, N. Teich, H. Varmus, and J. Coffin eds.) Cold Spring Harbor Laboratory, Cold Spring Harbor, New York, pp. 357–405.

Swift, R. A., Shaller, E., Witter, R. L., and Kung, H.-J. (1985). Insertional activation of c-*myc* by reticuloendotheliosis virus in chicken B lymphoma: Nonrandom distribution and orientation of the proviruses. *J. Virol. 54*: 869–872.

Swift, R. A., Boerkoel, N., Ridgeway, A., Fujita, D., Dodgson, J., and Kung, H. J. (1987). B-lymphoma induction by reticuloendotheliosis virus: Characterization of a mutated chicken syncytial virus provirus involved in c-*myc* activation. *J. Virol. 61*: 2084–2090.

Tabin, C. J., Bradly, S. M., Bergmann, C. I, Weinberg, R. A., Papageorge, A. G., Scolnick, E. M., Dhar, R., Lowy, D. L., and Change, E. H. (1982). Mechanism of activation of a human oncogene. *Nature 300*: 143–149.

Tsichlis, P. N., Strauss, P. G., and Fu Hu, L. (1983). A common region for proviral DNA integration of MoMuLV-induced rat thymic lymphomas. *Nature 302*: 445–449.

Ullrich, A., Coussens, L., Hayflick, J., Dull, T., Gray, A., Tam, A., Lee, J., Yarden, Y. Liberman, T., Schlessinger, J., Downward, J., Mayes, E., Whittle, N., Waterfield, M., and Seeberg, P. (1984). Human epidermal growth factor receptor cDNA sequence and aberrant expression of the amplified gene in A431 carcinoma cells. *Nature 309*: 418–525.

Vennstrom, B., and Bishop, J. M. (1982). Isolation and characterization of chicken DNA homologues to the two putative oncogenes of avian erythroblastosis virus. *Cell 28*: 135–143.

Walther, N., Jansen, H. W., Trachmann, C., and Bister, K. (1986). Nucleotide sequence of the CMII v-*myc* allele. *Virology 154*: 219–223.

Watson, D. K., Reddy, E. P., Duesberg, P. H., and Papas, T. S. (1983). Nucleotide sequence analysis of the chicken c-*myc* gene reveals homologous and unique coding regions by comparison with the transforming gene of avian myelocytomatosis virus MC29 delta-*gag-myc*. *Proc. Natl. Acad. Sci. U.S.A. 80*: 2146–2150.

Watts, S. L., and Smith, R. E. (1980). Pathology of chicken infected with avian nephroblastoma virus MAV-2(N). *Infect. Immun. 27*: 501–512.

Weinstein, Y., Ihle, J. N., Lavu, S., and Reddy, E. P. (1986). Truncation of the c-*myb* gene by a retroviral integration in an interleukin 3-dependent myeloid leukemia cell line. *Proc. Natl. Acad. Sci. U.S.A. 83*: 5010–5014.

Weinstein, Y., Cleveland, J. L., Askew, D. S., Rapp, U. R., and Ihle, J. N. (1987). Insertion and truncation of c-*myb* by murine leukemia virus in a myeloid cell line derived from cultures of normal hematopoietic cells. *J. Virol. 61*: 2339–2343.

Weiss, R. (1982). Experimental biology and assay of RNA tumor viruses. In *RNA Tumor Viruses.* (R. Weiss, N. Teich, H. Varmus, and J. Coffin, eds.) Cold Spring Harbor Laboratory, Cold Spring Harbor, New York, pp. 209–260.

Wendling, F., Fichelson, S., Heard, J. M., Gisselbrecht, S., Varet, B., and Tambourin, P. (1983). Induction of myeloid leukemias in mice by biologically cloned ecotropic F-MuLV. In *Tumor Viruses and Differentiation.* (E. Scolnick and E. Levine, eds.) Alan R. Liss, New York, pp. 357–362.

Westaway, D., Payne, G., and Varmus, H. (1984). Proviral deletions and oncogene base-substitutions in insertionally mutagenized c-*myc* alleles may contribute to the progression of avian bursal tumors. *Proc. Natl. Acad. Sci. U.S.A. 81*: 843–847.

Westaway, D., Papkoff, J. Moscovici, C., and Varmus, H. E. (1986). Identification of a provirally activated c-Ha-*ras* oncogene in an avian nephroblastoma via a novel procedure: cDNA cloning of a chimaeric viral-host transcript. *EMBO J. 5*: 301–309.

Wilhelmsen, K. C., Eggleton, K., and Temin, H. M. (1984). Nucleic acid sequences of the oncogene v-*rel* in reticuloendotheliosis virus strain T and its cellular homolog, the proto-oncogene c-*rel*. *J. Virol. 52*: 172–182.

Wiman, K. G., Clarkson, B., Hayday, A. C., Saito, H. Tonegawa, S., and Hayward W. S. (1984). Activation of a translocated c-*myc* gene: Role of structural alterations in the upstream region. *Proc. Natl. Acad. Sci. U.S.A. 81*: 6798–6802.

Witter, R. L., and Crittenden, L. B. (1979). Lymphomas resembling lymphoid leukosis in chickens inoculated with reticuloendotheliosis virus. *Int. J. Cancer 23*: 673–678.

Witter, R. L., Sharma, J. M., and Fadly, A. M. (1986). Nonbursal lymphomas induced by nondefective reticuloendotheliosis virus. *Avian Pathol. 15*: 467–486.

Wood, T. G., McGeady, M. L., Baroudy, B., Blair, D. G., and Vande Woude, G. F. (1984). Mouse c-*mos* oncogene activation is prevented by upstream sequences. *Proc. Natl. Acad. Sci. U.S.A. 81*: 7817–7821.

Yamamoto, T., Hihara, T., Mitajami, N., Kawai, S., Oboi, T., and Toyoshima, K. (1983). The *erb*B gene of avian erythroblastosis virus is a member of the *src* gene family. *Cell 35*: 71–78.

THREE

Cellular Oncogene Activation by Insertion of Retroviral DNA; Genes Identified by Provirus Tagging

Roel Nusse
The Netherlands Cancer Institute
Amsterdam, The Netherlands

Anton Berns
The Netherlands Cancer Institute
and The University of Amsterdam
Amsterdam, The Netherlands

INTRODUCTION

In this chapter, we shall give an overview of tumorigenesis by retroviruses that activate cellular oncogenes by insertional mutagenesis. This mechanism is used by a wide variety of retroviruses, including avian leukosis virus (ALV), murine leukemia virus (MLV), and mouse mammary tumor virus (MMTV), which can be grouped together because they all appear to lack viral genes directly responsible for tumorigenesis. Thereby, tumorigenesis by these viruses depends on host cellular oncogenes, transcriptionally activated, or otherwise mutated as a consequence of proviral integration. Mainly for historical reasons, these cellular genes can be divided in two classes: oncogenes previously known from other sources, most notably those cellular oncogenes first detected as viral sequences in transforming retroviruses; and cellular genes not identified before. Activation of known oncogenes by proviral insertion will be treated in Chapter 2, whereas here we shall review genes uniquely found as targets for inserted proviruses in tumors. Owing to this limitation, all genes discussed here have originally been found by an approach termed transposon tagging: molecular cloning of host cell DNA adjacent to integrated proviruses (reviewed in Goff, 1986; Nusse, 1986; Varmus, 1984). This strategy was initiated when it was found that the tumors caused by nontransforming retroviruses were clonal for the proviral integration sites, whereas infected but otherwise normal tissue was not. This finding, made in different systems, indicated that acquisition of proviral deoxyribonucleic acid (DNA) by itself is not sufficient for tumorigenic transformation. The clonal emergence of tumors from mass-infected cells gave a plausible hypothesis to explain the mechanism of viral oncogenesis by viruses lacking viral oncogenes: Proviral insertion causes a mutation in the host cell, and only mutations at sites predisposing to tumorigenic growth cause cell transformation. Evidently, the finding that the c-*myc* oncogene, previously found as a cellular progenitor of a retroviral transforming gene, is often activated by proviral insertion in ALV-induced leukosis (Hayward et al., 1981; Payne et al., 1982) gave much force to this model.

In case no known genes are rearranged, one has to resort to molecular cloning of inserted proviral DNA, thereby isolating the integration site. Molecular clones from the provirus linked to host cell sequences are isolated from tumor cell recombinant DNA libraries. The presence of novel, tumor-specific restriction fragments hybridizing with host cells as well as with viral probes is taken as evidence for a common integration site. The relevant gene within the integration domain can be identified by searching for tumor-specific transcripts and, ultimately, a biological assay in which the gene of interest is introduced into appropriate target cells, can provide formal evidence that indeed an oncogene has been uncovered. The assignment to a chromosomal location can indicate whether other genes are near or even identical to the integration domain.

This approach has been most successfully used in various murine tumor systems. A large series of integration domains has been found for leukemia viruses in diseases of the hemopoietic system, and for MMTV in mammary carcinomas.

LIMITATIONS AND POTENTIAL OF PROVIRUS TAGGING

We would like to emphasize a few aspects of oncogene activation by retroviral integration, which illustrate both the limitations and the enormous potential of provirus tagging:

1. The number of tissues in which retroviruses can efficiently replicate in vivo is limited. Proviral activations will be restricted accordingly.

2. The chromosomal regions containing proto-oncogenes have to be accessible for retroviral insertion. Since retroviral insertions might be less random than previously assumed (King et al., 1985; Rohdewohld et al., 1987; Vijaya et al., 1986), some proto-oncogenes might not or very infrequently be affected by proviral insertion.
3. The enhancer or promoter of the inserted proviruses should have the capacity to act dominantly in cis on regulatory sequences, or alternatively, the proviral insertion site has to affect specific characteristics of the mRNA of the activated oncogene (e.g., stability).
4. Proviral insertion can activate those proto-oncogenes that gain oncogenic potential by disregulated expression or by truncation of the protein; insertions can evidently not cause point mutations.
5. Provirus tagging can uncover genes contributing to any stage of the tumorigenic process, even if the contribution is relatively subtle.
6. Genes can be found that are not active in other assay systems for oncogene detection (e.g., by in vitro transformation assays). Therefore, the method might allow the detection of genes involved in activities as diverse as tumor initiation, promotion, progression, metastasis, and escape from immunosurveillance.

THE MOUSE MAMMARY TUMOR VIRUS

The mouse mammary tumor virus usually causes adenocarcinomas of mammary epithelial tissue, and has occasionally been associated with various types of other tumors, such as lymphomas and kidney carcinomas (reviewed in Weiss et al., 1982). Mammary tumor-inducing virus preparations can be isolated from the milk of several high cancer–incidence mouse strains like the C3H, the RIII, and the DBA. In these strains, the virus is naturally transmitted from mother to offspring, causing the high spontaneous tumor incidence. Foster nursing of other mice on mothers from milk-transmitting strains results in a similar high incidence of tumors.

This virus was one of the earliest tumor viruses discovered, being isolated as a milk factor that induces mammary tumors in mice (reviewed in Hilgers and Bentvelzen, 1979). Because of difficulties in handling the virus in in vitro cell systems and the lack of rapid and reliable assays for biologically active virus, MMTV is yet one of the less well-understood retroviruses. No viral mutants are available. Even the best virus preparations, which are highly oncogenic in susceptible mice, are very poorly infectious in cultured cells. Consequently, MMTV has never been biologically cloned. Additional difficulties arose when it appeared that MMTV proviral DNA was refractile to molecular cloning. Most attempts to isolate the

Table 1 Properties of Different *int* Genes

Gene	Mouse chromosome	Human chromosome	Transcript (kb)	Protein (kd)	Reference
int-1	15	12	2.6	41	Nusse and Varmus 1982
int-2	7	11	3.2, 3.0, 1.8, 1.4	27	Peters et al., 1983
int-3	17	?	2.4	?	Gallahan and Callahan, 1987
int-4	11	?	?	?	H. Roelink and R. Nusse, pers. comm.
int-41	?	?	5.2	?	Garcia et al., 1986

MMTV genome as recombinant DNA have yielded molecular clones lacking a part of the viral genome thought to contain a so-called poisonous sequence (cf. Brookes et al., 1986). These partial molecular clones were nevertheless very useful for studying the mechanism of viral tumorigenesis, using restriction enzyme analysis and blot hybridizations. Molecular hybridization techniques showed that in most strains of mice viral DNA was present in varying copy numbers, as endogenous, germ line–transmitted proviruses (Cohen et al., 1979). Tumors induced by MMTV had acquired additional MMTV sequences, as a consequence of integration of proviral DNA in the host cell genome, shown by restriction enzyme analysis to be integrated in a clonal fashion (Cohen et al., 1979; Groner and Hynes, 1980). After it was established that known oncogenes were not rearranged in MMTV-induced tumors, molecular cloning led to the discovery of various common integration areas. Three genes, called *int*-1, *int*-2, and *int*-3, have now been identified and characterized to a variable extent. The existence of several other genes has been inferred from less complete data. We shall discuss several aspects of these genes in varying detail, with emphasis on what is known of their function and action in tumorigenesis. Table 1 gives an overview of the *int* genes.

The *int*-1 Gene

The *int*-1 gene was the first cellular oncogene found by transposon tagging techniques (Nusse and Varmus, 1982; Nusse et al., 1984). In the C3H mouse strain, 70–80% of the tumors contain an MMTV provirus in the *int*-1 area, and a transcript of 2.6 kb is found in tumors but not in normal mammary tissue. The gene consists of four exons encoding a protein of 41,185 daltons (Van Ooyen and Nusse, 1984; Fung et al., 1985). This protein-encoding domain is always present in an intact configuration in tumors (Van Ooyen and Nusse,

1984), showing convincingly that the high frequency of insertions at *int*-1 is the consequence of selection for expression of the *int*-1 gene product and is not due to preferred integration as such.

Conspicuous properties of the *int*-1 protein, as deduced from the nucleotide sequence, are a hydrophobic leader sequence and a carboxyterminal half which is rich in cysteine residues (Fung et al., 1985; Van Ooyen and Nusse, 1984). These are features shared with growth factors and growth factor receptors, and may indicate that the *int*-1 protein functions in signaling between cells. The lack of a transmembrane domain in *int*-1 could be taken as evidence that the protein is secreted and functions as a ligand for a receptor. Assessment of the value of these predictions relies heavily on antisera to detect the actual site of the *int*-1 protein in the cell, but such sera have been hard to obtain. By synthesis of short peptides and bacterial fusion proteins containing *int*-1 sequences, several antisera of variable quality have been made (A. Brown, J. Papkoff, and H. E. Varmus, personal communication, and unpublished data from our own lab). These antibodies detect several forms of the *int*-1 protein of molecular weight between 36 and 42 kd, differing in extent of glycosylation, by immunoprecipitation from cells expressing the gene. The affinity of the antibodies is rather low, and not sufficient for localization studies by in situ techniques. By cell fractionation experiments, it has been shown that the *int*-1 protein enters the secretory pathway, but no *int*-1 species have been found outside cells (J. Papkoff et al., in preparation).

Recent findings have shed light on the biological properties of the *int*-1 gene. First, its nature as a genuine oncogene has been illustrated by an in vitro transformation assay. A cell line called C57MG, originally derived from normal mammary gland tissue of the C57/B1 mouse strain, becomes morphologically transformed by an *int*-1 retrovirus (Brown et al., 1986). The cells are also suitable for a focus assay in which groups of transformed cells can be detected on monolayers of flat epithelial cells. Transfection of another cell line, the RAC cells, with activated *int*-1 constructs leads to morphologically transformed cells that, unlike the transformed C57MG cells, are tumorigenic in syngeneic animals (Rijsewijk et al., 1987b). Fibroblastic cells cannot be transformed by *int*-1 (Brown et al., 1986; Rijsewijk et al., 1986).

These experiments demonstrate that *int*-1 is truly an oncogene, and underscore the validity of the approach taken to identify oncogenes by analysis of mutation sites in tumor cells. A point of concern, nevertheless, is that the cells transformed in vitro by *int*-1 are very different from mammary tumor cells in which the gene is activated by MMTV. The latter cells have usually retained many markers of mammary epithelial tissue, detected by monoclonal antibodies to cell surface or intermediate filament proteins (Sonnenberg et al., 1986, 1987). These markers are absent on the RAC cells transfected with *int*-1.

What about the normal fuction of *int*-1? In most adult tissues, the gene is not detectably expressed, except for the testis of mature mice, in postmeiotic round spermatids (Jakobovits et al., 1986). During embryogenesis of the mouse, *int*-1 is transiently expressed, between day 8 and day 14. By in situ ribonucleic acid (RNA) hybridizations and by dissection of embryos, it has been found that the site of expression is in the brain, most notably in the mid and hindbrain, but not in the forebrain (Shackleford and Varmus, 1987; Wilkinson et al., 1987). Expression is also detected at the site of closing of the neural tube. Although these findings do not give immediate clues, they indicate that the normal function of *int*-1 has to be sought in embryonic development of the nervous system.

More recently, a Drosophila homologue of *int*-1 has been cloned, and sequence analysis shows that the structure of the gene is conserved to a high degree in flies (Rijsewijk et al., 1987a). Moreover, the Drosophila *int*-1 gene is expressed in most stages of development, including embryos, larvae, pupae, but hardly detectable in adult files. This transient pattern of expression resembles that seen in the mouse. By in situ RNA hybridization experiments, a segmented pattern of expression in embryos is seen. The gene maps at position 28A and has been shown to be identical to the segmentation polarity gene *wingless*. The *wingless* gene is thought to be involved in pattern formation in segments (Baker, 1987; Cabrera et al., 1987), a hypothesis that fits with the structure of the D*int*-1/*wingless* protein, which is presumbly secreted from the cells. The full implications of these findings for the mechanism of mammary tumorigenesis are not clear yet; it can be imagined, however, that disregulated expression of a gene involved in pattern formation can cause abnormal growth of a tissue which, like the mammary gland, goes through cycles of development and regression in adult life.

The high degree of evolutionary conservation of *int*-1 is one of the most striking properties of the gene. A human homologue of *int*-1 has been cloned and sequenced, and shows only four amino acid differences with the mouse gene (Van Ooyen et al., 1985; Van't Veer et al., 1984). The changes are restricted to the amino terminal domain and do not affect the hydrophobic character of the leader. The gene has been mapped on chromosome 12 of man, probably at the cen-q14 region. Expression or rearrangements of *int*-1 in normal human tissue or in human tumors have not been found (M. van de Vijver and R. Nusse, unpublished data).

The *int*-2 Gene

The *int*-2 gene was discovered by Peters et al. (1983) in essentially the same way as *int*-1. The virus associated most frequently with *int*-2 insertions is from the RIII strain. The proviruses at *int*-2, with a few exceptions, point away from the gene, and are scattered over relatively large regions (Dickson et al., 1984). A common integration region for MMTV in some GR tumors (Schuermann and Michalides, 1987) that first appeared to represent a novel *int* gene, and was, like *int*-2, present on chromosome 7 (Peters et al., 1984a), has been shown to be located between 20 and 30 kb from *int*-2 (G. Peters and R. Michalides, personal communication). In between the two groups of insertions is the transcriptional unit of *int*-2, which appears to be quite complex (Moore et al., 1986). At least four different transcripts are detected in tumors and in normal tissue that arise through the use of different promoters and different polyadenylation signals (G. Peters and C. Dickson, personal communication). These transcripts are 3.2, 3.0, 1.8, and 1.4 kb long.

int-2 encodes 245 amino acids, predicting a protein of 27,000 daltons (Moore et al., 1986). Recently, this protein has been found to have considerable homology to basic and acidic fibroblast growth factor from bovine origin (Dickson and Peters, 1987), placing *int*-2 in the growth factor family of oncogenes. Good antisera to assay for the *int*-2 gene product are not available yet.

Peters et al. (1984b) have explored the biology of the mammary tumors in the BR6 strain to demonstrate that proviral activation of *int*-2 is an early event in the history of the tumor. When hormone-dependent BR6 tumors are followed during several cycles of pregnancy, leading to cycles of growth and disappearance of the tumor, it appears that successive tumors have the same *int*-2 rearrangement. The tumors can thus regress in spite of rearranged gene, indicating that the cells with the *int*-2 activation are present in a premalignant state in the non–hormone-stimulated mammary gland and need additional events to become hormone independent.

Indirect evidence for the oncogenicity of *int*-2 expression comes from the RAC mammary tumor cells (Sonnenberg et al., 1987). This line is clonal for insertion of MMTV near *int*-2, but sublines nevertheless show dramatic differences in expression of the gene and tumorigenicity. One variant grows as differentiated polygonal cells, which are tumorigenic, and express *int*-2. In culture, polygonal cells can convert to a nontumorigenic large cuboidal phenotype. The loss of tumorigenicity is accompanied by loss of *int*-2 expression. Direct assays for the oncogenic action of *int*-2 are not yet available.

The function of *int*-2 in normal physiology is probably in early development, but at a different stage that *int*-1. The gene is expressed in mouse embryos at day 7.5, and in several embryonic cell lines induced to differentiate into the endodermal lineage. *int*-2 is one of the few genes exclusively expressed during this type of differentiation (Jacobovits et al., 1986), indicating a key role for the gene in events occurring during early embryogenesis. The findings on expression of the *int* genes during development have attracted wide attention from developmental biologists.

A human homologue of *int*-2 has been isolated and mapped on chromosome 11, band q13 (Casey et al., 1986). Expression of *int*-2 in human tumors has not been reported. Restriction fragments hybridizing with *int*-2 probes are only detected in mammalian species and not in lower vertebrates, where mammary tumors do not occur.

The *int*-3 Gene

The *int*-3 gene was isolated from mammary tumors in the CzII strain by Gallahan and Callahan (1987). This CzII strain of mice is particularly suitable for studying MMTV insertions in tumors because it lacks endogenous MMTV proviral DNA. The strain has been isolated recently from the wild. Molecular cloning of a provirus from an *int*-1/*int*-2–negative tumor, and isolation of host cell probes showed that five out of 16 tumors contained a provirus at a new chromosomal area, called *int*-3. A tumor-specific *int*-3 transcript of 2.4 kb is found with probes upstream from the main cluster of insertions, which also appears to be conserved among mammalian species. *int*-3 has been mapped on mouse chromosome 17 and has no appreciable homology with other known genes by molecular hybridization (Gallahan et al., 1987). It is located in the proximity of the common insertion site *pim*-2 of MuLV (see below). Further cloning of the area is in progress, and may well reveal more insertions at the other side of the *int*-3 transcriptional unit.

The *int*-4 Gene

The characterization of the *int*-4 integration area is still in its infancy. Probes from a novel common insertion site have been obtained by molecular cloning of a single acquired provirus from a tumor in a Balb/c mice in which the GR virus was introduced. Four independent tumors showed insertions in the cloned area, called *int*-4. A transcript has hitherto not been found. *int*-4 has been mapped on chromosome 11 in the mouse (H. Roelink, J. Hilkens, and R. Nusse, in preparation).

Mutant MMTVs in Other Diseases; *int*-41

The tumorigenic spectrum of MMTV is not restricted to mammary oncogenesis. The virus is also associated with lymphomas and kidney carcinomas.

Garcia et al. (1986) have found an integration domain, called *int*-41, that originally was cloned from a mammary tumor in the C3H strain. No other mammary tumors contained an MMTV provirus near *int*-41, but, surprisingly, one kidney carcinoma had a rearranged *int*-41 allele, probably due to an MMTV insertion. In addition, probes from the region detected transcripts of various lengths, whose expression could be influenced by dexamethasone, indicating that they may have arisen as a consequence of an adjacent MMTV enhancer.

THE MURINE LEUKEMIA VIRUSES

A number of related murine leukemia viruses (MuLV) have been identified. They belong to the class of ecotropic (i.e., replicating exclusively in cells of mouse origin), xenotropic (i.e., replicating in cells of other species), and amphotropic viruses (i.e., replicating both in cells from mouse and in cells from other origin). Here we will refer only to characteristics of the ecotropic viruses, as members of this group cause tumors in the experimental systems described.

Two classes of ecotropic viruses can be discerned: the exogenously propagated FMR (Friend, Moloney, Rauscher) retroviruses, and the endogenous (AKV type) retrovirus (for review, see Weiss et al., 1985). These viruses are all closely related, but nevertheless exhibit significant differences in their capacity to cause tumors and in the type of disease; e.g., whereas Moloney and AKV viruses induce predominantly lymphoid tumors, Friend and Rauscher MuLV usually elicit erythroid and myeloid leukemias. Similarly, the AKV virus is only moderately leukemogenic, whereas its derivative, SL3, is highly tumorigenic. Different genetic factors appear to determine these characteristics, as has been shown by constructing hybrid viruses to map the disease determinants (Chatis et al., 1983; Evans and Morrey, 1987; Lenz et al., 1984). An important genetic determinant for both the leukemogenic potential and the tissue specificity appears to be the enhancer region located in the long terminal repeat (LTR) of MuLV (Davies et al., 1986; Holland et al., 1985; Short et al., 1987). Properties of the enhancer can cause variations in the tissue-specific replication of the virus and in the ability to activate proto-oncogenes by proviral insertion. The precise role of the different genetic determinants of MuLV is complicated further by the alterations these viruses can undergo during leukemogenesis. The alterations are found in the glycoprotein gene (env) of the virus and in the LTR. Recombination with endogenous proviral sequences in the mouse results in most cases in the generation of mink cell focus (MCF)–inducing viruses, which have an altered host range (Hartley et al., 1977; Vogt, 1979). The enhancer region in the viral LTR is also frequently altered, either by recombination with endogenous proviral sequences (Quint et al., 1984), or by rearrangements within the LTR itself (Berns et al., 1983). There is still dispute as to the exact role of MCF viruses in the leukemogenic process, as in some systems MuLV induces leukemogenesis without generating MCFs (Silver, 1984; Tsichlis et al., 1983).

Using murine leukemia viruses for transposon tagging, a variety of common integration sites have been defined. An overview of these common insertion sites is given in Table 2. The insertions have been found in tumors

Table 2 Properties of Common Insertion Sites of MuLV Proviruses

Insertion site	Chromosome mouse/rat	Chromosome human	Tumor	Transcription	Translocation	Reference
dsi-1	4 (m)	nd	T	—	—	Vijaya et al. 1987
evi-1	3 (m)	nd	M	—	—	N. Copeland, pers. comm.
evi-2	11 (m)	nd	M	—	?	N. Copeland, pers. comm.
fim-1	?	nd	M	?	?	Sola et al. 1986
fim-2 (CSF-1) receptor	?	nd	M	3.8	?	Sola et al. 1986; pers. comm.
fim-3	?	nd	M	?	?	Sola, pers. comm.
fis-1	7 (m)	nd	M/T	—	(+)	Silver and Buckler (1986) Silver and Kozak (1986)
gin-1	19 (m)	nd	T	—	?	Villemur et al. 1987
Mlvi-1	15 (m) 7 (r)	nd	T	—	(+)	Tsichlis et al. 1983
Mlvi-2	15 (m) 2 (r)	nd	T	—	?	Tsichlis et al. 1984
Mlvi-3	15 (r)	nd	T	—	?	Tsichlis et al. 1985a
Mlvi-4	15 (m) 7 (r)	nd	T	—	(+)	P. Tsichlis, pers. comm.
pim-1	17 (m)	6	T/B	2.8	(+)	Selten et al. 1986
pim-2	17 (m)	?	T	?	?	M. Breuer, pers. comm.
pvt-1/*mis*-1	15 (m)	8	B	—	+	Graham et al., 1985, Graham and Adams, 1986

derived from hematopoietic cell lineages, which is simply explained by the fact that hemopoietic cells constitute the major compartment for virus replication. Because of the presence of many cross-hybridizing endogenous proviruses in the mouse, many studies have been performed in the rat, which lacks proviruses cross-hybridizing with the murine leukemia viruses. Usually, a particular insertion site correlates to distinct disease pattern(s), but the frequency in which common integration sites are occupied depends on the genotype of both the host and the virus. An elegant study by the group of Jenkins and Copeland showed that the genetic background of the mouse strain can predispose for B, T, or myeloid lymphomas (Mucenski et al., 1986).

Although not addressed in this chapter, one should realize that activation of the c-*myc* gene plays a predominant role in the induction of hematopoietic neoplasias (reviewed by Alitalo et al., 1987). Analysis of T-cell lymphomas has shown that the majority of the tumors have elevated *myc* messenger RNA (mRNA) levels, in part mediated via proviral insertions near the c-*myc* proto-oncogene (Selten et al., 1984). The other common insertion sites are occupied generally in only some of the tumor cell clones, suggesting that alternative routes exist for similar tumorigenic processes. Furthermore, the different common insertion sites might be involved in different steps in the tumorigenic process. Insertions in up to three different common insertion sites within one tumor cell clone have been found (c-*myc*, *pim*-1, and *pim*-2 (M. Breuer et al., in preparation)), lending support to the notion that proviral insertions can cause sequential steps in tumor progression.

The *pim*-1 Locus

The *pim*-1 locus was indentified as a common insertion site in MuLV-induced T-cell lymphomas (Cuypers et al., 1984). The frequency of insertion in the *pim*-1 locus in these tumors can mount to 50%, and depends on the genetic background of the mouse and the strain of virus used. A relationship is observed between the latency of the disease and the frequency of proviral insertion in the *pim*-1 region; the latency time being inversely related to the incidence of insertion. Insertions in the *pim*-1 locus are not restricted to T-cell lymphomas; also in B-cell lymphomas insertions in this locus can be found (N. Copeland, personal communication). Within the same group of lymphomas, the incidence of insertions near *pim*-1 is somewhat lower than integrations near the c-*myc* gene (Selten et al., 1985). The majority of the proviruses at *pim*-1 cluster in the 3′ untranslated region of the gene in the same transcriptional orientation. These insertions separate a destabilizing (AUUUA)n motif (Shaw and Kamen, 1986) from the body of the *pim*-1 mRNA, and this accounts most likely for the higher steady-state levels of *pim*-1 mRNA in lymphomas (Domen et al., 1987; Selten et al., 1986). *pim*-1 transcription in these tumors terminates in the 5′ LTR of the inserted provirus. A small fraction of the insertions are found upstream (in both orientations) and downstream (same transcriptional orientation) of the gene. Mink cell focus-inducing (MCF) proviruses account for 80% of the insertions near *pim*-1, and for 50% of the insertions near c-*myc*. The remainder of the proviruses have an ecotropic genome organization. The *pim*-1 gene has been assigned to chromosome 17 (Hilkens et al., 1986) between the α-crystallin marker and tw12 at approximately 5 cM from H-2 (toward the centromere) (D. Bennett, unpublished results). The human *pim*-1 homolog has been assigned to the pter-q12 region of human chromosome 6 (Cuypers et al., 1986a; Nagarajan et al., 1986). The complete mouse *pim*-1 gene (7 kbp) and complementary DNA (cDNA) (2.6 kb) have been sequenced (Selten et al., 1986). Also, the sequence of the human *pim*-1 homologue has been determined (Domen et al., 1987; Meeker et al., 1987). From the 2.8-kb mRNA, a 313 acid–long protein is translated, which is conserved for more than 95% between mouse and man and which exhibits significant homology to both tyrosine and serine/threonine protein kinases. Antibodies have been raised against synthetic peptides, specifically recognizing the N-terminal and C-terminal region of the protein. These antisera precipitate a protein of the expected size from reticulocyte lysates primed with pSP6-synthesized *pim*-1 mRNA, but the *pim*-1 protein has as yet not been identified in vivo.

The *pim*-1 gene is expressed as a single 2.8-kb mRNA in mouse hemapoietic tissues and is easily detectable in bone marrow, spleen, thymus, and embryonic liver (Berns et al., 1987). Expression is also observed in placenta and adult testis. The mRNA levels in hematopoietic tissues are relatively high during fetal development and early life. Furthermore, the gene is highly inducible in lymphocytes by mitogens (Mally et al., 1985) with kinetics somewhat in between c-*fos* and c-*myc* (M. van Lohuizen et al., in preparation).

Gene transfer experiments both in vitro (cell culture) as well as in vivo (transgenic mice) have not yet provided clues to the function of *pim*-1 in the transformation process. In this respect it is interesting to mention the absence of selection of tumor cell clones with an insertion near *pim*-1 during tumor progression. When primary oligoclonal tumors carrying insertions in the *pim*-1 region were transplanted into syngeneic hosts, no preferential outgrowth of *pim*-1 positive subclones was seen; the fraction of transplanted tumors carrying an insertion near *pim*-1 remained essentially unchanged. This in contrast to subclones carrying a proviral insertion near c-*myc* or *pim*-2 (M. Breuer et al., in preparation). This might suggest that insertions in the *pim*-1 region is only advantageous during early stages of tumor outgrowth and might exert its effect even on neighboring, *pim*-1–negative, cells within the tumor.

The *pim*-2 Locus

The *pim*-2 locus has been identified as a proviral insertion site which is most frequently occupied in transplanted T-cell lymphomas (M. Breuer et al., in preparation). The transplanted tumors often carried additional proviral insertions which were almost undetectable in the primary lymphoma (Cuypers et al., 1986b). Molecular cloning of one of those additional integrated proviruses yielded probes for *pim*-2: Series of proviruses were found within approximately 10 kbp in this region, all with the same transcriptional orientation. The insertion sites were flanked by highly conserved sequences. The mouse *pim*-2 locus to chromosome 17 (at a large distance from *pim*-1, but in the neighborhood of *int*-3 [N. Jenkins, unpublished results]). No transcription unit has been defined in the *pim*-2 locus thus far.

A strong selection for cells with *pim*-2 rearranged was seen after transplantation of primary lymphomas. These transplantations are considered to lead to tumor progression, as a selection occurs for tumor cells with an increased invasive and metastatic capacity (Poste and Fidler, 1980). Whereas in the primary lymphomas insertions in the *pim*-2 locus were found only in less than 10% of the tumors, upon transplantation more than 65% of the tumors showed proviruses in the *pim*-2 locus, suggesting that cells with a *pim*-2 insertion are selected for during transplantation. As independent transplantations from the same primary tumor gave rise to secondary tumors with identical rearrangements at *pim*-2, these insertions preexisted in the primary tumor and cells with these insertions gained a predominant selective advantage upon transplantation. Thus, insertions at the *pim*-2 locus occur later than most other common proviral insertions (e.g., at *myc* and *pim*-1). Insertion at *pim*-2 is frequently seen in combination with an insertion near c-*myc*, and in a small number of the tumors, even three different common insertion sites are occupied by proviruses within the same cell clone; c-*myc*, *pim*-1, and *pim*-2. This example illuminates the potency of oncogene activation by proviruses, as it not only identifies a number of genes which can cooperate in the tumorigenic process, but also shows the order in which these genes act during tumor progression.

The *pvt*-1/*mis*-1 Locus

The *pvt*-1/*mis*-1 locus has been identified both as a recombination site in 6;15 variant translocations in murine plasmacytomas (Cory et al., 1985) and as a common proviral insertion site in MuLV-induced T-cell lymphomas (Graham et al., 1985; Lemay et al., 1984; Villeneuve et al., 1986). *pvt*-1 has been localized on mouse chromosome 15, downstream from the c-*myc* locus. The proviruses in MuLV-induced mouse lymphomas are distributed over a region of 5 kbp, all in the same transcriptional orientation (Graham et al., 1985). In the rat, the proviral insertions cluster in the same transcriptional orientation at approximately 10 kbp from the homologous region occupied by proviruses in the mouse (Graham and Adams, 1986). The structure of the 15^+ chromosome, found in the variant murine translocations, can be represented as centromere/*myc*/*pvt*-1/E-kappaC-kappa. The *pvt*-1 locus is more than 94 kbp downstream of the c-*myc* locus (Banerjee et al., 1985; Cory et al., 1985). In human Burkitt's lymphomas a region corresponding with the murine *pvt*-1 locus (based upon sequence homology) is found as breakpoint in the 2;8 variant translocation (Graham and Adams, 1986). Since *pvt*-1 is coamplified with c-*myc* in the ANN-1 cell line, the distance of *pvt*-1 from c-*myc* in the ANN-1 cell line is probably between 100 and 500 kbp. No specific transcript has been found in the *pvt*-1 locus in spite of extensive search. In addition, sequences in this locus are poorly conserved between mouse and man. Most data are compatible with a *cis*-acting effect on the c-*myc* gene, which is indeed overexpressed in tumors with a proviral insertion in (or translocation to) this region (see also below).

The Mlvi-1, Mlvi-2, Mlvi-3, and Mlvi-4 Loci

The Mlvi loci have been identified by Tsichlis and coworkers in Moloney MuLV–induced T-cell lymphomas in rat as preferential proviral insertion sites. Insertions in Mlvi-1 and Mlvi-2 are found in a significant fraction of the lymphomas. In both loci, proviruses cluster in region of less than 10 kbp of DNA (Tsichlis et al., 1983, 1984). Interestingly, Mlvi-1 and Mlvi-4 are found in close proximity of the c-*myc* gene, as shown by the low frequency of recombination between these loci in crosses between different mouse strains, and the coamplification of Mlvi-1 and c-*myc* in a cell line (P. Tsichlis, personal communication). Insertions in these loci might act in *cis* on the c-*myc* gene, as suggested for alterations at the *pvt*-1 locus Indeed, insertions in the Mlvi-1 and Mlvi-4 loci are associated with enhanced *myc* mRNA levels. No transcripts have been identified within the Mlvi-1 and Mlvi-2 loci. Interestingly, concerted DNA rearrangements in Mlvi-1 and Mlvi-2 are found frequently, suggesting that these two loci may act in a synergistic fashion during the tumorigenic process (Tsichlis et al., 1985b).

The *gin*-1 Locus

The *gin*-1 region has been found as a common proviral insertion region in Gross passage A MuLV-induced mouse thymomas by Villemur et al. (1987). Alterations in this locus were found in 11 out of 40 thymomas induced in the SIM.S inbred mouse strain. In thymomas induced by other MuLV in other mouse strains the frequency of insertion in this locus is much lower. Proviral integration at *gin*-1 was found in one out of three thymomas induced by Gross passage A virus in the outbred NIH/Swiss, whereas no insertions in this locus were found in 17 spontaneous AKR lymphomas and 11 SL3-induced thymomas in NFS mice. All proviruses found in the *gin*-1 locus are integrated as a cluster in the same transcriptional orientation within a 5-kbp region, and most of the proviruses have a MCF-like structure. No transcripts were detected from this locus using various *gin*-1 probes.

The *fim*-1/*fim*-2/*fim*-3 Locus

The *fim*-1 and *fim*-2 loci have been described by Sola et al. (1986) as common insertion sites in Friend MuLV-induced myeloblastic leukemias. Recently, the same group has identified a third common insertion site, *fim*-3 (B. Sola, personal communication). Myeloid leukemia is the predominant disease after inoculation of mice with Friend MuLV followed by erythroid and lymphoid leukemia. The proviruses appear to cluster within a region of approximately 5 kbp (*fim*-1 and *fim*-2) and 16 kbp (*fim*-3), all in the same transcriptional orientation. They have an ecotropic genome organization. *fim*-1 and *fim*-3 have not been further identified, but the *fim*-2 locus appears to correspond to the CSF-1 receptor gene (B. Sola, personal communication), which is identical to the *fms* oncogene (Sherr et al., 1985). Insertions upstream of the CSF-1 receptor gene have been found in 20% of the tumors. The insertions map in the 5′ region of the CSF-1 receptor gene, and are associated with overexpression of a normal-sized mRNA. Interestingly, a fraction of the tumor cell lines are lacking the CSF-1 receptor gene germ-line allele.

The *Dsi*-1 Locus

The *Dsi*-1 locus is defined by Vijaya et al. (1987) as a region of chromosomal DNA that has undergone proviral insertion in three of 24 Moloney MuLV-induced rat thymomas. The proviruses were located in the same transcriptional orientation within a 2-kbp long region. The region downstream from the insertion site is highly conserved in various species (including chicken), whereas a region upstream of the integration sites is less conserved but still detectable in mouse and human DNA. This conserved region is not expressed in MuLV-induced rat thymoma cell line RCC2-1M.

The *fis*-1 Locus

The *fis*-1 locus has been identified by Silver and Kozak (1986) as a common insertion site for Friend MuLV in mouse myeloid and lymphoid tumors. Four insertions were found in 34 tumors induced by this virus in C57BL/6 mice. The insertions cluster in a region of 1.5 kbp in the same transcriptional orientation. Insertions in the *fis*-1 domain were also found in four out of 116 spontaneously arisen T-cell lymphomas in AKXD recombinant inbred mice, which express the endogenous AKV virus (N. Copeland, personal communication). No transcripts have been found hybridizing to the *fis*-1–specific probes. The *fis*-1 locus is closely linked to the *int*-2 gene, since no segregation is observed in over 50 recombinant inbred strains (Silver and Buckler, 1986). Molecular cloning of the region flanking the *fis*-1 proviral insertion sites indicate that the two regions are at least 30 kbp apart. Although this situations is reminiscent of the common insertions sites near the c-*myc* gene, a major difference is observed: Insertions in the *fis*-1 region do not affect transcription of the *int*-2 gene.

The *evi*-1 and *evi*-2 Loci

The *evi*-1 locus has been identified as a predominant proviral insertion site in myeloid tumors found in some AKXD recombinant inbred strains by the group of Copeland and Jenkins (personal communication) (see also Mucenski et al., 1986). Nine out of nine myeloid tumors carry a provirus in this locus, whereas no insertions are found near c-*myc*, *pim*-1, *pvt*-1/*mis*-1, and *fis*-1. The high association of myeloid tumors in the AKXD RI strains with insertions at *evi*-1 is rather unique for MuLV-induced hematopoietic neoplasias. Integrations in *evi*-1 were found in various myeloid cell lines.

evi-2 has been found by the same group in 11 out of 99 MuLV-induced tumors in the BXH-2 recombinant inbred strain. More than 90% of the tumors in this strain were classified as granulocytic leukemias. In these tumors no insertions were found in any of the other loci mentioned above.

COMPLEMENTATION BETWEEN DIFFERENT GENES

Peters et al. (1986) have reported that in the BR6 strain many mammary tumors actually have MMTV insertions at both *int*-1 and *int*-2, in a clonal fashion. Thus, the genes can act within the same cell, and can perhaps cooperate in transformation. It is, however, not yet clear whether MMTV-induced tumors in other strains have the same frequency of concerted activation of different genes.

A different form of complementation between the *int* genes is suggested by the behavior of early, hormone-dependent mammary tumors in the GH strains. Many of these tumors appear to be oligoclonal for insertions near the different *int* genes, and consist of balanced populations of cells with one or the other gene rearranged (Gray et al., 1986; Mester et al., 1987). The retention of oligoclonality is highly suggestive for interdependent complementation between cells expressing various *int* genes.

Insertions in more than one common integration site has also been reported for MuLV-induced hematopoietic neoplasiás; Mlvi-1, Mlvi-2, and Mlvi-3 (Tsichlis 1985b), c-*myc* and *pim*-1 (Cuypers et al., 1986b), *pvt*-1 and *pim*-1 (Sola et al., 1986), and c-*myc*, *pim*-1, and *pim*-2 (Breuer et al., in preparation). The occurrence of these activated loci within the same tumor cell clones strongly suggests that the different combinations can act in a synergistic fashion. Reconstitution experiments in vitro and in vivo (transgenic mice) seem most appropriate to further define these cooperative interactions.

THE MECHANISM OF ACTIVATION OF CELLULAR ONCOGENES BY INSERTION OF RETROVIRUSES

The mechanism of transcriptional activation by proviral insertion is rather diverse. In Chapter 2, it is discussed how ALV can activate c-*myc* usually through promoter insertion but sometimes, more indirectly, by enhancement over variable distances. In other cases of insertions near known oncogenes, other types of activation are found, including insertions leading to deletions or fusions of the oncogene proteins (reviewed in Nusse, 1986).

In the group of genes described here, promoter insertions are rare, invoking enhancers on the provirus as responsible for transcriptional activation. In the cases where the structure of the activated oncogene is known in sufficient detail (*int*-1, *int*-2, and *pim*-1) the provirus is usually at a distance from the promoter. The restricted orientation of the provirus near the *int* and *pim* genes—usually pointing away from the gene—could be a consequence of the inability of enhancers to act beyond the first promoter encountered, as documented for the SV40 enhancer (Wasylyk et al., 1983). The orientation generally seen avoids a viral promoter in between the viral enhancer and the *int/pim* promoter.

The high incidence of MLV insertions in the 3′ untranslated region of the *pim*-1 gene, leading to hybrid transcripts, suggests that another selective mechanism operates, involving stabilization of the *pim*-1 mRNA. It has indeed been found that the untranslated tail of *pim*-1 contains various copies of the AU-rich sequence that has been shown to destabilize mRNAs for several gene products (Shaw and Kamen 1986). By insertion of MLV upstream of the (AUUUA)n motif these sequences are removed from the *pim*-1 mRNA molecule, as transcription prematurely terminates in the 5′ LTR of the inserted provirus.

CONCLUSIONS

We have described that provirus tagging has yielded a large and rapidly growing family of common integration domains in various animal tumor systems. In some members of this group, genes have been found that are of considerable interest because of their involvement in embryogenesis or their predicted enzymatic function. Further characterization of these genes is now in progress. These findings should encourage a search for additional oncogenes by the same method.

Nonetheless, the majority of the common insertion domains, in particular for MLVs, have not been shown to contain a gene or even a transcriptional unit. It is possible that these regions reflect preference of retroviruses for integration in selected cellular targets, and not so much selection for activation of oncogenes in the course of tumorigenesis. We then have to assume that there is a limited number of possible integrations sites for a provirus in a cell, and that the clonal outgrowth of the cell with a provirus in these sites is actually due to mutations unrelated to the proviral insertion. In our view, however, preferential integration as such plays a minor role in tumorigenesis by retroviruses. We consider it is more likely that the occurrence of common insertion domains indicates some form of selection for the integration site during tumor formation, and thus points to the presence of an important gene near the insertion. It is possible that expression of this gene has only contributed to initial phases of tumor growth, and is absent when the tumor is detectable. It has indeed been observed that expression of *int*-2 is not required for progression of a mouse mammary tumor line (Sonnenberg et al., 1987).

Another explanation for the absence of transcripts from the direct vicinity of the insertion sites is perhaps given by some variant chromosome translocations that appear to affect expression of c-*myc*, but at a considerable distance. Interestingly, one of those translocation breakpoint sites, *pvt*-1, is also a common insertion site (*mis*-1) for MLV, although it has not been proven that these proviral insertions affect c-*myc* transcription. Even more striking is the observation that Mlvi-1 and Mlvi-4 also cluster in the same region. The association between insertion in either Mlvi-1, Mlvi-4, or *pvt*-1 and a high level of c-*myc* expression seems more than coincidental. One can image that proviruses, like translocations of chromosomes, can have long-range effects on transcription and that the common insertion sites, which lack a nearby gene, are actually at a relatively large distance from oncogenes. This poses the question as to how a provirus can disregulate the transcription of genes at such large distances. The chromosomal structure of the region could play a role in the mechanism of activation; it has been proposed that the nuclear matrix is an important factor in the regulations of transcription (Gasser and Laemmli, 1987), and that active genes are part of rather large domains on chromosomes, separated by matrix attachment sites. Proviruses could interfere with the matrix attachment sites, either by disruption or by introduction of new sites, thereby influencing the transcriptional activity over a large distance. Clustering of insertions in regions as large as 1000 kbp might also explain the low incidence of insertions in a particular common site, as one now may consider certain insertions (e.g., at c-*myc*, *pvt*-1, Mlvi-1, and Mlvi-4) as functionally one and the same. Recent technological advances, like pulse-field gradient electrophoresis, Restriction Fragment Length Polymorphism (RFLP) analysis, and the cloning of very large DNA fragments in yeast, can perhaps be successful in resolving these issues.

ACKNOWLEDGMENT

We would like to thank Drs. M. Breuer, A. Brown, N. Copeland, C. Dickson, N. Jenkins, R. Michalides, J. Papkoff, G. Peters, H. Roelink, B. Sola, P. Tsichlis, M. van Lohuizen, and H. Varmus for the communication of unpublished results and our colleagues for critically reading the manuscript.

REFERENCES

Alitalo, K., Koskinen, P., Makela, T. P., Saksela, K., Sistonen, L., and Winqvist R. (1987). *Myc* oncogenes: Activation and amplification. *Biochim. Biophys. Acta 907*: 1–32.

Baker, N. E. (1987. Molecular cloning of sequences from *wingless*, a segment polarity gene in *Drosophila*: The spatial distribution of a transcript in embryos. *EMBO J. 6* 1765–1773.

Banerjee, M., Wiener, F., Spira, J., Babonits, M., Nilsson, M. G., Sumegi, J., and Klein, G. (1985). Mapping of the c-*myc* and *pvt*-1 and immunoglobulin kappa genes in relation to the mouse plasmacytoma-associated variant (6;15) translocation breakpoint. *EMBO J. 4*: 3183–3188.

Berns, A., Robanus-Maandag, E., van der Putten, H., and Quint, W. (1983). The role of the long terminal repeat of retroviruses in integration and expression. In The Fifth John Innes Symposium (Chater, K., Cullis, C., Hopwood, D., and Johnston, A. W. B., eds.). London, pp. 93–106.

Berns, A., Cuypers, H. T., Selten, G., and Domen, J. (1987). *pim*-1 activation in T-cell lymphomas. In *Proceedings Benzon Symposium on Viral Carcinogenesis* [Kjeldgaard, N. O., and Forchhammer, J. eds.]. Munskgaard, Copenhagen, pp. 211–224.

Brookes, S., Placzek, M., Moore, R., Dickson, C., and Peters, G. (1986). Insertion elements and transitions in cloned mouse mammary tumour virus DNA: Further delineation of the poison sequences. *Nucl. Acids Res. 14*: 8231–8245.

Brown, A. M. C., Wildin, R. S., Prendergast, T. J., and Varmus, H. E. (1986). A retrovirus vector expressing the putative mammary oncogene *int*-1 causes partial transformation of a mammary epithelial cell line. *Cell 46*: 1001–1009.

Cabrera, C. V., Alonso, M. C., Johnston, P., Phillips, R. G., and Lawrence, P. A. (1987). Phenocopies induced with antisense RNA identify the wingless gene. *Cell 50*: 659–663.

Casey, G., Smith R., McGillivray, D., Peters, G., and Dickson, C. (1986). Characterization and chromosome assignment of the human homolog of *int*-2, a potential proto-oncogene. *Mol. Cell. Biol. 6*: 502–510.

Chatis, P. A., Holland, C. A., Hartley, J. W., Rowe, W. P., and Hopkins, N. (1983). Role for the 3′ end of the genome in determining disease specificity of Friend and Moloney murine leukemia viruses. *Proc. Natl. Acad. Sci. U.S.A. 80*: 4408–4411.

Cohen, J. C., Shank, P. R., Morris, V. L., Cardiff, R., and Varmus, H. E. (1979). Integration of the DNA of mouse mammary tumor virus in viru-infected normal and neoplastic tissues of the mouse. *Cell 16*: 333–345.

Cory, S., Graham, M., Webb, L., Corcoran, L., and Adams, J. (1985). Variant (6;15) translocation in murine plasmacytomas involve a chromosome 15 locus at least 72 kb from the c-*myc* oncogene. *EMBO J. 4*: 675–681.

Cuypers, H. T., Selten, G., Quint, W., Zijlstra, M., Robanus-Maandag, E., Boelens, W., van Wezenbeek, P., Melief, C., and Berns, A. (1984). Murine leukemia virus-induced T-cell lymphomagenesis: Integration of proviruses in a distinct chromosomal region. *Cell 37*: 141–150.

Cuypers, H. T., Selten, G., Berns, A., and Geurts van Kessel, A. (1986a). Assignment of the human homolog of *pim*-1, a mouse gene implicated in leukemogenesis, to the pter-12 region of chromosome 6. *Human Genet. 72*: 262–265.

Cuypers, H. T., Selten, G., Zijlstra, M., de Goede, R., Melief, C., and Berns, A. (1986b). Tumor progression in MuLV induced T-cell lymphomas: Monitoring of clonal selections with viral and cellular probes. *J. Virol. 60*: 230–241.

Davis, B. R., Chandy, K. G., Brightman, B. K., Gupta, S., and Fan, H. (1986). Effects of nonleukemogenic and wild-type Moloney murine leukemia virus on lymphoid cells "in vivo": Identification of a preleukemia shift in thymocyte subpopulations. *J. Virol. 60*: 423–430.

Dickson, C., and Peters, G. (1987). Potential oncogene product related to growth factors. *Nature 326*: 833.

Dickson, C., Smith, R., Brookes, S., and Peters, G. (1984). Tumorigenesis by mouse mammary tumor virus: Proviral activation of a cellular gene in the common integration region *int*-2. *Cell 37*: 529–536.

Domen, J., von Lindern, J., Hermans, A., Breuer, M., Grosveld, G., and Berns, A. (1987). Comparison of the human and mouse *pim*-1 cDNAs: Nucleotide sequence and immunological identification of the 'in vitro' synthesized *pim*-1 protein. *Oncogene Res. 1*: 103–112.

Evans, L. H., and Morrey, J. D. (1987). Tissue-specific replication of Friend and Moloney murine leukemia viruses in infected mice. *J. Virol. 61*: 1350–1357.

Fung, Y. K. T., Shackleford G. M., Brown, A. M. C., Sanders, G. S., and Varmus, H. E. (1985). Nucleotide sequence and expression "in vitro" of cDNA derived from mRNA of *int*-1, a provirally activated mouse mammary oncogene. *Mol. Cell. Biol. 5*: 3337–3344.

Gallahan, D., and Callahan, R. (1987). Mammary tumorigenesis in feral mice: Identification of a new *int* locus in mouse mammary tumor virus (Czech II)-induced mammary tumors. *J. Virol. 61*: 66–74.

Gallahan, D., Kozak, C., and Callahan, R. (1987). A new common integration region (*int*-3) for mouse mammary tumor virus on mouse chromosome 17. *J. Virol. 61*: 218–220.

Garcia, M., Wellinger, R., Vessaz, A., and Diggelmann, H. (1986). A new site of integration for mouse mammary tumor virus proviral DNA common to BALB/cf(C3H) mammary and kidney adenocarcinomas. *EMBO J. 5*: 127–134.

Gasser, S. M., and Laemmli, U. K. (1987). A glimpse at chromosomal order. *Trends Genet. 3*: 16–22.

Goff, S. P. (1986). Retroviral integration and insertional mutagenesis. In *Gene Tranfer*. (Kucherlapati, R. ed.). Plenum Press, New York. pp. 325–361.

Graham, M., and Adams, J. M. (1986). Chromosome 8 breakpoint for 3′ of the c-*myc* oncogene in a Burkitt's lymphoma 2;8 variant translocation is equivalent to the murine *pvt*-1 locus *EMBO J. 5*: 2845–2851.

Graham, M., Adams, J. M., and Cory, S. (1985). Murine T lymphomas with retroviral inserts in the chromosomal 15 locus for plasmacytoma variant translocations. *Nature 314*: 740–743.

Gray, D. A., Jackson, D. P., Percy, D. H., and Morris, V. L. (1986). Activation of *int*-1 and *int*-2 loci in GRf mammary tumors. *Virology 154*: 271–278.

Groner, B., and Hynes, N. (1980). Number and location of mouse mammary tumor virus proviral DNA in mouse DNA of normal tissue and of mammary tumors. *J. Virol. 33*: 1013–1025.

Hartley, J. W., Wolford, N. K., Old, L. J., and Rowe, W. P. (1977). A new class of murine leukemia virus associated with development of spontaneous lymphomas. *Proc. Natl. Acad. Sci. U.S.A. 74*: 789–792.

Hayward, W. S., Neel, B. G., and Astrin, S. M. (1981). Activation of a cellular onc gene by promoter insertion in ALV-induced lymphoid leukosis. *Nature 290*: 475–480.

Hilgers, J., and Bentvelzen, P. (1979). Interaction between viral and genetic factors in murine mammary cancer. *Adv. Cancer Res. 26*: 143–195.

Hilkens, J., Cuypers, H. T., Selten, G., Kroezen, V., Hilgers, J., and Berns, A. (1986). Genetic mapping of *pim*-1 putative oncogene to mouse chromosome 17. *Somat. Cell. Mol. Genet. 12*: 81–88.

Holland, C. A., Wozney, J., Chatis, P. A., Hopkins, N., and Hartley, J. W. (1985). Construction of recombinants between molecular clones of murine retrovirus MCF 247 and Akv: Determinant of an "in vitro" host range property that maps in the long terminal repeat. *J. Virol. 53*: 152–157.

Jakobovits, A., Shackleford, G. M., Varmus, H. E., and Martin, G. R. (1986). Two proto-oncogenes implicated in mammary carcinogenesis, *int*-1 and *int*-2, are independently regulated during development. *Proc. Natl. Acad. Sci. U.S.A. 83*: 7806–7810.

King, W., Patel, M. D., Lobel, L. I., Goff, S. P., and Nguyen-Huu, M. C. (1985). Insertion mutagenesis of embryonal carcinoma cells by retroviruses. *Science 228*: 554–558.

Lemay, G., and Jolicoeur, P. (1984). Rearrangement of a DNA sequence homologous to a cell-virus junction fragment in several Moloney murine leukemia virus-induced rat thymomas. *Proc. Natl. Acad. Sci. U.S.A. 81*: 38–42.

Lenz, J., Celander, D., Crowther, R. L., Patarca, R., Perkins, D. W., and Haseltine, W. A. (1984). Determination of the leukaemogenicity of a murine retrovirus by sequences within the long terminal repeat. *Nature 308*: 467–470.

Mally, M. I., Vogt, M., Swift, S. E., and Haas, M. (1985). Oncogene expression in murine splenic T cells and in murine T-cells neoplasma. *Virology 144*: 115–126.

Meeker, T. C., Nagarajan, L., Ar-Rushdi, A., Rovera, G., Huebner, K., and Croce, C. M. (1987). Characterization of the human *pim*-1 gene: A putative proto-oncogene coding for a tissue specific member of the protein kinase family. *Oncogene Res. 1*: 87–101.

Mester, J., Wagenaar, E., Sluyser, M., and Nusse, R. (1987). Activation of the *int*-1 and *int*-2 mammary oncogenes in hormone-dependent and -independent mammary tumors of GR mice. *J. Virol. 61*: 1073–1078.

Moore, R., Casey, G., Brookes, S., Dixon, M., Peters, G., and Dickson, C. (1986). Sequence, topography and protein coding potential of mouse *int*-2: A putative oncogene activated by mouse mammary tumor virus. *EMBO J. 5*: 919–924.

Mucenski, M. L., Taylor, B. A., Jenkins, N. A., and Copeland, N. G. (1986). AKXD recombinant inbred strains: Models for studying the molecular genetic basis of murine lymphomas. *Mol. Cell. Biol. 6*: 4236–4243.

Nagarajan, L., Tsujimoto, Y., ar-Rushdi, A., Huebnes, K., and Croce, C. M. (1986). Localization of the human *pim* oncogene (PIM) to a region of chromosome 6 involved in translocations in acute leukemias. *Proc. Natl. Acad. Sci. U.S.A. 83*: 2556–2560.

Nusse, R. (1986). The activation of cellular oncogenes by retroviral insertion. *Trends Genet. 2*: 244–247.

Nusse, R., and Varmus, H. E. (1982). Many tumors induced by the mouse mammary tumor virus contain a provirus integrated in the same region of the host genome. *Cell 31*: 99–109.

Nusse, R., van Ooyen, A., Cox, D., Fung, Y., and Varmus, H. (1984). Mode of proviral activation of a putative mammary oncogene (*int*-1) on mouse chromosome 15. *Nature 307*: 131–136.

Payne, G. S., Bishop, J. M., and Varmus, H. E. (1982). Multiple arrangements of viral DNA and an activated host oncogene in bursal lymphomas. *Nature 295*: 209–213.

Peters, G., Brookes, S., Smith, R., and Dickson, C. (1983). Tumorigenesis by mouse mammary tumor virus: Evidence for a common region for provirus integration in mammary tumors. *Cell 33*: 369–377.

Peters, G., Kozak, C., and Dickson, C. (1984a). Mouse mammary tumor virus integration regions *int*-1 and *int*-2 map on different mouse chromosomes. *Mol. Cell. Biol. 4*: 375–378.

Peters, G., Lee, A. E., and Dickson, C. (1984b). Activation of cellular gene by mouse mammary tumor virus may occur early in tumor development. *Nature 309*: 273–275.

Peters, G., Lee, A. E., and Dickson, C. (1986). Concerted activation of two potential proto-oncogenes in carcinomas induced by mouse mammary tumor virus. *Nature 320*: 628–631.

Poste, G., and Fidler, I. J. (1980). The pathogenesis of cancer metastasis. *Nature 283*: 139–146.

Quint, W., Boelens, W., Van Wezenbeek, P., Cuypers, H. T., Robanus-Maandag, E., Selten, G., and Berns, A. (1984). Generation of AKR focus-forming viruses: A conserved single copy xenotropic-like provirus provides recombinant long terminal repeat sequences. *J. Virol. 50*: 432–438.

Rijsewijk, F. A. M., Van Lohuizen, M., van Ooyen, A., and Nusse, R. (1986). Construction of a retroviral cDNA version of the *int*-1 mammary oncogene and its expression "in vitro". *Nucl. Acids Res. 14*: 693–702.

Rijsewijk, F., Schuermann, M., Wagenaar, E., Parren, P., Weigel, D., and Nusse R. (1987a). The *Drosophila* homologue of the mammary oncogene *int*-1 is identical to the segment polarity gene *wingless*. *Cell 50*: 649–657.

Rijsewijk, F., van Deemter, L., Wagenaar, E., Sonnenberg, A., and Nusse, R. (1987b). Transfection of the *int*-1 mammary oncogene in cuboidal RAC mammary cell line results in morphological transformation and tumorigenicity. *EMBO J. 6*: 127–131.

Rohdewohld, H., Weiher, H., Freik, W., Jaenisch, R., and Breindl, M. (1987). Retrovirus integration and chromatin structure: Moloney murine leukemia proviral integration sites map near DNase I-hyersensitive sites. *J. Virol. 61*: 336–343.

Schuermann, M., and Michalides, R. (1987). A rare common integration site of proviruses of the mouse mammary tumor virus in P-type mammary tumors of mouse strain GR. *Virology 156*: 229–238.

Selten, G., Cuypers, H. T., Zijlstra, M., Melief, C., and Berns, A. (1984). Involvement of c-*myc* in MuLV-induced T cell lymphomas in mice: Frequency and mechanisms of activation. *EMBO J. 3*: 3215–3222.

Selten, G., Cuypers, H. T., and Berns, A. (1985). Proviral activation of the putative oncogene *pim*-1 in MuLV-induced T-cell lymphomas. *EMBO J. 4*: 1793–1798.

Selten, G., Cuypers, H. T., Boelens, W., Robanus-Maandag, E., Verbeek, J., Domen, J., van Beveren, C., and Berns, A. (1986). The primary structure of the putative oncogene *pim*-1 shows extensive homology with protein kinase. *Cell 46*: 603–611.

Shackleford, G. M., and Varmus, H. E. (1987). Expression of the proto-oncogene *int*-1 is restricted to postmeiotic male germ cells and the neural tube of midgestation embryos. *Cell 50*: 89–95.

Shaw, G., and Kamen, R. (1986). A conserved AU sequence from the 3′ untranslated region of GM-CSF mRNA mediates selective mRNA degradation. *Cell 46*: 659–667.

Sherr, C. J., Rettenmier, C. W., Sacca, R., Roussel, M. F., Look, A. T., and Stanley, E. R. (1985). The c-*fms* proto-oncogene product is related to the receptor of the mononuclear phagocyte growth factor, CSF-1. *Cell 41*: 665–676.

Short, M. K., Okenquist, S. A., and Lenz, J. (1987). Correlation of leukemogenic potential of murine retroviruses with transcriptional tissue preference of the viral long terminal repeats. *J. Virol. 61*:1067–1072.

Silver, J. (1984). Role of mink cell focus-forming virus in leukemias induced by Friend ecotropic virus. *J. Virol. 50*: 872–877.

Silver, J., and Buckler, C. E. (1986). A preferred region for integration of Friend murine leukemia virus in hematopoietic neoplasmsis closely linked to the *int*-2 oncogene. *J. Virol. 60*: 1156–1158.

Silver, J., and Kozak, C. (1986). Common proviral integration region on mouse chromosome 7 in lymphomas and myelogenous leukemias induced by Friend murine leukemia virus. *J. Virol. 57*: 526–533.

Sola, B., Fichelson, S., Bordereaux, D., Tambourin, P. E., and Gisselbrecht, S. (1986). *fim*-1 and *fim*-2: Two new integration regions of Friend Murine Leukemia Virus in myeloblastic leukemias. *J. Virol. 60*: 718–725.

Sonnenberg, A., Daams, H., Calafat, J., and Hilgers, J. (1986). "In vitro" differentiation and progression of mouse mammary tumor cells. *Cancer Res. 46*: 5913–5922.

Sonnenberg, A., van Balen, P., Hilgers, J., Schuuring, E., and Nusse, R. (1987). Oncogene expression during progression of mouse mammary tumor cells; activity of a proviral enhancer and the resulting expression of *int*-2 is influenced by the state of differentiation. *EMBO J. 6*: 121–125.

Tsichlis, P. N., Strauss, P. G., and Hu, L. F. (1983). A common region for proviral DNA integration in MoMuLV-induced rat thymic lymphomas. *Nature 302*: 445–449.

Tsichlis, P. N., Strauss, P. G., and Kozak, C. A. (1984). Cellular DNA region involved in induction of thymic lymphomas (Mlvi-2) maps to mouse chromosome 15. *Mol. Cell. Biol. 4*: 997–1000.

Tsichlis, P. M., Lohse, M. A., Szpirer, C., Szpirer, J., and Levan, G. (1985a). Cellular DNA regions involved in the induction of rat thymic lymphomas (Mlvi-1, Mlvi-2, Mlvi-3 and c-*myc*) represent independent loci as determined by their chromosomal map location in the rat. *J. Virol. 50*: 938–942.

Tsichlis, P. M., Strauss, P. G., and Lohse, M. A. (1985b). Concerted DNA rearrangement in Moloney Murine Leukemia Virus-induced thymomas: A potential synergistic relationship in oncogenesis. *J. Virol. 56*: 258–267.

Van Ooyen, A., and Nusse, R. (1984). Structure and nucleotide sequence of the putative mammary oncogene *int*-1; proviral insertions leave the protein-encoding domain intact. *Cell 39*: 233–240.

Van Ooyen, A., Kwee, V., and Nusse, R. (1985). The nucleotide sequence of the human *int*-1 mammary oncogene; evolutionary conservation of coding and noncoding sequences. *EMBO J. 4*: 2905–2909.

Van't Veer, L. J., Geurts van Kessel, A., van Heerikhuizen, H., van Ooyen, A., and Nusse, R. (1984). Molecular cloning and chromosomal assignment of the human homolog of *int*-1, a mouse gene implicated in mammary tumorigenesis. *Mol. Cell. Biol. 4*: 2532–2534.

Varmus, H. E. (1984). The molecular genetics of cellular oncogenes. *Ann. Rev. Genet. 18*: 553–612.

Vijaya, S., Steffen, D. L., and Robinson, H. L. (1986). Acceptor sites for retroviral integrations map near DNase I-hypersensitive sites in chromatin. *J. Virol. 60*: 683–692.

Vijaya, S., Steffen, D. L., Kozak, C., and Robinson, H. L. (1987). *Dsi*-1, a region with frequent proviral insertions in Moloney murine leukemia virus-induced rat thymomas. *J. Virol. 61*: 1164–1170.

Villemur, R., Monczak, Y., Rassart, E., Kozak, C., and Jolicoeur, P. (1987). Identification of a new common provirus integration site in Gross passage A murine leukemia virus-induced mouse thymoma DNA. *Mol. Cell. Biol. 7*: 512–522.

Villeneuve, L., Rassart, E., Jolicoeur, P., Graham, M., and Adams, J. M. (1986). Proviral integration site *Mis*-1 in rat thymomas corresponds to the *pvt*-1 translocation breakpoint in murine plasma cytomas. *Mol. Cell. Biol. 6*: 1834–1837.

Vogt, M. (1979). Properties of "mink cell focus-inducing" (MCF) virus isolated from spontaneous lymphoma lines of BALB/c mice carrying Moloney murine leukemia virus as an endogenous virus. *Virology 93*: 226–236.

Wasylyk, B., Wasylyk, C., Augereau, P., and Chambon, P. (1983). The SV40 72 bp repeat preferentially potentiates transcription starting from proximal natural or substitute promoter elements. *Cell 32*: 503–514.

Weiss, R., Teich, N., Varmus, H. E., and Coffin, J. (1982). RNA Tumor Viruses. The Molecular Biology of Tumor Viruses. Cold Spring Harbor Laboratory, Cold Spring Harbor. New York.

Weiss, R., Teich, N., Varmus, H., and Coffin, J. (1985). RNA Tumor Viruses. The Molecular Biology of Tumor Viruses. Cold Spring Harbor Laboratory, Cold Spring Harbor. New York.

Wilkinson, D. G., Bailes, J. A., and McMahon, A. P. (1987). Expression of the proto-oncogene *int*-1 is restricted to specific neural cells in the developing mouse embryo. *Cell 50*: 79–88.

FOUR

ras Oncogenes in Human and Carcinogen-Induced Animal Tumors

Mariano Barbacid
National Cancer Institute
Frederick Cancer Research Facility
Frederick, Maryland

INTRODUCTION

ras genes are an ubiquitous eukaryotic gene family. They exist in mammals, birds, insects, mollusks, plants, fungi, and yeast (reviewed in Ref. 1). To date, three *ras* genes, designated H-*ras*-1, K-*ras*-2, and N-*ras*, have been identified in the mammalian genome (2–8). In addition, two pseudogenes, H-*ras*-2 and K-*ras*-1, have been found in rats and humans and are likely to exist in most, if not all, mammals (2,3,9,10). Several mouse and hamster subspecies possess additional *ras* pseudogenes, probably due to a relatively recent germ-line amplification (11). The *ras* gene family may be part of a larger supergene family. Genes exhibiting limited sequence homology to *ras* genes have been recently identified in a variety of eukaryotic organisms. These *ras*-related genes include the mammalian R-*ras* (12), *ral* (13), *rab* (A. Tavitian, personal communication) and *rho* (14) genes, the D*ras*3 gene present in fruit flies (15), and the yeast YP2 (16) and *rho* (14) genes.

Evidence that these cellular genes could become activated as oncogenes was first provided by the transduction of two mammalian *ras* loci, H-*ras*-1 and K-*ras*-2, into acute transforming retroviruses, the Harvey and Kirsten strains of murine sarcoma virus (MSV) (2,3). The H-*ras*-1 oncogene has also been found as the transforming principle of two additional MSVs, the BALB strain of mouse sarcoma virus (17), and the Rasheed strain of rat sarcoma virus (18). More recently, *ras* oncogenes have been found in tumors induced by retroviruses that lack oncogene sequences. These viruses can integrate in the vicinity of cellular genes, disrupting their normal regulatory elements. Activation of *ras* genes by retroviral insertional mutagenesis has been occasionally observed in tumors of both avian and mammalian origin (19,20; J. Ihle, personal communication).

ras genes have been the focus of intense research since 1982 when their transforming alleles were identified in a significant fraction of human tumors (4–8). Subsequently, *ras* oncogenes have been found in a large percentage of animal tumors induced by chemical and physical carcinogens (reviewed in Ref. 21). Indeed, the members of the *ras* gene family are the most prevalent oncogenes found in nonvirally induced tumors of both animal and human origin. Unveiling the role that these oncogenes play in neoplastic development should have a major impact on our understanding of the pathogenesis of human cancer.

ras GENE FUNCTION

Although the basic function of *ras* genes remains to be determined, a great deal of information about the structural and biochemical properties of their gene products has been obtained in the last few years (1). Mammalian *ras* genes code for highly related proteins of 189 amino acid residues generically known as p21 (22). The p21 coding sequences of each of these genes are equally distributed in four exons except for the K-*ras*-2 locus, which possesses two alternative fourth coding exons that allow it to synthesize two isomorphic p21 proteins of 188 and 189 residues (10,23,24). Although the spliced junctions of all mammalian *ras* genes correspond precisely, suggesting a common origin from one ancestral gene, their intron sequences vary greatly. As a consequence, *ras* genes exhibit distinct genetic complexity, ranging from the 4.5 kbp size of H-*ras*-1 to the 50 kbp of K-*ras*-2. Mammalian *ras* genes contain an additional 5′ noncoding exon (10,23,25,26) located immediately downstream from their respective promoters (27,28). These promoters do not possess the characteristic TATA and CAT boxes commonly found in other eukaryotic genes. Instead, they are rich in G/C boxes which are presumably involved in the binding of Spl-like proteins, a characteristic of the promoters of housekeeping genes.

Comparison of the deduced amino acid sequences of mammalian H-*ras*-1, K-*ras*-2, and N-*ras* p21 proteins has helped to define four domains within these molecules (Fig. 1). The first domain encompasses their amino terminal third and is a highly conserved region. For instance, the first 85 amino acid residues of mammalian p21 *ras* proteins are identical. The next 80 amino acid residues define a second domain where the structures of the different mammalian p21 *ras* proteins diverged slightly from each other. A highly variable region encompasses the rest of the molecule except for the last four amino acids where the sequence Cys-A-A-X-COOH (where A is any aliphatic amino acid) is present in all members of the *ras* gene family (Fig. 1). This carboxyterminal sequence has been shown to be responsible for the membrane attachment of p21 proteins (reviewed in Ref. 29).

The *ras* gene products of other eukaryotic *ras* genes also conform to this basic structure, although some of those present in yeasts have additional aminoterminal sequences and longer carboxyterminal variable domains (Fig. 1). Most significantly, genetic studies have shown that mammalian *ras* gene products can support the growth of *ras*-defective yeasts, and *ras* proteins of yeasts can transform mammalian cells (30,31). These results illustrate the high degree of structural as well as functional conservation of *ras* gene proteins during millions of years of evolution.

ras proteins, independently of their phylogenetic origin, have been shown to bind the nucleotides guanine triphosphate (GTP) and guanine diphosphate (GDP), and possess intrinsic GTPase activity (32–39). In addition, certain *ras* proteins (those carrying Thr in position 59) exhibit an autophosphorylating activity of an as yet unknown biological significance (33). Biochemical properties of *ras* proteins closely resemble those of G proteins involved in the modulation of signal transduction through membrane signaling systems (reviewed in Ref. 40). In fact, *ras* proteins exhibit significant sequence homology with the α subunit of G proteins such as G_s, a protein that activates adenylate cyclase in response to β-adrenergic stimuli; G_i which inhibits this enzyme and perhaps activates phospholipase C; G_0, a protein of an as yet unknown function; and transducin, a protein that regulates cyclic guanosine monophosphate (cGMP) phosphodiesterase activity in visual signal transduction (40). In addition to G proteins, p21 *ras* proteins also share limited sequence homology with other nucleotide-binding proteins such as the bacterial elongation factor T_u, the β subunit of adenine triphosphate (ATP) synthetase, phosphofructokinase, and tubulin (1).

```
                                              1                  20                  40                  60                  80                 100
HUMAN/RAT     H-ras-1                         MTEYKLVVVGAGGVGKSALTIQLIQNHFVDEYDPTIEDSYRKQVVIDGETCLLDILDTAGQEEYSAMRDQYMRTGEGFLCVFAINNTKSFEDIHQYREQI
CHICKEN       H-ras-1                         ----------------------------------------------------------------------------------------------------
HUMAN         K-ras-2A                        ----------------------------------------------------------------------------------------------H-----
MOUSE         K-ras-2A                        ----------------------------------------------------------------------------------------------H-----
HUMAN         K-ras-2B                        ----------------------------------------------------------------------------------------------H-----
MOUSE         K-ras-2B                        ----------------------------------------------------------------------------------------------H-----
HUMAN         N-ras                           --------------------------------------------------------------------------------------S---A--NL-----
MOUSE         N-ras                           --------------------------------------------------------------------------------------S---A--NL-----
Drosophila    Dras1                           ----------P------------------------------RS------------------------------------L-----SA------GT-----
Drosophila    Dras2/64B                    MQ -QT-------G-------I---F--SY--TD---------T--CN--DVPAK-----------F----E----S-----L---L-DHS--DE-PKFQR--
Dyctiostelium Ddras                           -------I--G-----------------I---------------S--D-----------------------Q-----YS-TSRS-YDE-ASF----
S.cerevisiae  RAS1                    MQGNKST IR---I----G-----------F--SY--------------------DKVSI---------------E----------L-YSVTSRN--DELLS-YQ--
S.cerevisiae  RAS2                    MPLNKSN IR--------G------------T-S---------------------D-VSI---------------E----N-----L-YS-TSKS-LDELMT-YQ--
S.pombe       SPRAS                     MRSTY LR--------D--------------S----------------KCE----GA---V-------------E----------L-YN-TSRS--DE-STFYQ--
```

```
                                             120                 140                 160                 180          189
HUMAN/RAT     H-ras-1    KRVKDSDDVPMVLVGNKCDLAARTVESRQ AQDLARSYGIPYIETSAKTRQGVEDAFYTLVREIRQHKLRKLNPPDESGPGCMSCK          CVLS
CHICKEN       H-ras-1    --------------------P-----T-- -----------------------------------------------------N--          --I-
HUMAN         K-ras-2A   ------E-------------PS---DTK- -----------F---------R--------------YR-K-ISKEEKTPGCVKIK-          -IIM
MOUSE         K-ras-2A   ------E-------------PS---DTK- --E--------F---------R--------------YR-K-ISKEEKTPGCVKIK-          --IM
HUMAN         K-ras-2B   ------E-------------PS---DTK- -----------F-----------D-----------K--EKMSKDGKKKKKKSK T-          --IM
MOUSE         K-ras-2B   -•----E-------------PS---DTK- --E--------F-----------D-----------K--EKMSKDGKKKKKKSR TR          -TVM
HUMAN         N-ras      --------------------PT---DTK- -HE--K-----F------------------------YRMK---SS-DGTQ---GLP          --VM
MOUSE         N-ras      --------------------PT---DTK- -HE--K-----F------------------------YR-K---SS-DGTQ---GSP          ---M
Drosophila    Dras1      -H---AEE-----A-------SWN-NNE- -REV-KQ-------------M--D-----------KD-DN-GRRGRKMNKPNCRF-          -KML
Drosophila    Dras2/64B  L----R-EF--LM-------KHQQQV-LEE--NTS-NLM-----C---L-VN-DQ--HE---IV-KFQIAERPFIEQDYKKKGKR-          -C-M
Dyctiostelium Ddras      L----K-R--LI-----A--DHERQV-VNEG-E--KDSLS FH-S---S-IN--E---S------KELKGDQSSGKAQKKKKQ           -LIL
S.cerevisiae  RAS1       Q------YI-V-V----L--ENERQV-YEDGLR--KQLNA-FL-----QAIN-DE---S-I-LV-DDGGKYNSMNRQLDNTNEIRD(111 aa)-IIC
S.cerevisiae  RAS2       L----T-Y--I-V----S--ENEKQV-Y-DGLNM-KQMNA-FL-----QAIN--E-----A-LV-DEGGKYNKTLT-NDNSKQTSQ(114 aa)-II-
S.pombe       SPRAS      L----K-TF-V---A-----E-ER-V--REGEQ--K-MHCL-V-----L-LN--E---S---T--RYNKSEEKGFQNKQAVQIAQV( 24 aa)--IC
```

Figure 1 Comparative amino acid sequence of *ras* proteins. Residues identical to the human H-*ras*-1 gene product are designated by a dash.

The biochemical and biological properties of *ras* proteins, along with their strong resemblance to G proteins, have led to the proposal that p21 *ras* proteins may be involved in signal transduction (1). It has been hypothesized that *ras* proteins exist in equilibrium between an active and an inactive state. Most of the *ras* molecules in a resting cell would exist in their inactive state which is characterized by a conformation that allows the binding of GDP. Normal *ras* proteins will remain in their inactive state until they receive a stimulus from another protein, likely a transmembrane receptor. This stimulus will result in the exchange of GDP for GTP, which in turn will cause a conformational change to the activated state. The unique conformation of active *ras* proteins would enable them to interact with their putative effector molecules to continue the pathway of signal transduction. Once the interaction between the activated GTP-bound *ras* proteins with their putative effector molecules has taken place, they would be immediately deactivated. This can be accomplished by their intrinsic GTPase activity which by catalyzing the hydrolysis of GTP will induce the return of *ras* proteins to their inactive GDP-bound state.

During the last 3 years, a great deal of effort has been dedicated to identifying the signal transduction pathways in which *ras* proteins may participate. Most available information has been obtained in the budding yeast *Saccharomyces cerevisiae*. *S. cerevisiae* contains two *ras* loci, designated *RAS1* and *RAS2*. Whereas mutants defective in either locus are viable, *ras*1$^-$ *ras*2$^-$ mutants are not (41). Genetic and biochemical studies strongly support the concept that in this microorganism, *ras* proteins participate in a pathway that controls the activation of adenylate cyclase (42). Whether *S. cerevisiae RAS* proteins are indeed the G proteins that interact directly with adenylate cyclase remains to be established. Unfortunately, these observations do not appear to be applicable to other eukaryotic organisms. For instance, in the fission yeast *Schizosaccharomyces pombe*, their single *ras* gene, *SPRAS*, appears to play a different physiological role. Genetic studies in which the *S. pombe SPRAS* locus has been disrupted, the cells are viable, although they lose their ability to mate (43). In addition, this mutation does not appear to affect the intracellular levels of cyclic adenosine monophosphate (cAMP), the product of adenylate cyclase.

Lack of association between *ras* genes and adenylate cyclase has also been reported in other systems. For instance, human *ras* proteins can induce maturation of frog oocytes without affecting their cAMP levels (44). Moveover, mammalian epithelial and fibroblastic cells lines transformed with retroviral *ras* oncogenes exhibit reduced adenylate cyclase activity (45). These observations represent an evolutionary puzzle. It is impossible that *ras* proteins function at a pivotal crossroads of signal transduction pathways. If so, selection of one pathway over another may have changed during evolution depending on the peculiar physiological necessities of each organism. In support of this view is the observation that *S. cerevisiae* depends on its intracellular levels of cAMP to exit from G_1 into the S phase, and to switch from G_1 into the sporulation pathway. In contrast, there is not evidence for the involvement of cAMP in the control of the life cycle of *S. pombe*. Thus, if *ras* proteins were to be involved in the regulation of cell proliferation, it is likely that in *S. cerevisiae* they do so by interacting with adenylate cyclase. However, other organisms in which cAMP does not play such a role in the control of cell growth may not require that their *ras* products interact with the adenylate cyclase pathway.

In mammalian cells, there is preliminary evidence suggesting that *ras* genes may participate in the phosphatidylinositol pathway. Rodent fibroblasts transformed by different *ras* oncogenes exhibit elevated steady-state levels of phosphatidylinositol-4,5-biphosphate (PIP_2) and their breakdown products, the second messengers 1,2-diacylglycerol (DAG) and inositol-1,4,5-triphosphate (IP_3) (46). Similar results have been obtained when NIH3T3 cells carrying an inducible N-*ras* proto-oncogene were treated with several growth factors such as bombesin and bradykinin, but not with epidermal growth factor (EGF) or platelet-derived growth factor (PDGF) (47). These observations have led to the proposal that N-*ras* p21 proteins may be identical to G_p, the putative G protein that mediates the activation of phospholipase C, the enzyme responsible for the breakdown of PIP_2 into DAG and IP_3 (47). However, in related experiments in which *ras* p21 proteins were microinjected into REF52 rat fibroblasts, stimulation of phospholipase A_2, an enzyme involved in a completely different pathway, was observed instead (48). Additional experiments are needed to determine whether these observations reflect the physiological role of *ras* proteins or they represent an indirect consequence of cell transformation, since cells transformed by unrelated oncogenes were not used as controls in any of these experiments.

Finally, the importance of *ras* genes in cell proliferation has been illustrated by experiments in which antibodies capable of recognizing all known *ras* proteins have been microinjected into the cytoplasm of NIH3T3 cells. Microinjected cells were blocked from leaving G_0 and entering the S phase as a response to serum stimulation (49). Time-course experiments suggest that *ras* proteins are not required once the cells have entered the S phase. The validity of these observations has been confirmed by showing that NIH3T3 cells transformed by a *ras* mutant that cannot bind this monoclonal antibody are not prevented from entering the S phase (50). Studies utilizing antibodies specific for each of the mammalian *ras* products may provide additional information of the specific role of each of these proteins and the proliferation of mammalian cells.

ras ONCOGENES: MECHANISM OF ACTIVATION

ras genes can acquire transforming properties by qualitative and quantitative mechanisms. Most *ras* oncogenes, including those transduced into acute transforming retroviruses and those present in human and animal tumors, owe their transforming properties to single point mutations within their coding sequences (1). However, increased expression (10- to 100-fold) of normal *ras* genes can also induce certain manifestations of the malignant phenotype (1). In general terms, the neoplastic properties induced by highly overexpressed *ras* proto-oncogenes are more limited than those induced by normal expression levels of their mutated alleles. Combination of qualitative and quantitative alterations within *ras* genes results in oncogenes (e.g., retroviral v-*ras* oncogenes) capable of inducing a more complete spectrum of neoplastic phenotypes.

Mutations in naturally occurring *ras* oncogenes have been localized in codons 12, 13, 59, and 61 (1). In vitro mutagenesis studies have shown that missense mutations in codons 63, 116, and 119 can also confer comparable transforming properties to *ras* genes (1). Among these mutations, those occurring at codon 12 and 61 are the most abundant in both human and carcinogen-induced animal tumors (1). Normal *ras* gene proteins contain glycine at position 12, a residue that appears to be necessary for their normal function (Fig. 1). Substitution of ^{12}Gly by any other amino acid results in the oncogenic activation of *ras* molecules (51–53). An exception to this rule is proline, an amino acid known to disrupt a helical structures (54). Based on sequence homology between *ras* proteins and EF-T_u, it has been proposed that the critical ^{12}Gly residue might be part of the phosphoryl-binding loop of guanine nucleotides (55). Thus, replacement or elimination of ^{12}Gly is likely to create a rigid domain that cannot efficiently interact with GTP, thus reducing the intrinsic GTPase activity of *ras* oncogene proteins. Oncogenic activation of *ras* proteins also occurs if ^{12}Gly is deleted, or if additional amino acids are inserted between ^{11}Ala and ^{12}Gly (56).

Substitution of its neighboring amino acid, ^{13}Gly, also has transforming consequences for the harboring cells, although in this case not all substitutions appear to have the same activating effect (57,58). Whereas ^{13}Val, ^{13}Asp, and ^{13}Cys substitutions yield *ras* oncogenes, replacement of Gly^{13} by ^{13}Ser has little effect on the transforming activity of *ras* proteins

(57). Miscoding mutations in the domain surrounding codon 61 also play a very important role in the generation of *ras* oncogenes. Substitution of ^{61}Gln by any other amino acid residue except ^{61}Pro or ^{61}Glu yields *ras* oncogenes (59–62). Substitutions in residue 59 have only been observed in retroviral or in vitro mutagenized *ras* oncogenes (57,63,64). In all cases, substitution of the normal ^{59}Ala by ^{59}Thr has been observed.

The products of *ras* oncogenes exhibit either a dramatically decreased ability to hydrolyze GDP (mutations in codons 12 and 61) (35–39), or a very limited affinity to bind guanine nucleotides (mutations in codons 116 and 119) (65,66). These biochemical properties of *ras* oncogene proteins fit within the context of the proposed model for *ras* protein function described above. Since *ras* proteins exist in a equilibrium between inactive (GDP-bound) and active (GTP-bound) forms, mutations that lead to the stabilization of *ras* proteins in their active state should cause a continuous flow of signal transduction which may result in malignant transformation. This process can be achieved by mutations that inhibit the intrinsic GTPase activity of *ras* proteins, since they could not become efficiently deactivated. Similarly, mutations that cause an increased exchange rate between GDP and GTP would also favor the formation of the active *ras*. GTP complex owing to the higher availability of GTP molecules in the cell. Therefore, it appears that any missense mutations that will favor the active GTP-bound state of *ras* proteins should lead to the malignant activation of these genes as oncogenes (1).

This model also takes into account that overexpression of normal *ras* proteins might also lead to malignant transformation. Since activation of the *ras*-signaling pathway requires a certain amount of activated *ras* proteins, significant overexpression of normal *ras* proteins may create the necessary concentration of *ras* proteins in an active state to cause malignant transformation without necessarily altering the equilibrium between their active and inactive states.

ras ONCOGENES: BIOLOGICAL PROPERTIES

Cellular *ras* oncogenes transform established rodent cell lines in vitro in a dominant fashion. *ras* oncogenes are necessary not only for initiation, but also for maintenance of the transformed phenotype. Neither the resident *ras* genes nor cotransfection with their respective normal alleles affects the transformation efficiencies of *ras* oncogenes. However, the levels of expression of mutated *ras* proteins appear to modulate their transforming potency (1).

Cellular *ras* oncogenes cannot transform rat primary embryo cells in vitro (67–69). Transformation of these cells requires either the cooperation of nuclear oncogenes (e.g., c-*myc*, adenovirus E1A, polyoma large T, N-*myc*, p53) (1), or the elimination of the surrounding cells by co-transfecting the *ras* oncogene with a dominant selectable marker such as the bacterial neo^{R} gene (70). Linkage of *ras* oncogenes to transcriptional enhancers increases the percentage of cells that become transformed under either of these experimental conditions (71). Evaluation of the neoplastic properties of *ras* oncogenes in cells other than cultured fibroblasts has been somewhat hampered by the limited cell types that can be efficiently transfected by these oncogenes. The use of retroviruses carrying *ras* oncogenes has somewhat circumvented this problem. *ras*-containing retroviruses efficiently transform rodent cells of hematopoietic origin, including those of erythroid, lymphoid, and myeloid lineages (1).

Neither cellular nor retroviral *ras* oncogenes have been able to induce stable transformation of normal human fibroblasts in vitro (72). Recently, transfection of normal human bronchial epithelial cells by a DNA clone of the Harvey murine sarcoma virus (MSV) *ras* oncogene has yielded colonies of transformed cells (73). These cells are obtained at very low frequencies and after careful and long-term culture. Other authors have been able to transform human epidermal karotinocytes (74), embryonic kidney cells (75), and normal fibroblasts by *ras*-containing retroviruses (76). However, transformation of these cells requires prior acquisition of indefinite life span by either infection with DNA tumor viruses (74,75), or by treatment with ^{60}Co α-rays (76). In addition, *ras* oncogenes can confer tumorigenic properties to cell lines derived from human tumors that cannot induce tumors when injected into suitable hosts such as nude mice (77).

Recent studies indicate that in addition to their transforming properties, *ras* oncogenes can also induce terminal differentiation of the rat pheochromocytoma cell line PC12 (78–80). PC12 cells can differentiate into neuronlike cells if infected with *ras*-containing retroviruses or microinjected with oncogene p21 *ras* proteins. Differentiation of PC12 cells induced by *ras* oncogenes exhibit differentiation markers very similar to those induced by nerve growth factor (NGF), thus raising the possibility that *ras* oncogenes may participate in a signal transduction pathway commonly used by NGF (78–80). This hypothesis has been strengthened by a recent report showing that microinjection of PC12 cells with antibodies that block *ras* protein function inhibited neurite formation induced by NGF (81).

RETROVIRAL VERSUS CELLULAR *ras* ONCOGENES

The tumorigenic properties of retroviral *ras* oncogenes have been extensively studied (reviewed in Ref. 82). It has been well documented that each of the four strains of acute transforming retrovirus that carry *ras* oncogenes can induce a variety of tumors when inoculated into newborn rodents. The highly malignant properties of retroviral oncogenes contrast with the limited tumorigenic properties of cellular *ras* oncogenes. Their differential carcinogenic spectrum cannot be explained by qualitative mechanisms, since retroviral *ras* oncogenes are activated by the same missense mutations as those found in *ras* oncogenes of human and carcinogen-induced animal tumors. In other words, retroviral and cellular *ras* oncogenes produce identical p21 proteins. However, retroviral *ras* oncogenes can target a much larger number of cells and cell types than their cellular counterparts whose oncogenic activation is restricted to their harboring cells. In addition, owing to the more efficient enhancer and promoting activity of retroviral regulatory elements, the higher levels of expression of retroviral *ras* oncogenes is likely to contribute to the more prominent neoplastic properties of retroviral *ras* oncogenes.

In addition to their distinct promoters, retroviral *ras* oncogenes differ from their cellular counterparts in their 5′ noncoding sequences and in their polyadenylation signals (24,26). However, since these structural changes do not affect the nature of their corresponding gene products, it is unlikely that they play any significant role in the differential oncogenic properties of cellular and retroviral *ras* oncogenes. Experimental demonstration that cellular oncogenes are intrinsically identical to their retroviral counterparts except for the qualitative differences indicated above has been recently obtained. Introduction of the human H-*ras*-1 oncogene isolated from the T24/EJ bladder carcinoma cell line into appropriate retroviral vectors has yielded acute transforming retroviruses (83). These viruses have been shown to induce erythroleukemias and sarcomas when injected into newborn mice, thus illustrating the similar oncogenic properties of human and retroviral *ras* oncogenes when expressed under comparable environments.

ras ONCOGENES IN HUMAN CANCER

ras oncogenes have been identified in a larger variety of human cancers (1). They have been found in carcinomas of the bladder, breast, colon, kidney, liver, lung, ovary, pancreas, and stomach; in hematopoietic tumors of lymphoid (acute lymphocytic leukemia, B-cell lymphoma, Burkitt's lymphoma, non-Hodgkin's lymphoma) and myeloid (acute and chronic myelogenous leukemias, promyelocytic leukemia) lineage; and in tumors of mesenchymal origin such as fibrosarcomas and rhabdomyosarcomas. Other tumors, including melanomas, neuroblastomas, gliomas, and teratocarcinomas, have also been shown to possess *ras* oncogenes (reviewed in Ref. 84). On the average, *ras* oncogenes are estimated to occur in 10–15% of human malignancies. However, the relative incidence of *ras* oncogenes varies greatly. Whereas, *ras* oncogenes have seldom been found in certain common malignancies such as breast carcinomas, they have been identified in as many as 30% of acute myelogenous leukemias (AML) (58) and in 40–50% of colon carcinomas (85,86). Overall *ras* oncogenes are by far the most frequent transforming genes found in human cancer.

The incidence of *ras* oncogene activation in human neoplasia may have been underestimated. For the most part, detection of *ras* oncogenes has relied on biological assays of limited sensitivity. The recent development of more sophisticated and sensitive methodologies suggests that, at least in certain types of neoplasia, *ras* oncogenes are even more prevalent than previously suspected. One of these new diagnostic methodologies is the polymerase chain reaction, a technique that amplifies small segments of cellular sequences by using flanking oligonucleotide primers followed by incubation with DNA polymerase (87). These amplified sequences can be subsequently assayed with oligonucleotide probes of defined sequence capable of identifying the point mutations responsible for the activation of *ras* oncogenes. A related methodology based on the ability of RNase A to cleave RNA:RNA hybrids exhibiting base pair mismatches has also been developed (88). Both experimental approaches have been recently utilized to establish that at least 40% of human colon carcinomas carry K-*ras*-2 oncogenes activated by single point mutations within their twelfth codon (85,86). This incidence is about four-fold greater than the one previously estimated based on gene transfer assays (84).

Another important development in our understanding of the involvement of *ras* oncogenes in human cancer has been their identification in preneoplastic lesions. K-*ras*-2 oncogenes have been found in seven out of eight benign colonic tumors originating from villous adenomas and villoglandular polyps (86). These benign tumors emerge directly from the colonic mucosa as superficial neoplasms and are not considered malignant unless they acquire infiltrating activity. In related studies, five out of eight residual adenomatous regions isolated from cryostat sections of frozen colon carcinomas have been found to also contain K-*ras*-2 oncogenes (85). These results indicate that these oncogenes were present before carcinoma development. Only in one of the eight cases analyzed was the mutated K-*ras*-2 oncogene present in the carcinoma, but not in the preneoplastic adenoma.

Additional examples of the role of *ras* oncogenes in the early stages of human neoplastic development has been provided by the identification of transforming *ras* oncogenes in a keratoacanthoma (H-*ras*-1) (J. Leon and A. Pellicer, personal communication) and in three patients with myelodysplastic syndrome (MDS) (N-*ras*) (89). Keratoacanthomas are benign tumors of the skin that undergo complete spontaneous regression. Myelodysplastic syndrome is a preneoplastic condition with a high risk of developing into AML. Interestingly, only those MDS patients in which the N-*ras* oncogene was present (three out of eight) developed malignant AML within a year (89).

In addition to the frequent involvement of mutated *ras* oncogenes in human cancer, it has been suggested that *ras* genes may contribute to human malignancy by quantitative mechanisms not involving the occurrence of missense mutations (1). Expression of *ras* genes is often increased in tumors relative to normal tissues. Careful quantitative analysis has indicated that the levels of *ras* transcripts in about 50% of human tumors are two- to 10-fold higher than in control tissues (90–92). Similar results have been obtained by either immunoblotting or immunohistochemical analysis of p21 *ras* expression in a variety of primary carcinomas (93–98). The biological significance of these results is not clear. Transformation of immortal rodent cells in culture requires at least 30- to 100-fold increased in the level of p21 *ras* expression (99,100). No such increases have been observed in human tumors except in a small number of cases in which their *ras* genes have been found to be amplified (100–102). Moreover, increases in *ras* transcripts of up to eightfold can be associated with normal proliferative processes such as regenerating rat liver (103). Therefore, there is not sufficient experimental basis at the present time to implicate moderate variations of nonmutated *ras* gene expression in the development of human tumors.

ras ONCOGENES IN CARCINOGEN-INDUCED ANIMAL TUMORS

Understanding the role that *ras* oncogenes play in human neoplasia requires the development of appropriate in vivo model systems in which these oncogenes can be reproducibly activated under controlled experimental conditions. Evidence accumulated during the last few years has indicated that *ras* oncogenes are frequently activated in a variety of carcinogen-induced animal tumor systems (Table 1). In rats, induction of mammary carcinomas by a

Table 1 Activation of *ras* Oncogenes in Carcinogen-Induced Animal Tumors

Species	Tumor	Carcinogen	Oncogene	Incidence (%)	Ref.
Rat	Mammary carcinoma	NMU	H-*ras*-1	86	104, 105
		DMBA	H-*ras*-1	23	105
	Kidney mesenchymal	NMU	K-*ras*-2	60	a
		DMN	K-*ras*-2	40	106
	Lung carcinoma	TNM	K-*ras*-2	74	107
	Hepatocellular carcinoma	AFB_1	K-*ras*-2	25	108
	Skin carcinoma	x-rays	K-*ras*-2	50	109
Mouse	Skin carcinoma	DMBA	H-*ras*-1	90	110–112
		DBACR	H-*ras*-1	80	112
	Mammary carcinoma	DMBA	H-*ras*-1	75	113
	Lymphoma	x-rays	K-*ras*-2, N-*ras*	57	114
		NMU	K-*ras*-2, N-*ras*	85	114
	Thymic lymphoma	MCA	K-*ras*-2	83	115
	Fibrosarcoma	MCA	K-*ras*-2	50	116
	Lung carcinoma	TNM	K-*ras*-2	100	107
	Hepatocellular carcinoma	HOAAF	H-*ras*-1	100	118
		EC	H-*ras*-1	100	b
		VC	H-*ras*-1	100	118
		HODE	H-*ras*-1	100	118
		HOAB	H-*ras*-1	100	b
		Vinthionine	H-*ras*-1	100	b
		Safrole	H-*ras*-1	100	b
		Estragole	H-*ras*-1	100	b
		Furfural	H-*ras*-1	85	c
		Aflatoxin B_1	H-*ras*-1, K-*ras*-2	85	b
		B(*a*)P	K-*ras*-2, H-*ras*-1	80	b
Rabbit	Keratoacanthoma	DMBA	H-*ras*-1	60	d

[a]Our unpublished results.
[b]R. W. Wiseman, personal communication.
[c]S. Reynolds and M. W. Anderson, personal communication.
[d]J. Leon and A. Pellicer, personal communication.

single dose of nitrosomethylurea (NMU) during puberty leads to the activation of H-*ras*-1 oncogenes in over 85% of the tumors (104,105). Substitution of this carcinogen by dimethylbenz(a)anthracene (DMBA) also results in the malignant activation of the H-*ras*-1 locus, although in only 25% of the tumors

(105). At least four other rat tumor systems have been shown to contain transforming K-*ras*-2 oncogenes. They include induction of kidney mesenchymal tumors by single doses of either NMU (our unpublished observations) or methyl (methoxymethyl)nitrosamine (DMN) (106), induction of carcinomas of the lung by chronic exposure to tetranitromethane (TNM) (107), and induction of carcinomas of the liver by aflatoxin B_1 (AFB_1) treatment (108). Finally, carcinomas of the skin induced by exposure to gamma radiation have also been shown to contain K-*ras*-2 oncogenes (109).

The frequency of oncogene activation in these tumors varies. Whereas in lung carcinomas induced by TNM 75% of the animals exhibited activated K-*ras*-2 oncogenes (107), only 25% of the hepatocellular carcinomas induced by AFB_1 appeared to contain this oncogene (108). Since K-*ras*-2 is a large locus (see previous section) it is likely that the incidence of K-*ras*-2 oncogenes present in these tumors is an underestimate. Routine use of the polymerase chain reaction technique in these model systems will allow a better assessment of the real incidence of K-*ras*-2 oncogene activation in these tumors. *ras* oncogenes have been found to be randomly (<10% incidence) identified in certain animal model systems such as rat fibrosarcomas induced by either 1,6- or 1,8-dinitropyrene. Similar results have been obtained in liver (five out of 93 tumors) and intestinal epithelial (two out of 51) tumors of F344 rats induced by either DMN-OMe or DMN-OAc, respectively (J. Rice, personal communication).

In mice, the list of carcinogen-induced animal tumor systems possessing *ras* oncogenes is even more extensive than in rats (Table 1). H-*ras*-1 oncogenes have been found to be reproducibly activated in over 90% of skin papillomas and carcinomas of Sencar mice initiated by either DMBA or dibenz(c,h)acridine (DBACR) treatment followed by promotion with phorbol esters (110–112). Similarly, H-*ras*-1 oncogenes have been found in three out of four mammary tumors arising from hyperplastic alveolar nodules implanted in mice treated with DMBA (113). Tumors of hematopoietic origin induced by chronic exposure to either x-rays (114), NMU (114), or 3-methylcholantrene (MCA) (115) have been shown to contain *ras* oncogenes. In the case of lymphomas induced by x-rays or NMU, K-*ras*-2 is the oncogene most frequently activated (114). However, N-*ras* oncogenes are occasionally observed (114). The overall incidence of *ras* oncogenes in these tumors varies between 60% for those induced with x-rays to 85% for those induced by NMU. A similar percentage of K-*ras*-2 oncogenes have been observed in thymic lymphomas induced by MCA (115).

Tumors of mesenchymal and epithelial origin have also been shown to contain activated K-*ras*-2 oncogenes. For instance, 50% of fibrosarcomas induced by subcutaneous injection of MCA have been found to contain K-*ras*-2 oncogenes (116). Reproducible activation of K-*ras*-2 oncogenes was also seen in lung carcinomas induced by TMN (107). Induction of hepatocellular carcinomas in B6C3F$_1$ mice, a strain often used in toxicology tests, has been the tumor system most extensively used to study the activation of *ras* oncogenes by various chemical carcinogens (117,118). The different carcinogens used are listed in Table 1. The H-*ras*-1 oncogene was detected in most of the tumors, independently of the carcinogen utilized (117,118). However, occasional activation of K-*ras*-2 oncogenes has been found in tumors induced by estragole, AFB$_1$, and benz(*a*)pyrene (B[*a*]P) (S. Reynolds, M. W. Anderson, and R. Wiseman, personal communication).

ras oncogenes have also been found in spontaneous tumors known to arise in old animals of certain strains of mice (Table 2). H-*ras*-1 oncogenes exist in 80% of hepatocellular carcinomas and 30% benign hepatocellular adenomas of 2.5-year-old B6C3F$_1$ mice (117). Similarly, K-*ras*-2 oncogenes occurred in most (nine out of 10) spontaneous lung tumors of the A strain of mice (M. W. Anderson, personal communication). Finally, *ras* oncogenes have also been found to be reproducibly activated in carcinogen-induced tumors of nonrodent species. Repeated application of DMBA on the skin of rabbit ears leads to the induction of keratoacanthomas, a benign cell-regressing skin tumor very similar to those observed in humans (see previous section). About 60% of the DNAs isolated from these rabbit tumors induced the appearance of transformed foci when transfected into NIH3T3 cells (J. Leon and A. Pellicer, personal communication). Each of these foci has been found to contain the same transforming gene, H-*ras*-1.

The availability of such variety of animal model systems is makes it possible to design experimental approaches to investigate the relationship between the carcinogenic action of known carcinogens and the molecular pathways that lead to neoplasia. Indeed, emerging evidence indicates that *ras* oncogenes can be activated during the initiation of carcinogenesis as a direct consequence of the mutagenic action of the carcinogen. These observations are derived from experiments in which the known mutagenic spectrum of certain chemical carcinogens have been compared with the nature

Table 2 Reproducible Activation of *ras* Oncogenes in Spontaneous Animal Tumors

Species	Strain	Tumor	Oncogene	Incidence %	Ref.
Mouse	B6C3F$_1$	Hepatocellular carcinoma	H-*ras*-1	80	117
	B6C3F$_1$	Hepatocellular carcinoma	H-*ras*-1	30	117
	A	Lung carcinoma	K-*ras*-2	90	a

[a]M. W. Anderson, personal communication.

of the activating missense mutations present in *ras* oncogenes. These studies are summarized in the next section.

ras GENES AS TARGETS OF CARCINOGENS

Most carcinogens are known to be active mutagens. A significant number of chemical carcinogens form adducts with DNA bases either directly or after metabolic activation (reviewed in Ref. 119). Some of these adducts are highly mutagenic owing to their miscoding properties. Others can lead to mutations owing to the generation of apurinic sites, or because of the limited fidelity of repair polymerases (119). Whereas most of these mutations have no consequence to the host, a small number of them presumably located in critical genes, can trigger neoplastic development.

The reproducible activation of *ras* oncogenes in carcinogen-induced tumors has made it possible to correlate their activated mutations with the known mutagenic effects of certain carcinogens (Table 3). For instance, each of the H-*ras*-1 oncogenes present in rat mammary carcinomas induced by NMU became activated by G to A transitions (105), the most common mutation induced by this carcinogen (120,121). In contrast, DMBA, a carcinogen whose activated form reacts preferentially with adenine residues (122), induced activation of H-*ras*-1 oncogenes by missense mutations affecting deoxyadenosine residues (105). Similar results have been obtained with a variety of animal tumor systems. Induction of skin carcinomas in mice by DMBA involves the specific activation of H-*ras*-1 oncogenes by A to T transitions in the second base of codon 61 (112, 123). In contrast, each of the four H-*ras*-1 oncogenes present in skin papillomas induced by the direct-acting carcinogen *N*-methyl-*N*′-nitrosoguanidine (MNNG) were activated by G to A transitions, precisely the type of mutation known to be induced by this methylating agent (A. Balmain, personal communication).

The reproducible activation of H-*ras*-1 oncogenes in hepatocellular carcinomas of B6C3F$_1$ mice has become a fruitful system to analyze the correspondence between the known mutagenic activity of carcinogens with the type of missense mutations found in the activated H-*ras*-1 oncogenes (Table 3). For instance, H-*ras*-1 oncogenes present in spontaneous tumors of old age mice carry random mutations in the first two nucleotides of codon 61 (S. Reynolds and M. W. Anderson, personal communication). Whereas half of these H-*ras*-1 oncogenes (15 out of 25) exhibit G to A transitions, the others carry A to T transversions (six tumors) or A to G transitions (three tumors). However, induction of hepatocellular carcinomas by carcinogenic treatment completely changes the pattern of activating mutations. Treatment of B6C3F$_1$ mice with a single dose of either *N*-hydroxy-2-acetyl-aminofluoride (HOAAF) or *N*-hydroxy-4-aminoazobenzene (HOAB) generates H-*ras*-1 oncogenes activated by C to A transversions in the first base of codon 61 (118).

Table 3 Activation of H-*ras*-1 Oncogenes by Specific Missense Mutations in Chemically Induced Tumors

Species	Tumor	Carcinogen	Expected mutation	Activating mutation	Incidence	Ref.
Rat	Mammary carcinoma	NMU	G → A	G^{35} → A	61/61	105
		DMBA	A → N	A^{182}, A^{183} → N	5/5	105
Mouse	Skin papilloma or carcinoma	DMBA	A → N	A^{182} → T	33/37	112, 123
		MNNG	G → A	G^{35} → A	4/4	a
Mouse	Hepatocarcinoma	None		C^{181} → A	15/25	b
				A^{182} → T	6/25	b
				A^{182} → G	3/25	b
		HO-AAF	C → A	C^{181} → A	8/10	118
		HOAB	C → A	C^{181} → A	9/10	c
		VC, EC	?	A^{182} → T	13/16	118, c
		DMBA	A → N	A^{182} → T	10/10	c

[a] A. Balmain, personal communication.
[b] S. Reynolds, M. W. Anderson, and R. Wiseman, personal communication.
[c] R. W. Wiseman, personal communication.

Although the mutagenic specificity of these two compounds are not known, in vitro studies with the related carcinogens *N*-hydroxy-*N*-2-aminofluorene and *N*-acetoxy-acetylaminofluorene (AAAF) revealed that they preferentially induce C to A transversions (124,125). In contrast, H-*ras*-1 oncogenes present in hepatocellular carcinomas induced by carbamate derivatives exhibit a different mutagenic spectrum. Both vinyl and ethyl carbamates (VC and EC) preferentially (85%) induced A to T transversions in the second base of codon 61 (118; R. W. Wiseman, personal communication).

These findings strongly support the concept that *ras* oncogenes can be directly activated by the mutagenic action of the initiating carcinogen. Since most of these tumors are induced by a single carcinogenic insult, activation of *ras* oncogenes must be concomitant with, and presumably responsible for, the initiation of neoplastic delvelopment.

ras ONCOGENES AND MULTISTAGE CARCINOGENESIS

Several lines of evidence suggest that activation of *ras* oncogenes is not sufficient to trigger tumorigenesis and must cooperate with secondary genetic events and/or specific developmental programs in order to elicit neoplastic development. For instance, it has been shown that the active stage of proliferation of the developing mammary gland at the time of the carcinogen insult plays a fundamental role in tumor development (reviewed in Ref. 126). A similar situation may occur in the skin carcinogenesis model of mice. Initiated cells are known to remain dormant in the skin of DMBA-treated mice for long periods of time until they are treated with tumor promoters (127). Considering that most of the papillomas and carcinomas generated in this model system contain H-*ras*-1 oncogenes (111–123), it is likely that these initiated cells already carry such oncogenes. Direct support for this hypothesis has been recently obtained (128). Infection of mouse epidermal skin cells with Harvey MSV results in the generation of initiated cells that do not express discernible neoplastic properties unless they are treated with TPA. These results indicate that in this model system *ras* oncogenes also require cooperation with cellular proliferation to allow expression of their neoplastic properties.

Induction of skin carcinomas by Harvey MSV has provided direct experimental evidence for the existence of secondary genetic events in *ras*-induced tumors (128). Whereas Harvey MSV–induced papillomas appear to be polyclonal, the malignant carcinomas are clonal in origin. Papillomas are known to regress to small hyperkeriotic lesions before a few of them begin their invasive growth characteristic of skin carcinomas. Therefore, a second genetic event distinct and independent from *ras* oncogene activation is required for development of skin carcinomas. Recently, it has been shown that skin grafts of cultured keratinocytes infected with Harvey MSV lead to the generation of papillomas but not carcinomas (129), thus adding further evidence to the concept that *ras* oncogenes are not sufficient for the development of the full malignant phenotype.

ras ONCOGENES IN TRANSGENIC MICE

Another experimental approach that is making it possible to study the tumorigenic properties of *ras* oncogenes in vivo is the development of transgenic mice carrying *ras* oncogenes under the transcriptional control of either tissue-specific or inducible promoters. To date, three independent classes of transgenic mice carrying *ras* oncogenes have been described (130–132). In one case, the activated human H-*ras*-1 oncogene was placed under the control of the promoter for the murine whey acidic protein (*Wap*) gene (130). This gene is specifically expressed in mammary epithelial cells of lactating mothers. Five transgenic *Wap-ras* mice (four females and one male) were obtained, of which only two of the females and the male founders expressed human H-*ras*-1 transcripts. In these two female lines, expression of the chimeric *Wap-ras* gene was restricted to the lactating mammary epithelial cells and to a lesser extend to brain tissue. In contrast, *Wap-ras* expression in mice derived from the male founders was exclusively found in the salivary gland.

Tumor development in these animals occurred late in life and corresponded with the occurrence of *Wap-ras* expression (130). In one of the female founders, tumors of the mammary gland appeared after 2 years and five pregnancies. Adenocarcinomas of the salivary gland also appeared after 9 months in five animals derived from the founder male. In each case, levels of expression of the *Wap-ras* gene was elevated in tumor versus control tissue (130). These studies illustrate the tumorigenic potential of *ras* oncogenes based on the correlation between *ras* oncogene expression and tumor development. However, their low frequency and long latency suggest that *ras* oncogenes are not sufficient to induce the neoplastic phenotype, and that additional changes must occur during the genesis of these neoplasms.

A similar situation occurs in transgenic mice carrying a retroviral H-*ras* oncogene under the transcriptional control of the long terminal repeat (LTR) of mouse mammary tumor viruses (MMTVs) (131). In these animals, *ras* oncogene expression was reproducibly observed in the mammary and salivary glands and occasionally in other organs such as the Harderion gland, spleen, thymus, lung, and seminal vesicle. Ten out of 13 strains developed adenocarcinomas of the mammary and salivary gland as well as occasional lymphomas. The adenocarcinomas appeared as focal tumors surrounded by normal epithelium, thus suggesting a clonal origin. Tumor clonality was unambiguously demonstrated in the lymphomas (131). Therefore, tumor development in these transgenic mice must also require additional genetic changes.

Interestingly, mating of MMTV-*ras* transgenic mice with MMTV-*myc* transgenic strains (133) resulted in hybrid mice that exhibited a synergistic incidence of tumor formation (131). Neoplastic development in these animals is greatly accelerated, and they all have developed tumors by 5 months of age. Yet, tumors also appear to be monoclonal, and coexpression of both *ras* and *myc* oncogenes could be observed in nonmalignant mammary epithelium adjacent to tumor tissue. These observations suggest that in spite of carrying two transcriptionally active oncogenes, tumored cells may require additional genetic changes in order to achieve their full neoplastic potential (131).

A somewhat different picture has been observed in the third *ras* transgenic system in which the human H-*ras*-1 oncogene was placed under the regulatory control of the rat elastase I gene (132). Previous studies have indicated that heterologous genes driven by this promoter are expressed specifically in pancreatic acinar cells starting at day 14 of embryonal development. Transgenic fetuses carrying the chimeric elastase I–*ras* oncogene almost invariably exhibited neoplastic growth of their pancreatic acinar cells as early as 16 days of gestation (132). The abnormal proliferation and morphogenesis of these cells appeared to be polyclonal. These observations along with their rapid phenotypic manifestation strongly supports the concept that they are the direct consequence of the onset of *ras* oncogene expression. Moreover, this dramatic description of pancreatic development was not observed in similar transgenic mice carrying the normal H-*ras*-1 proto-oncogene (132). However, it should be noted that the abnormal morphology of the fetal pancreas in these transgenic mice might not be equated with full neoplastic development. For instance, no evidence of aneuploidity, invasiveness, or metastasis was observed. These findings were not too surprising, since these characteristic properties of tumor cells are often associated with the late stages of tumor progression. However, pancreatic cells carrying *ras* oncogenes have failed so far to induce tumors, thus raising the possibility that further genetic changes are also required in these cells to acquire full tumorigenic properties (132).

In summary, results obtained with transgenic mice carrying activated *ras* oncogenes support the concept that these oncogenes are intimately associated with neoplastic development, although they are not sufficient to confer full tumorigenic properties to the harboring cells (130–132). More importantly, availability of these strains should make it possible to investigate the precise role of *ras* oncogenes in in vivo neoplasia and perhaps to identify those additional genetic changes required for tumor development.

ACKNOWLEDGMENTS

Research sponsored by the National Cancer Institute, Department of Health and Human Services, under contract No. N01-CO-23909 with Bionetics

Research, Inc. The contents of this publication do not necessarily reflect the views or policies of the Department of Health and Human Services, nor does mention of trade names, commercial products, or organizations imply endorsement by the U.S. government.

REFERENCES

1. Barbacid, M. (1987). *Ann. Rev. Biochem., 56*: 779–827.
2. DeFeo, D., Gonda, M. A., Young, H. A., Chang, E. H., Lowy, D. R., Scolnick, E. M., and Ellis, R. W. (1981). *Proc. Natl. Acad. Sci. U.S.A. 78*: 328–3332.
3. Ellis, R. W., DeFeo, D., Shih, T. Y., Gonda, M. A., Young, H. A., Tsuchida, N., Lowy, D. R., and Scolnick, E. M. (1981). *Nature 292*: 506–511.
4. Der, C. J., Krontiris, T. G., and Cooper, G. M. (1982). *Proc. Natl. Acad. Sci. U.S.A. 79*: 3637–3640.
5. Parada, L. F., Tabin, C. J., Shih, C., and Weinberg, R. A. (1982). *Nature 297*: 474–478.
6. Santos, E., Tronick, S. R., Aaronson, S. A., Pulciani, S., and Barbacid, M. (1982). *Nature 298*: 343–347.
7. Shimizu, K., Goldfarb, M., Perucho, M., and Wigler, M. (1983). *Proc. Natl. Acad. Sci. U.S.A. 80*: 383–387.
8. Hall, A., Marshall, C. J., Spurr, N. K., and Weiss, R. A. *Nature* (1983). *303*: 396–400.
9. Miyoshi, J., Kagimoto, M., Soeda, E., and Sakayi, Y. (1984). *Nucleic Acids Res. 12*: 1821–1828.
10. McGrath, J. P., Capon, D. J., Smith, D. H., Chen, E. Y., Seeburgh, P. H., Goeddel, D. V., and Levinson, A. D. (1983). *Nature 304*: 501–506.
11. Chattopadhyay, S. K., Chang, E. H., Lander, M. R., Ellis, R. W., Scolnick, E. M., and Lowy, D. R. (1982). *Nature 296*: 361–363.
12. Lowy, D. R., Capon, D. J., Delwart, E., Sakaguchi, A. Y., Naylor, S. L., and Goeddel, D. V. (1987). *Cell 48*: 137–146.
13. Chardin, P., and Tavitian, A. (1986). *EMBO J. 5*: 2203–2208.
14. Madaule, P., and Axel, R. (1985). *Cell 41*: 31–40.
15. Schejter, E. D., and Shilo, B. Z. (1985). *EMBO J. 4*: 407–412.
16. Gallwitz, D., Donath, C., and Sander, C. (1983). *Nature 306*: 704–707.
17. Anderson, P. R., Devare, S. G., Tronick, S. R., Ellis, R. W., Aaronson, S. A., and Scolnick, E. M. (1981). *Cell 26*: 129–134.
18. Rasheed, S., Norman, G. L., and Heidecker, G. (1981). *Science 221*: 155–157.
19. Westaway, D., Papkoff, J., Moscovici, C., and Varmus, H. E. (1986). *EMBO J. 5*: 301–309.
20. George, D. L., Glick, B., Trusko, S., and Freeman, N. *Proc. Natl. Acad. Sci. U.S.A. 83*: 1651–1655.
21. Barbacid, M. (1986). *Trends Genet. 2*: 188–192.
22. Shih, T. Y., Weeks, M. O., Young, H. A., and Scolnick, E. M. (1979). *Virology 96*: 64–79.

23. Shimizu, K., Birnbaum, D., Ruley, M. A., Fasano, O., Suard, Y., Edlund, L., Taparowsky, E., Goldfarb, M., and Wigler, M. (1983). *Nature 304*: 497–500.
24. Capon, D. J., Seeburg, P. H., McGrath, J. P., Hayflick, J. S., Edman, U., Levinson, A. D., and Goeddel, D. V. (1983). *Nature 304*: 507–513.
25. Nakano, H., Yamamoto, F., Neville, C., Evans, D., Mizuno, T., and Perucho, M. (1984). *Proc. Natl. Acad. Sci. U.S.A. 81*: 71–75.
26. Cichutek, K., and Duesburg, P. H. (1986). *Proc. Natl. Acad. Sci. U.S.A. 83*: 2340–2344.
27. Ishii, S., Merlino, G. T., and Pastan, I. (1985). *Science 230*: 1378–1381.
28. Jordano, J., and Perucho, M. (1986). *Nucleic Acids Res. 14*: 7361–7378.
29. Lowy, D. R., and Willumsen, B. M. (1986). *Cancer Surv. 5*: 275–289.
30. DeFeo-Jones, D., Tatchell, K., Robinson, L. C., Sigal, I. S., Vass, W. C., Lowy, D. R., and Scolnick, E. M. (1985). *Science 228*: 197–184.
31. Kataoka, T., Powers, S., Cameron, S., Fasano, O., Goldfarb, M., Broach, J., and Wigler, M. (1985). *Cell 40*: 19–26.
32. Scolnick, E. M., Papageorge, A. G., and Shih, T. Y. (1979). *Proc. Natl. Acad. Sci. U.S.A. 76*: 5355–5359.
33. Shih, T. Y., Papageorge, A. G., Stokes, P. E., Weeks, M. O., and Scolnick, E. M. (1980). *Nature 287*: 686–691.
34. Tamanoi, F., Walsh, M., Kataoka, T., and Wigler, M. (1984). *Proc. Natl. Acad. Sci. U.S.A. 81*: 6924–6928.
35. Temeles, G. L., Gibbs, J. B., D'Alonzo, J. S., Sigal, I. S., and Scolnick, E. M. (1985). *Nature 313*: 700–703.
36. Gibbs, J. B., Sigal, I. S., Poe, M., and Scolnick, E. M. (1984). *Proc. Natl. Acad. Sci. U.S.A. 81*: 5704–5708.
37. McGrath, J. P., Capon, D. J., Goeddel, D. V., and Levinson, A. D. (1984). *Nature 310*: 644–649.
38. Sweet, R. W., Yokoyama, S., Kamata, T., Feramisco, J. R., Rosenberg, M., and Gross, M. (1984). *Nature 311*: 273–275.
39. Manne, V., Bekesi, E., and Kung, H. F. (1985). *Proc. Natl. Acad. Sci. U.S.A. 82*: 376–380.
40. Gilman, A. G. (1987). *Ann. Rev. Biochem. 56*: 615–649.
41. Kataoka, T., Powers, S., McGill, C., Fasano, O., Strathern, J., Broach, J., and Wigler, M. (1984). *Cell 37*: 437–445.
42. Toda, T., Uno, I., Ishikawa, T., Powers, S., Kataoka, T., Broek, D., Cameron, S., Broach, J., Matsumoto, K., and Wigler, M. (1985). *Cell 40*: 27–36.
43. Fukui, Y., Kozasa, T., Kaziro, Y., Takeda, T., and Yamamoto, M., (1986). *Cell 44*: 329–336.
44. Birchmeier, C., Broek, D., and Wigler, M. (1985). *Cell 43*: 615–621.
45. Beckner, S. K., Hattori, S., and Shih, T. Y. (1985). *Nature 317*: 71–72.
46. Fleischman, L. F., Chahwala, S. B., and Cantley, L. (1986). *Science 231*: 407–410.
47. Wakelam, M. J. O., Davies, S. A., Houslay, M. D., McKay, I., Marshall, C. J., and Hall, A. (1986). *Nature 323*: 173–176.

48. Bar-Sagi, D., and Feramisco, J. R. (1986). *Science 223*: 1061–1068.
49. Mulcahy, L. S., Smith, M. R., and Stacey, D. W. (1985). *Nature 313*: 241–243.
50. Papageorge, A. G., Willumsen, B. M., Johnsen, M., Kung, H.-F., Stacey, D. W., Vass, W. C., and Lowy, D. R. (1986). *Mol. Cell. Biol. 6*: 1843–1846.
51. Tabin, C. J., Bradley, S. M., Bargmann, C. I., Weinberg, R. A., Papageorge, A. G., Scolnick, E. M., Dhar, R., Lowy, D. R., and Chang, E. H. (1982). *Nature 300*: 143–149.
52. Reddy, E. P., Reynolds, R. K., Santos, E., Barbacid, M., (1982). *Nature 300*: 149–152.
53. Taparowsky, E., Suard, Y., Fasano, O., Shimizu, K., Goldfarb, M., and Wigler, M. (1982). *Nature 300*: 762–765.
54. Seeburg, P. H., Colby, W. W., Capon, D. J., Goeddel, D. V., and Levinson, A. D. (1984). *Nature 312*: 71–75.
55. McCormick, F., Clark, B. F., la Cour, T. F., Kjeldgaard, M., Norskov-Lauritsen, L., and Nyborg, J. (1985). *Science 230*: 78–82.
56. Chipperfield, R. G., Johnes, S. S., Lo, K.-M., Weinberg, R. A. (1985). *Mol. Cell. Biol. 5*: 1809–1818.
57. Fasano, O, Aldrich, T., Tamanoi, F., Taparowsky, E., Furth, M., and Wigler, M. (1984). *Proc. Natl. Acad. Sci. U.S.A. 81*: 4008–4012.
58. Bos, J. L., Toksov, D., Marshall, C. J., Verlaan-de Vries, M., Veeneman, G. H., van der Eb, A. J., van Boom, J. H., Janssen, J. W., and Steenvoorden, A. C. (1985). *Nature 315*: 726–730.
59. Yuasa, Y., Srivastava, S. K., Dunn, C. Y., Rhim, J. S., Reddy, E. P., and Aaronson, S. A., (1983). *Nature 303*: 775–779.
60. Taparowsky, E., Shimizu, K., Goldfarb, M., and Wigler, M. (1983). *Cell 34*: 581–586.
61. Brown, R., Marshall, C. J., Pennie, S. G., and Hall, A. (1984). *EMBO J. 3*: 1321–1326.
62. Der, C. J., Finkel, T., and Cooper, G. M. (1986). *Cell 44*: 167–176.
63. Dhar, R., Ellis, R. W., Shih, T. Y., Oroszlan, S., Shapiro, B., Maizel, J., Lowy, D, and Scolnick, E. (1982). *Science 217*: 934–936.
64. Tsuchida, M., Ohtsubo, E., and Ryder, T. (1982). *Science 217*: 937–939.
65. Walter, M., Clark, S. G., and Levinson, A. D. (1986). *Science 223*: 649–652.
66. Sigal, I. S., Gibbs, J. B., D'Alonzo, J. S., Temeles, G. L., Wolanski, B. S., Socher, S. H., and Scolnick, E. M. (1986). *Proc. Natl. Acad. Sci. U.S.A. 83*: 952–956.
67. Land, H., Parada, L. F., and Weinberg, R. A. (1983). *Nature 304*: 596–602.
68. Ruley, H. E. (1983). *Nature 304*: 602–606.
69. Newbold, R. F., and Overell, R. W. (1983). *Nature 304*: 648–651.
70. Pozzatti, R., Muschel, R., Williams, J., Padmanabhan, R., Howard, B., Liotta, L., and Khoury, G. (1986). *Science 232*: 223–227.
71. Spandidos, D. A., and Wilkie, N. M. (1984). *Nature 310*: 469–475.
72. Sager, R., Tanaka, K., Lau, C. C., Ebina, Y., and Anisowicz, A. (1983). *Proc. Natl. Acad. Sci. U.S.A. 80*: 7601–7605.

73. Yoakum, G. H., Lechner, J. F., Gabrielson, E. W., Korba, B. E., Malan-Shibley, L., Willey, J. C., Valerio, M. G., Shamsuddin, A. M., Trump, B. F., and Harris, C. C. (1985). *Science 227*: 1174–1179.
74. Rhim, J. S., Jay, G., Arnstein, P., Price, F. M., Sanford, K. K., and Aaronson, S. A. (1985). *Science 227*: 1250–1252.
75. Pater, A., and Pater, M. M. (1986). *J. Virol. 58*: 680–683.
76. Namba, M., Nishitani, K., Fukushima, F., Kimoto, T., and Nose, K. (1986). *Int. J. Cancer 37*: 419–423.
77. Rhim, J. S., Cho, H. Y., Vernon, M. L., Arnstein, P., Huebner, R. J., and Gilden, R. V. (1975). *Int. J. Cancer 16*: 840–849.
78. Noda, M., Ko, M., Ogura, A., Liu, D. G., Amano, T., Takano, T., and Ikawa, Y. (1985). *Nature 318*: 73–75.
79. Bar-Sagi, D., and Feramisco, J. R. (1985). *Cell 42*: 841–848.
80. Guerrero, I., Wong, H., Pellicer, A., and Burstein, D. (1986). *J. Cell. Physiol. 129*: 71–76.
81. Hagag, N., Halegoua, S., and Viola, M. (1986). *Nature 319*: 680–682.
82. Weiss, R., Teich, N., Varmus, H., and Coffin, J. (eds.). In *RNA Tumor Viruses,* 2nd ed. vol. 1. Cold Spring Harbor, New York, Cold Spring Harbor Laboratory.
83. Tabin, C. J., and Weinberg, R. A. (1985). *J. Virol. 53*: 260–265.
84. Barbacid, M. (1986). In *Important Advances in Oncology 1986* (DeVita, V., Hellman, S., and Rosenberg, S. eds.). Philadelphia, Lippincott, pp. 3–22.
85. Bos, J. L., Fearon, E. R., Hamilton, S. R., Verlaan-de Vries, M., van Boom, J. H., van der Eb, A. J., and Vogelstein, B. (1987). *Nature 327*: 293–297.
86. Forrester, K., Almoguera, C., Han, K., Grizzle, W. E., and Perucho, M. (1987). *Nature 327*: 298–303.
87. Saiki, R. K., Schart, S., Faloona, F., Mullis, K. B., Horn, G. T., Erlich, H. A., Arnheim, N. (1985). *Science 230*: 1350–1354.
88. Winter, E., Yamamoto, F., Almoguera, C., and Perucho, M. (1985). *Proc. Natl. Acad. Sci. U.S.A. 82*: 7575–7579.
89. Hirai, H., Kobayashi, Y., Mano, H., Hagiwara, K., Maru, Y., Omine, M., Mizoguchi, H., Nishida, J., and Takaku, F. (1987). *Nature 327*: 430–432.
90. Slamon, D. J., deKernion, J. B., Verma, I. M., and Cline, M. J. (1984). *Science 224*: 256–262.
91. Spandidos, D. A., and Agnantis, N. J. (1984). *Anticancer Res. 4*: 269–272.
92. Spandidos, D. A., and Kerr, I. B. (1984). *Br. J. Cancer 49*: 681–688.
93. Gallick, G. E., Kurzrock, R., Kloetzer, W. S., Arlinghaus, R. B., and Gutterman, J. U. (1985). *Proc. Natl. Acad. Sci. U.S.A. 82*: 1795–1799.
94. Kurzrock, R., Gallick, G. E., and Gutterman, J. U. (1986). *Cancer Res. 46*: 1530–1534.
95. Tanaka, T., Slamon, D. J., Battifora, H., and Cline, M. J. (1986). *Cancer Res. 46*: 1465–1470.
96. Hand, P. H., Thor, A., Wunderlich, D., Muraro, R., Caruso, A., and Schlom, J. (1984). *Proc. Natl. Acad. Sci. U.S.A. 81*: 5527–5231.
97. Thor, A., Horan Hand, P., Wunderlich, D., Caruso, A., Muraro, R., and Schlom, J. (1984). *Nature 311*: 562–565.

98. Viola, M. V., Fromowitz, F., Oravez, S., Deb, S., and Schlom, J. (1985). *J. Exp. Med. 161*: 1213–1218.
99. Chang, E. H., Furth, M. E., Scolnick, E. M., and Lowy, D. R. (1982). *Nature 297*: 479–483.
100. Pulciani, S., Santos, E., Long, L. K., Sorrentino, V., and Barbacid, M. (1985). *Mol. Cell. Biol. 5*: 2836–2841.
101. Fujita, J., Srivastava, S. K., Kraus, M. H., Rhim, J. S., Tronick, S. R., and Aaronson, S. A. (1985). *Proc. Natl. Acad. Sci. U.S.A. 82*: 3849–3853.
102. Yokota, J., Tsunetsugu-Yokota, Y., Battifora, H., LeFevre, C., and Cline, M. J. (1986). *Science 231*: 261–265.
103. Goyette, M., Petropoulos, C. J., Shank, P. R., and Fausto, N. (1983). *Science 219*: 510–512.
104. Sukumar, S., Notario, V., Martin-Zanca, D., and Barbacid, M. (1983). *Nature 306*: 658–661.
105. Zarbl, H., Sukumar, S., Arthur, A. V., Martin-Zanca, D., and Barbacid, M. (1985). *Nature 315*: 382–385.
106. Sukumar, S., Perantoni, A., Reed, C., Rice, J. M., and Wenk, M. L. (1986). *Mol. Cell. Biol. 6*: 2716–2720.
107. Stowers, S. J., Glover, P. L., Reynolds, S. H., Boone, L. R., Maronpot, R. R., and Anderson, M. W. (1987). *Cancer Res. 47*: 3212–3219.
108. McMahon, G., Hanson, L., Lee, J. J., and Wogan, G. N. (1986). *Proc. Natl. Acad. Sci. U.S.A. 83*: 9418–9422.
109. Sawey, M. J., Hood, A. T., Burns, F. J., and Garte, S. J. (1987). *Mol. Cell. Biol. 7*: 932–935.
110. Balmain, A., and Pragnell, I. B. (1983). *Nature 303*: 72–74.
111. Balmain, A., Ramsden, M., Bowden, G. T., and Smith, J. (1984). *Nature 307*: 658–660.
112. Bizub, D., Wood, A. W., and Skalka, A. M. (1986) *Proc. Natl. Acad. Sci. U.S.A. 83*: 6048–6052.
113. Dandekar, S., Sukumar, S., Zarbl, H., Young, L. J., and Cardiff, R. D. (1986). *Mol. Cell. Biol. 6*: 4104–4108.
114. Guerrero, I., Calzada, P., Mayer, A., and Pellicer, A. (1986). *Proc. Natl. Acad. Sci. U.S.A. 81*: 202–205.
115. Eva, A., and Trimmer, R. W. (1986). *Carcinogenesis 7*: 1931–1933.
116. Eva, A., and Aaronson, S. A. (1983). *Science 220*: 955–956.
117. Reynolds, S. H., Stowers, S. J., Maronpot, R. R., Anderson, M. W., and Aaronson, S. A. (1986). *Proc. Natl. Acad. Sci. U.S.A. 83*: 33–37.
118. Wiseman, R. W., Stowers, S. J., Miller, E. C., Anderson, M. W., and Miller, J. A. (1986). *Proc. Natl. Acad. Sci. U.S.A. 83*: 5825–5829.
119. Singer, B., and Kusmierek, J. T. (1982). *Ann. Rev. Biochem. 51*: 655–693.
120. Eadie, J. S., Conrad, M., Toorchen, D., and Topal, M. D. (1984). *Nature 308*: 201–203.
121. Loechler, E. L., Green, C. L., and Essigmann, J. M. (1984). *Proc. Natl. Acad. Sci. U.S.A. 81*: 6271–6275.
122. Bigger, C. A., Sawicki, J. T., Blake, D. M., Ramond, L. G., and Dipple, A. (1983). *Cancer Res. 43*: 5647–5651.

123. Quintanilla, M., Brown, K., Ramsden, M., and Balmain, A. (1986). *Nature 322*: 78–80.
124. Bichara, M., and Fuchs, R. P. (1985). *J. Mol. Biol. 183*: 341–351.
125. Foster, P. L., Eisenstadt, E., and Miller, J. H. (1983). *Proc. Natl. Acad. Sci. U.S.A. 80*: 2695–2698.
126. Welsch, C. W. (1985). *Cancer Res. 45*: 3415–3443.
127. Van Duuren, B. L., Sivak, A., Katz, C., Seidman, I., and Melchionne, S. (1975). *Cancer Res. 35*: 502–505.
128. Brown, K., Quintanilla, M., Ramsden, M., Kerr, I. B., Young, S., and Balmain, A. (1986). *Cell 46*: 447–456.
129. Roop, D. R., Lowy, D. R., Tambourin, P. E., Strickland, J., Harper, J. R., Balaschak, M., Spangler, E. F., and Yuspa, S. H. (1986). *Nature 323*: 822–824.
130. Andres, A. C., Schonenberger, C. A., Groner, B., Henninghausen, L., LeMeur, M., and Gerlinger, P. (1987). *Proc. Natl. Acad. Sci. U.S.A. 84*: 1299–1303.
131. Sinn, E., Muller, W., Pattengale, P., Tepler, I., Wallace, R., and Leder, P. (1987). *Cell 49*: 465–475.
132. Quaife, C. J., Pinkert, C. A., Ornitz, D. M., Palmiter, R. D., and Brinster, R. L. (1987). *Cell 48*: 1023–1034.
133. Stewart, T. A., Pattengale, P. K., and Leder, P. (1984). *Cell 38*: 627–637.

FIVE

Activation of Proto-Oncogenes Coding for Growth Factors or Growth Factor Receptors

Bengt Westermark
University of Uppsala
Uppsala, Sweden

Carl-Henrik Heldin
Ludwig Institute for Cancer Research
Uppsala, Sweden

INTRODUCTION

Studies of polypeptide growth factors and their receptors and mechanism of action have been particularly rewarding during the last years as they have provided important information, both on normal growth control and the molecular processes involved in transformation and neoplastic development. The first indication of a direct molecular link between normal mitogenesis and transformation was provided by the finding that the epidermal growth factor (EGF) receptor catalyzes tyrosine phosphorylation when activated by its ligand (Ushiro and Cohen, 1980); shortly previous to this finding, the transforming gene product of Rous sarcoma virus, pp60$^{v\text{-}src}$, was found to be a tyrosine-specific protein kinase (Hunter and Sefton, 1980).

Subsequent studies which demonstrated that also the platelet-derived growth factor (PDGF) receptor is endowed with a tyrosine kinase activity (Ek et al., 1982) further strengthened the notion of tyrosine phosphorylation as a common denominator of normal growth stimulation and transformation.

Direct evidence for a link between normal mitogenesis and transformation was provided by the finding of a structural homology between the B chain of PDGF and p28^{sis} of simian sarcoma virus (SSV) (Devare et al., 1983; Doolittle et al., 1983; Waterfield et al., 1983). Subsequent to this finding, the normal cellular homologues of a number of retroviral oncogenes have been identified as structural genes for proteins which are proven or thought to have a role in mitogenesis. The corresponding oncogenes products are therefore thought to cause transformation by subverting the mitogenic pathway (Heldin and Westermark, 1984; Heldin et al., 1987).

Acutely transforming retroviruses have provided an enormously valuable source of information on the structure and function of oncogenes; their role in the development of naturally occurring cancer is, however, infinitesimal. In "spontaneous" neoplasia, other genetic mechanisms, such as point mutation, rearrangement, and amplification, operate in the conversion of proto-oncogenes to transforming elements. In this chapter, we will focus on the transforming potential of genes encoding growth factors and their receptors.

GROWTH FACTORS AS TRANSFORMING PROTEINS

Temin (1967) was one of the first to consider the possibility that autonomous growth of transformed cells may be attributed to self-stimulation by an endogenous growth factor. This idea was later revived by Todaro and collaborators, and has become known as the autocrine concept of cell growth (Sporn and Todaro, 1980), which is generally thought to be one of the causes of unrestrained growth of tumor cells in vitro and in vivo.

Evidence for autocrine mechanisms in transformation and tumorigenesis remained circumstantial for a long time, as the concept was largely based on findings of growth factors in conditioned media of tumor cells. A more stringent demonstration of autocrine stimulation requires direct proof for the coexpression of a growth factor and its cognate receptor, and conclusive evidence has to be based on a growth inhibitory effect of specific antagonists, such as growth factor antibodies or receptor-blocking antibodies. In fact, many types of transformed cells have been shown to produce growth-promoting factors. Not as many have been shown to coexpress the corresponding receptor, and even fewer have been shown to be mitogenically stimulated by an autocrine pathway. Finally, in only a minority of cases, an autocrine growth stimulation is a proven part of the transformation process per se.

Platelet-Derived Growth Factor and the c-*sis* Proto-Oncogene

Human PDGF is an M_r 30,000 protein made up as dimers of A and B chains (Johnsson et al., 1982) which are encoded by separate genes (Betsholtz et al., 1986a; Swan et al., 1982). Because of the extensive amino acid sequence homology between the two chains (Johnsson et al., 1984; Betsholtz et al., 1986a), the genes have apparently evolved through duplication of a common ancestral gene. The possible evolutionary advantage of the development of two closely related PDGF chains is poorly understood. As will also be apparent below, all three possible dimers (AA, AB, BB) appear to occur naturally and seem to bind to PDGF receptors; however, with some possible differences in biological activity. Human platelet PDGF is probably assembled as a heterodimer, although the presence of homodimers has not been ruled out (Hammacher et al., 1988). Porcine PDGF is a homodimer of peptides, closely related to the human B chain (Stroobant and Waterfield, 1984), whereas the factors found in the conditioned media of various cell types in culture in general have been identified as homodimers of A chains (see below).

The transforming potential of the B chain of PDGF became apparent through the finding of a structural homology with the v-*sis* oncogene product $p28^{sis}$ of simian sarcoma virus (Devare et al., 1983; Doolittle et al., 1983; Johnsson et al., 1984; Waterfield et al., 1983) such that the B chain sequence is essentially identical to the mid portion of $p28^{sis}$. Molecular cloning of the human proto-oncogene c-*sis* from complementary deoxyribonucleic acid (cDNA) libraries (Collins et al., 1985; Josephs et al., 1984a) and genomic libraries (Chiu et al., 1984; Johnsson et al., 1984; Rao et al., 1986) clearly established an identity with the structural gene encoding a PDGF B chain precursor. The oncogene of yet another retrovirus; namely, Parodi-Irgens feline sarcoma virus, has also been found to be a transduced version of c-*sis* (Besmer et al., 1983).

A body of evidence has been presented in favor of the notion that SSV transformation in culture is mediated by a PDGF-like growth factor that stimulates the growth of the infected cells by an autocrine mechanism (reviewed by Westermark et al., 1987). The primary translation product $p28^{sis}$ is thus dimerized and trimmed in both ends to yield an apparently stable end product ($p24^{sis}$) (Robbins et al., 1983) which is structurally very similar to a homodimer of PDGF B chains. Moreover, lysates (Deuel et al., 1983) and conditioned media (Johnsson et al., 1985) of SSV-transformed cells contain PDGF-like activity. The autocrine hypothesis is further strengthened by the target cell specificity of SSV; the virus seems only to transform PDGF-responsive cells (Leal et al., 1985). Finally, SSV-transformation can be blocked and reverted by specific and nonspecific PDGF antagonists, such as PDGF antibodies (Johnsson et al., 1985) or suramin, (Betsholtz et al. 1986b) the latter being a chemical agent that displaces PDGF from its receptor (Williams et al., 1984).

A transforming potential of the human c-*sis* gene has been shown in transfection experiments using NIH 3T3 cells as recipients. In such experiments, constructs have been made using either genomic (Gazit et al., 1984) or cDNA (Clarke et al., 1984; Josephs et al., 1984b) sequences placed under the control of viral promoters. This finding raises the important question whether an unscheduled expression of the c-*sis*/PDGF B chain gene (or the A chain gene) is involved in the genesis of "spontaneous" tumors. Several human sarcoma and glioma cell lines which are presumably derived from PDGF-responsive tissues have been found to produce PDGF-like growth factors (Betsholtz et al., 1983, 1986a; Heldin et al., 1980, 1986; Nist′ er et al., 1984, 1986, 1988a; Pantazis et al., 1985). The growth factors produced by osteosarcoma (Heldin et al., 1986), melanoma (Westermark et al., 1986), and glioma (Hammacher et al., submitted) cells were purified to homogeneity and were all found to be homodimers of PDGF A chains, irrespective of the fact that both the A and B chain genes were found to be expressed at the messenger ribonucleic acid (mRNA) level in the osteosarcoma (Betsholtz et al., 1986a) and glioma (Nistér et al., 1988a) cell lines. Concordant results have been obtained by immunoprecipitation of lysates and conditioned media of metabolically labeled cells.

Although the bulk of PDGF-like growth factor secreted by tumor cells is thus constituted by A chain homodimers, traces of B chain–containing material have been found in the conditioned medium of glioma cells (Hammacher et al., submitted); whether this is in the form of B chain homodimers (i.e., homologous to the product of SSV-transformed cells) or assembled as heterodimers (like platelet PDGF) is not known. It thus seems as if the c-*sis*/B chain mRNA is indeed translated in glioma cells albeit with a low net efficiency. In this context, it is interesting that the c-*sis* transcripts contains three AUGs in the 5′ untranslated region (Collins et al., 1985; Rao et al., 1986). These could possibly have a regulatory function and repress translation (c.f. Kozak, 1986; Mueller and Hinebusch, 1986). Indeed, deletion of these sequences increases the rate of translation in an in vitro system (Collins and Pober, 1986). It is noteworthy that the entire first exon, where the corresponding ATGs are located, is deleted in v-*sis* (Devare et al., 1983; Rao et al., 1986). This structural alteration may thus increase the translation efficiency of the v-*sis* mRNA compared to the c-*sis* transcript, and thereby contribute to the transforming activity of SSV.

Although the A chain homodimer purified from glioma cells binds to the PDGF receptor on fibroblasts, it is considerably less mitogenic on these cells than PDGF (Nistér et al., 1988b), whereas the B chain–containing material purified from the same cells was found to display a high mitogenic activity. This finding is the first indication of a functional difference between the possible dimeric forms of PDGF-related molecules, the physiological implication of which remains to be elucidated.

The actual role of PDGF-like growth factors in the pathogenesis of spontaneous tumors is as yet poorly understood. The putative autocrine loop was dissected in U-2 OS osteosarcoma cells, which have been found to express PDGF receptor mRNA (Levéen et al., in preparation) and to display high-affinity PDGF receptors (Betsholtz et al., 1984; Graves et al., 1985) which are functional inasmuch as they become autophosphorylated upon binding of PDGF (Betsholtz et al., 1984). Moreover, a 115-kd cellular component in U-2OS cells was found to be constitutively phosphorylated on tyrosine residues, which may be taken as a sign of constitutive receptor activation; a similar component is phosphorylated in normal cells only after PDGF stimulation (Ek and Heldin, 1984). However, the addition of PDGF antibodies to U-2 OS cells has no effect on their growth rate in serum-free medium, in contrast to the effect on SSV-transformed fibroblasts. Studies on other sarcoma or glioma cells that concomitantly express a PDGF-like growth factor and PDGF receptors have given the same results. These findings do not immediately invalidate the autocrine hypothesis in the pathogenesis of sarcoma and glioma. It is possible that an autocrine growth stimulation is an early event in tumor development and that subsequent changes in the cell genome abolish the requirement for the endogenously produced factors (see also below). Notably, PDGF antibodies have no or only marginal effect on the growth rate of serially passaged SSV-transformed immortalized cell lines (Huang et al., 1984) in contrast to the marked effect on acutely transformed human diploid fibroblasts (Johnsson et al., 1985).

Expression of the genes encoding the subunits of PDGF and the production of PDGF-like growth factors may also occur in tumor cells that do not express PDGF receptors, such as melanoma cells (Westermark et al., 1986), mammary carcinoma cells (Perez et al., 1987; Rozengurt et al., 1985), lung carcinoma cells (Betsholtz et al., 1987), and certain glioma cells (Nistér et al., 1986, 1988a). In these instances, the role of the produced factor in vivo may be to mediate stroma development.

Transforming Growth Factor-α

Transforming growth factor-α (TGF-α) is a member of the epidermal growth factor (EGF) family of mitogens, with an about 40% sequence similarity with EGF (Marquardt et al., 1983, 1984). It is produced by certain retrovirus-transformed cells (DeLarco and Todaro, 1978; Ozanne et al., 1980; Todaro et al., 1979; Twardzik et al., 1982, 1983). In these cases, cellular TGF-α production is controlled by the retroviral oncogene product (*abl, mos, fes, ras*), and is thus not a product of the oncogene per se. Transforming growth factor–α production may also occur in cells transformed by DNA viruses (Kaplan and Ozanne, 1982; Ozanne et al., 1980) and cell lines established from human tumors (Derynck et al., 1984; Nistér et al., 1988; Todaro et al., 1980). The factor binds to the EGF receptor (Carpenter et al., 1983; Reynolds et al., 1981) and induces autophosphorylation of the receptor (Pike et al., 1982). Most, if not all, of the cellular effects of TGF-α are probably mediated via the EGF receptor. The term "transforming" growth factor–α is somewhat of a misnomer, and is based on its ability to provoke anchorage independent growth of certain cells in synergy with TGF-β (Anzano et al., 1983; Derynck et al., 1984). Such an effect is also exerted by EGF in cooperation with TGF-β, and probably represents a physiological function.

The role of TGF-α in virus transformation and tumorigenesis is enigmatic, and no successful attempts to block the growth of transformed cells by interfering with the autocrine loop have been presented. Circumstantial evidence for an autocrine receptor activation have been obtained using cells transformed by temperature-sensitive mutants of Moloney and Kirsten sarcoma virus (Kaplan et al., 1982; Todaro et al., 1979). Binding of EGF at the permissive temperature is markedly reduced, implying that the endogenously produced growth factor causes a blockade and down-regulation of the EGF receptors; at this temperature, the cells have a low serum requirement and do not respond to exogenous EGF. At the nonpermissive temperature, the cells bind and respond to exogenously added EGF. Although this finding clearly shows that TGF-α production is regulated by the oncogene product, it cannot be taken as an indication of an autocrine stimulation as a mechanism of transformation. This question was addressed by McKay et al. (1986), who found that *ras* transformation is independent of the expression of functional EGF receptors, as it occurs even in cells that constitutively lack EGF receptors.

Whereas studies on virus-transformed and spontaneously transformed cells have given no indication of a mechanistic role of TGF-α in transformation, studies of genetic transfer of TGF-α or EGF expression vectors have shown that an autocrine EGF receptor activation may to some extent confer transforming properties on suitable recipients. Transfer of a TGF-α cDNA sequence under the control of the simian vacuolating virus (SV40) early promoter into Rat 1 cells gave rise to growth factor–independent clones, the anchorage independent growth of which was inhibited by TGF-α

antibodies (Rosenthal et al., 1986). These cells also formed small tumor nodules when transplanted into athymic mice. Similar results were obtained using retrovirus constructs containing a synthetic gene encoding TGF-α (Watanabe et al., 1987) or EGF (Stern et al., 1987).

Whereas TGF-α is commonly found to be produced by tumor cells, EGF production has only been found in a salivary gland adenocarcinoma cell line, in which it probably only represents a normal cell trait (Sato et al., 1985).

Fibroblast Growth Factor and Related Oncogenes (*hst, int*-2)

Two forms of fibroblast growth factor (FGF) have been purified; namely, acidic FGF and basic FGF (Gospodarowicz et al., 1986). The two factors are extensively homologous and show the same repertoire of biological responses, and are likely to exert their function via the same receptor. Acidic as well as basic FGF has been isolated from a variety of sources, including tumor cells. Because of its mitogenic activity on endothelial cells in culture and angiogenic effect in vivo (Folkman and Klagsbrun, 1987), tumor cell-derived FGF is thought to be part of the tumor angiogenesis factor, the production of which is considered to be a prerequisite for neovascularization of the tumor tissue. Although this may be an important function of FGF, it is likewise possible that the factor mediates an autocrine growth response in the producing tumor cell. Thus, human glioma cells have recently been found to produce acidic FGF in culture and to be responsive to exogenous FGF (Libermann et al., 1987). A similar situation prevails in the rhabdomyosarcoma cell line A-204 (Schweigerer et al., 1987), which produces basic FGF to which they also respond. Conceivably, tumor cell-derived FGF may have the dual function of stimulating the producer cells by an autocrine mechanism as well as inducing neovascularization of the tumor by a paracrine route.

Interestingly, two oncogenes have recently been found to encode proteins with an amino acid sequence homology to FGF. The oncogene *hst* was identified in the DNA of a human gastric cancer through its ability to induce focus formation in NIH 3T3 cells in gene transfer experiments (Sakamoto et al., 1986). The cDNA nucleotide sequence predicts a peptide with an about 40% amino acid sequence homology with basic FGF (Taira et al., 1987). As the predicted translation product has a leader peptide, these data indicate that the transforming protein of *hst* is a secreted FGF-like factor. Recently, the predicted protein product of *int*-2 also has been found to have an extensive amino acid sequence homology with basic FGF (Dickson and Peters, 1987). By inference from the FGF-like structure of their products, both *hst* and *int*-2 may thus be assumed to transform cells via an autocrine mechanism, and thus belong to the same functional category of oncogenes as *sis*.

Bombesin as a Mediator of Autocrine Stimulation of Growth in Small Cell Lung Carcinoma

Human small cell lung carcinoma cells secrete (Moody et al., 1981; Wood et al., 1981) and respond (Weber et al., 1985) to bombesinlike peptides. Evidence for a function of bombesinlike peptides as autocrine growth factors was presented by Cuttitta et al. (1985). A monclonal antibody directed against the C-terminal of bombesin was found to inhibit the growth of some small cell lung carcinoma cell lines in culture and to abolish their growth as xenografts in athymic mice. The results of Cuttitta et al. (1985) have, however, not been confirmed or extended. Probably, an autocrine state only represents a transient feature along the progression of small cell lung carcinoma which is overridden by other events, such as c-*myc* amplification (Little et al., 1983). It is remarkable that several of the xenografted animals in the study of Cuttitta et al. (1985) developed progressively growing tumors in the presence of antibodies. This phenomenon probably reflects a progression into a nonautocrine malignant phenotype (see below).

Interleukins and Colony-Stimulating Factors

A number of growth factors with defined target cell specificities in the bone marrow and in the lymphoid organ have been identified, isolated, and molecularly cloned. This group of growth factors include colony-stimulating factors and interleukins. Although there is so far no example of an oncogene that encodes an interleukin or a colony-stimulating factor, it is becoming increasingly clear that an aberrant expression of such growth factors may play a role in the genesis of leukemias and lymphomas. As a complete review is beyond the scope of this chapter, this field of research will be highlighted by a few representative examples.

Human interleukin-2 (IL-2) (TCGF) is a major stimulus to T-cell proliferation (Cantrell and Smith, 1984; Taniguchi et al., 1986). A transient coexpression of IL-2 and its receptor is a physiological event in antigen-stimulated T cells. Exogenously added IL-2 promotes long-term growth of normal as well as of human T-cell leukemia type I (HTLV I)–transformed T cells in culture (Gootenberg et al., 1981; Morgan et al., 1976). Human T-cell leukemia type I–transformed cell lines may progress to IL-2 independence upon long-term culture, most likely as a function of an autocrine production of IL-2 (Gootenberg et al., 1981). However, as some IL-2 independent HTLV I–transformed T-cell lines lack expression of IL-2 (Arya et al., 1984), nonautocrine mechanisms for growth factor independence also must exist. Further evidence for an involvement of an IL-2–dependent autocrine stimulation of neoplastic T cells has been derived from studies on the human T-cell lymphoma cell line IARC 301 (Duprez et al., 1985), and on T-cell leukemia cells in primary culture (Arima et al., 1986). In both instances, a blockade of the autocrine pathway resulted in growth retardation.

The question whether transformed B cells may be subject to autostimulation by B-cell growth factors has been addressed by Gordon et al. 1984a,b; 1985. The impetus for these studies was the finding that B cells transformed by Epstein-Barr virus (EBV) do not require exogenous growth factors unless growing in diluted cultures. An autostimulatory factor can indeed be harvested from the conditioned medium of such cells (Blazar et al., 1983; Gordon et al., 1984a). Although this factor has not been characterized, it is probably a B-cell growth factor proper, since conditioned medium of EBV-transformed cells can also stimulate primed B cells (Gordon et al., 1984b). A survey of B lymphocytic cell lines in culture showed that the production of B-cell growth factors is a common phenomenon (Gordon et al., 1985). However, the tumor-derived cell lines differed from EBV-transformed lymphoblastoid cells in their total or partial lack of requirement for their own growth factor.

Normal hematopoiesis requires and is regulated by growth factors. These are collectively called colony-stimulating factors (CSF) because they have been identified by their ability to support clonal growth on bone marrow cells in semisolid media (Metcalf, 1985). Only rarely does autocrine stimulation by CSF:s seem to be involved in the pathogenesis of "spontaneous" leukemia; studies on myeloid leukemia cells in culture have shown that they are in general as dependent on the addition of exogenous CSF as normal myeloid cells (reviewed by Gough, 1986; Metcalf, 1985). The finding of an autocrine response to CSF in acute myeloblastic leukemia (Young and Griffin, 1986) may thus be regarded as an exception to the rule.

Experimental manipulation of myeloid cells in culture may, however, convert them from a nonautocrine, nontumorigenic to an autocrine, tumorigenic state. This may occur by spontaneous mutation of long-term cultured normal bone marrow cells (Schrader and Crapper, 1983), or experimentally by introducing a suitable CSF cDNA expression vector into immortal cell lines (Laker et al., 1987; Lang et al., 1985). In the study by Lang et al. (1985), a recombinant retrovirus encoding granulocyte-macrophage-CSF (GM-CSF) was used to infect a factor-dependent promyelocytic cell line. Expression of the GM-CSF cDNA vector resulted in factor secretion, autonomous growth in culture, and tumorigenicity.

Surprisingly, the growth of these cells in culture could not be inhibited by GM-CSF antibodies. Using another GM-CSF cDNA recombinant retrovirus, Laker et al. (1987) have recently shown that the total emancipation of growth factor requirement probably occurs in two steps, the first through a true autocrine stimulation (which can be blocked by antibodies), and the second probably through secondary, mutational events which cause an abolition of growth factor dependence by a nonautocrine mechanism.

Mechanisms of Growth Factor Gene Activation in Transformed Cells

There is a growing understanding that autocrine growth stimulation does not only occur in transformed cells, but is also a physiological growth stimulatory pathway. The coexpression of a growth factor and its cognate receptor is in these cases tightly controlled and is likely to occur only as a transient phenomenon in a proliferative phase in the development of a specific cell lineage. Typical examples are found in the immune system, in which autocrine loops are involved in the expansion of antigen-stimulated lymphocytes. An interesting finding is that growth factors may induce a transient expression of their own genes in nontransformed cells: PDGF induces PDGF A chain synthesis (Paulsson et al., 1987), and TGF-α induces production of TGF-α. This phenomenon may reflect a positive autocrine feedback loop in growth stimulation.

When we discuss the pathogenetic role of an autocrine loop in transformation and tumorigenesis and the mechanism by which its occurs, the following two possibilities have to be considered:

1. The coordinate expression of a growth factor and its receptor is a normal feature of the progenitor cell in which it occurs as a developmentally regulated phenomenon. The autocrine loop simply persists in the transformed cell and may or may not be of importance for its proliferative capacity. Even if self-stimulation occurs in the transformed cell, it is to be considered a result of transformation rather than the cause of it.
2. The coordinate expression of a growth factor and its receptor is an unscheduled phenomenon and constitutes an important feature of the transformed phenotype. An autocrine stimulation may also in this case be a feature of the normal progenitor cell. In contrast to point 1 above, lack of down-regulation of the autocrine pathway, e.g., through mutations in the growth factor gene itself, is a direct cause of transformation rather than the result of it.

In a few cases, a defined genetic alteration has been found to be the cause of an unscheduled growth factor synthesis in transformed cells. The only example of a retrovirally transduced growth factor gene is v-*sis*, which is found as an oncogene in SSV and in a strain of feline sarcoma virus (see above). Activation of a growth factor gene by insertional mutagenesis is also a rare phenomenon. A nearby insertion of retroviral DNA is probably the cause of the constitutive expression of the IL-3 gene in WEHI-3B leukemia cells (Ymer et al., 1985), and the activation of the IL-2 gene in a T-cell lymphoma cell line (Chen et al., 1985). Moreover, the putative growth factor gene *int*-2 is activated by the insertion of mouse mammary tumor virus (MMTV) proviral DNA (Nusse, 1986).

In the aforementioned cases, normal regulatory functions are lost and the growth factor gene expression is driven by *cis*-acting retroviral elements (promoters/enhancers), whereas a *trans*-activating mechanism is likely to be involved in the expression of IL-2 and IL-2 receptors in HTLV-transformed cells. Thus, the tat_{II} gene (of HTLV-II) induces a coexpression of IL-2 and IL-2 receptors when transferred into Jurkat T-lymphoma cells (Greene et al., 1986). A *trans*-activation mechanism of unknown nature is also likely to be involved in the expression of TGF-α in cells transformed by *abl, mos, fes,* and *ras* (see above). Similarly, autocrine production of chicken myelomonocytic growth factor is induced by the v-*src* and v-*mil* oncogenes (Adkins et al., 1984; Graf et al., 1986; von Weizäcker et al., 1986) Analogous mechanisms may also operate in B-cell growth factor-producing EBV-transformed cells (Gordon et al., 1984a).

In the vast majority of cases, constitutive growth factor synthesis in tumor cells has been found to occur without any noticeable changes in gene structure or gene dosage. In those instances, it may be impossible to determine whether growth factor production is reminiscent of the phenotype of the normal progenitor cell, or if it is directly involved in the transformation process, perhaps through a subtle change in gene structure or gene control. Studies on the production of PDGF-like growth factors in tumor cells may exemplify this matter. In no instance has the expression of the PDGF B chain/c-*sis* or A chain gene has been shown to be associated with rearrangement or an amplification of the PDGF B chain/c-*sis* or A chain gene (Nistér et al., 1988a, and unpublished observations).

We also know that the genes are constitutively expressed or inducible in several systems of nontransformed cells. The function of such cellularly produced PDGF may either be to stimulate cell growth by an autocrine mechanism, when produced by a responsive cell, or to stimulate responsive bystanders when produced by a cell that lacks PDGF receptors. Placental cytotrophoblasts (Goustin et al., 1985) and vascular smooth muscle cells (Nilsson et al., 1985; Seifert et al., 1984; Sejersen et al., 1986) belong to the former group, whereas endothelial cells (Barrett et al., 1985; Collins et al., 1987) and macrophages (Martinet et al., 1986; Shimokado et al., 1985) are examples of the latter.

It is thus clear that we need much more information on the involvement of PDGF-like growth factors in autocrine stimulation of normal growth, its developmental control, and the molecular mechanism of PDGF gene expression in order to properly estimate findings in tumor cells. Similar arguments may, in fact, be raised with regard to any of the growth factors mentioned in the previous sections. Thus, TGF-α is normally expressed in embryonic tissue (Lee et al., 1985; Twardzik, 1985).

GROWTH FACTOR RECEPTORS AS TRANSFORMING PROTEINS

As discussed in previous chapters, the production of a growth factor in a cell that carries the cognate receptor will cause an autocrine loop which drives cell multiplication. Likewise, the expression of a growth factor receptor in a cell that has as its normal function the secretion of the corresponding growth factor, would result in autocrine stimulation of growth. While no such example is known today, there are several examples of perturbations of growth factor receptors leading to a constitutive activation in the absence of ligand.

Growth factor receptors are transmembrane proteins with an aminoterminal ligand-binding domain on the outside of the cell and a carboxyterminal effector domain facing the interior of the cell. Many growth factor receptors are endowed with protein tyrosine kinases which become activated after ligand binding (Table 1). The fact that also a number of oncogene products are protein tyrosine kinases indicates that tyrosine phosphorylation is important in cell growth (reviewed in Hunter and Cooper, 1985). Some oncogene products are clearly mutated versions of growth factor receptors, like *erb*B and *fms*, which correspond to the EGF receptor and the CSF-1 receptor, respectively. Others, like *neu, trk, ros, met, kit,* and *ret*, are most likely also derived from growth factor receptors, since they are transmembrane proteins with receptorlike structures (Table 1) (reviewed in Heldin et al., 1987).

There are, however, also tyrosine kinase oncogene products that are not derived from growth factor receptors, since their normal counterparts are not transmembrane proteins. Examples include *abl, fes/fps*, and the *src* family. The *src* family is a group of homologous proteins which show

Table 1 Protein Tyrosine Kinases

Genes encoding protein tyrosine kinases with transmembrane domain	Genes encoding protein tyrosine kinases without transmembrane domain
EGF receptor gene/*erb*B	*src*
CSF-1 receptor gene/*fms*	*yes*
PDGF receptor gene	*fgr*
insulin receptor gene	*hck*
IGF-I receptor gene	*lyn*
neu	*fyn*
trk	*lck*
met	*abl*
ros	*fes/fps*
ret	

For references, see text and Heldin et al. (1987).

specific tissue distributions. Since e.g., the *src* product in normal cells is mainly found in nonproliferating cell types, like neurons (Cotton and Brugge, 1983) and platelets (Golden et al., 1986), it is possible that the normal functions of the members of the *src* family are related to cell differentiation rather than to cell proliferation.

Activation of the tyrosine kinases of growth factor receptors induces autophosphorylation of the receptor as well as phosphorylation on tyrosine residues of specific cellular substrates (Hunter and Cooper, 1985). Such substrates may be involved in the mitogenic pathway. However, to date it has not been possible to link any tyrosine kinase substrate to such a function. Other cellular effects of growth factors include elevations of cytoplasmic pH and Ca^{2+} concentration, and expression of specific genes. The two former effects may be due to the stimulatory effect of certain growth factors on turnover of phosphatidylinositol, leading to the release of inositoltrisphosphate, which mobilizes Ca^{2+} from internal stores, and diacylglycerol, which activates protein kinase C. This protein kinase phosphorylates serine or threonine residues in certain substrates, e.g., the Na^+/H^+ carrier protein, leading to the extrusion of protons from the cell (reviewed by Rozengurt, 1986).

A constitutive activation of a growth factor receptor would lead to the continuous generation of the abovementioned signals in the absence of the corresponding ligand. Several different mechanisms for oncogene activation of growth factor receptor genes have been found (Table 2). Some oncogenes arise after deletion of regulatory domains of growth factor receptors, and there is at least one example of a truncated growth factor

Table 2 Mechanism of Activation of Growth Factor Receptorlike Oncogenes

Mechanisms	Examples
Truncation	*erb*B, *fms*
Point mutation	*neu*
Chimeric molecule	*trk, ret*
Amplification	*erb*B, *neu, met*
Insertional mutagenesis	*erb*B

For references, see text and Heldin et al. (1987).

receptor that has been fused to another protein yielding a chimeric product. Another oncogene carries a single point mutation which apparently locks the protein in a constitutivelly active form. There are also examples of anomalous expression of growth factor receptors after insertional mutagenesis and amplification of growth factor receptor genes. This may lead to the expression of too high levels of the receptor, which may trigger a mitogenic response either through a low background activity of each receptor, or through an extreme sensitivity to stimulation by low concentrations of ligand present in the cell environment. Some examples of growth factor receptorlike proteins as transforming proteins will be discussed below.

*erb*B/EGF Receptor

The EGF receptor is one of the most well-characterized growth factor receptors. Its entire amino acid sequence is known through cloned cDNA (Ullrich et al., 1984). The human receptor has 1186 amino acids, and is split into two approximately similar-sized parts by a hydrophobic membrane spanning region. The external ligand-binding domain contains two regions rich in cysteine residues. Similar cysteine-rich regions are found also in other receptors, e.g., the insulin (Ullrich et al., 1985) and insulinlike growth factor I (Ullrich et al., 1986) receptors. The internal domain contains a stretch of amino acids with homology to other tyrosine kinases, and tyrosine acceptor sites for autophosphorylation near the carboxyterminal. An indication that mutated forms of the EGF receptor can have transforming activity came from the observation of an amino acid sequence homology to the v-*erb*B product of avian erythroblastosis virus (AEV) (Downward et al., 1984).

In fact, AEV has aquired a part of the chicken EGF receptor, comprising a short external sequence and most of the internal part with the tyrosine kinase domain, but lacking a short stretch in the carboxyterminal, including the major autophosphorylation site (Ullrich et al., 1984; Yamamoto et al., 1983). The carboxyterminal deletion is of importance in the conversion of the normal growth factor receptor to a transforming protein. Thus, a chimaer of an intact extra cellular domain of the EGF receptor and the intracellular portion of the v-*erb*B product retains transforming potential (Ried et al., 1987). The absence of this, and possibly other, regulatory sequences results in an aberrant activation of the *erb*B product. It has been demonstrated that the *erb*B product has a constitutively active tyrosine kinase (Gilmore et al., 1985; Kris et al., 1985), which may be involved in a continuous and uncontrolled stimulation of cell growth.

Avian erythroblastosis virus carries two oncogenes, *erb*A and *erb*B (Frykberg et al., 1983), which cooperate in the transformation of chicken erythroblasts. The *erb*A product is homologous to the thyroxin receptor (Sap et al., 1986; Weinberger et al., 1986), and it is possible that the combination of perturbations of the erythroid differentiation process, via *erb*A, and of the mitogenic pathway of EGF, via *erb*B, gives a particularly powerful transforming effect on erythroblasts. This notion is supported by the finding that fibroblasts are much less dependent on *erb*A for transformation (Kahn et al., 1986).

Activation of the cellular EGF receptor gene may also occur by proviral integration. In a large number of cases of avian leukosis virus–induced erythroblastosis examined, most of the proviral integration sites were clustered within a few hundred bases in the middle of the EGF receptor gene, leading to the expression of a truncated receptor of similar size as the v-*erb*B product (Miles and Robinson, 1986; Nilsen et al., 1985; Raines et al., 1985). Interestingly, the *erb*B products of avian leukosis virus–induced leukemias appeared to contain intact carboxyterminals (Lax et al., 1985; Nilsen et al., 1985). Since these retroviruses were found to be inefficient in transforming fibroblasts (Beug et al., 1986), it is possible that the carboxyterminal truncation in the v-*erb*B product is important for the transformation of fibroblasts, but not required for erythroblast transformation.

There are several indications that the EGF receptor may be involved in the growth of human tumors. Thus, about 30% of human glioblastomas show overexpression of EGF receptors and amplification of the EGF receptor gene (Bigner et al., 1987; Libermann et al., 1985). No amplification of has been found in astrocytomas of higher differentiation grade.

How can the overexpression of a normal growth factor receptor contribute to excessive cell growth? Although the answer to this question is not known, there are several possibilities. Each receptor may have a low background activity in the absence of ligand, and an excess of receptor could then push the cell over the threshold for mitogenic stimulation. It is also likely that a cell with an excess of EGF receptors are more sensitive to stimulation by minute quantities of ligand that may be present in the environment. Alternatively, the tumor cells may produce a small amount of TGF-α, the autocrine response to which is augmented by an increased receptor number.

fms/CSF-1 Receptor

CSF-1 (also called M-CSF) stimulates growth and maturation of the macrophage cell lineage from hematopoietic stem cells (Stanley et al., 1983).

The CSF-1 receptor is of similar size as the EGF receptor, but differs slightly in its overall organization. Thus, the external domain does not contain any cluster of cysteine residues, but rather 10 evenly distributed cysteine residues (Coussens et al., 1986). In addition, the tyrosine kinase domain contains an insert without homology to other tyrosine kinases. Structurally, the CSF-1 receptor is most homologous to the PDGF receptor (Yarden et al., 1986).

By analogy with the EGF receptor gene, the CSF-1 receptor gene has also been transduced by a retrovirus (Sherr et al., 1985). The corresponding oncogene has been designated v-*fms*. It is translated into a *gag*-*fms* fusion product which is then cleaved to generate a v-*fms* glycoprotein of M_r 140,000 (Wheeler et al., 1986a). In contrast to the v-*erb*B product, the v-*fms* product seems to retain an intact ligand-binding domain. However, the carboxyterminal 40 amino acids in the CSF-1 receptor has been substituted by 11 unrelated residues in v-*fms*; a distal tyrosine residue (^{969}Tyr) found in the CSF-1 receptor, which constitute a potential autophosphorylation site, is thereby lacking in the v-*fms* protein (Coussens et al., 1986; Verbeek et al., 1985; Wheeler et al., 1986b). There is some experimental support for the assumption that the carboxyterminal truncation of the CSF-1 receptor is important for its activation to an oncogene, since replacement of the carboxyterminal end of v-*fms* with normal c-*fms* sequences reduces the transforming potential (Browning et al., 1986). Moreover, in cotransfection experiments with CSF-1 cDNA, a c-*fms* gene containing ^{969}Phe is more active than one containing the native ^{969}Tyr, implying an autoregulatory role of the C-terminal tyrosine residue (Roussel et al., 1987). As in the case of the v-*erb*B product, the tyrosine kinase activity of the v-*fms* product appears to be constitutive (Sacca et al., 1986). Based on the finding that v-*fms* induces factor independence in CSF-1–dependent macrophage cell lines, it has been suggested that the v-*fms* product provides growth stimulatory signals in the absence of ligand (Wheeler et al., 1986b).

neu

The *neu* oncogene was identified in neuroglioblastoma cell lines derived from intracranial tumors induced in rats by ethylnitrosourea. The *neu* product is a 185-kd receptorlike protein, which is structurally and immunologically related to the EGF receptor (Bargmann et al., 1986a; Coussens et al., 1985; Yamamoto et al., 1986). A potential ligand for the *neu* encoded protein has not been identified.

Interestingly, a single point mutation can covert c-*neu* to a transforming gene; e.g., a substitution of a valine residue in the transmembrane region to a glutamic acid (Bargmann et al., 1986b). This implies that the transmembrane region has a critical role in the transduction of the mitogenic signal from the ligand-binding external domain to the intracellular effector domain. It is possible that the introduction of a charged amino acid in this domain locks the receptor in a constitutively activated form.

Another mechanism of activation of *neu* involves amplification of the gene. This has been found in mammary carcinoma cell lines (King et al., 1985; Slamon et al., 1987) and in a salivary gland adenocarcinoma (Semba et al., 1985); in human mammary carcinomas amplification was seen in as many as 20% of the tumors (Slamon et al., 1987). As discussed for the EGF receptor above, it is conceivable that overexpression of a putative growth factor receptor can lead to excessive unregulated cell growth.

met

The *met* oncogene was identified in human osteosarcoma cells treated with the carcinogen methylnitrosurea (Cooper et al., 1984). The activation of *met* in this particular cell line is caused by gene rearrangement such that the 5′ end of the transforming gene consists of a segment from chromosome 1, and the 3′ end of a truncated c-*met* gene (Park et al., 1986). The protein expressed from the *met* oncogene is a tyrosine phosphorylated doublet of 60/65 kd, whereas components of 165 and 140 kd can be immunoprecipitated from cells containing an amplified c-*met* gene (Tempest et al., 1986). It is possible that c-*met* codes for a growth factor receptor for an unknown ligand, which becomes activated by an aminoterminal truncation.

Evidence for a transforming capacity of an amplified c-*met* gene has been derived from transfection experiments with normal cellular DNA using NIH 3T3 cells as recipients. A high proportion of such spontaneously occurring foci was shown to have a four- to eightfold amplification of c-*met* and at least a 20-fold overexpression of an apparently normal c-*met* transcript (Cooper et al., 1986). No reports on a rearranged or amplified c-*met* in spontaneously occurring tumors have so far been published.

ros

v-*ros* was identified as the transforming sequence of avian sarcoma virus UR2 (Balduzzi et al., 1981). The corresponding normal gene is expressed at highest levels in the kidney (Neckameyer et al., 1986; Shibuya et al., 1982). A putative ligand remains to be identified.

kit

The oncogene v-*kit* represents the transforming sequence of a feline sarcoma virus; its product encodes a protein tyrosine kinase with an insert in the kinase domain at the same position as those found in the receptors for CSF-1 and PDGF (Besmer et al., 1986). Apparently, c-*kit* encodes a protein similar to the CSF-1 receptor and PDGF receptor; its putative ligand remains to be elucidated.

trk

The oncogene *trk* was isolated from a human colon carcinoma, as a hybrid between a tyrosine kinase with a transmembrane domain and a nonmuscle tropomyosine molecule (Martin-Zanca et al., 1986). It is conceivable that the extracellular ligand-binding domain of a receptor for an unidentified growth factor in this case has been replaced by the tropomyosin molecule by somatic rearrangement.

ret

The activation of the *ret* oncogene involved a recombination of two unlinked sequences of human DNA, which most likely occurred during transfection of NIH 3T3 cells (Takahashi and Cooper, 1987). This resulted in a fusion protein consisting of an aminoterminal part from a protein with a sequence unrelated to other known proteins, and a carboxyterminal part of a tyrosine kinase with a transmembrane domain. As in the case of the *trk* protein, the regulatory domain of a growth factor receptor might have been replaced by another sequence, presumably causing a constitutively activated growth factor receptor.

AUTOCRINE GROWTH STIMULATION AND CONSTITUTIVE GROWTH FACTOR RECEPTOR ACTIVATION IN MULTISTEP CARCINOGENESIS

An unscheduled activation of a growth factor receptor by an autocrine mechanism or by qualitative or quantitative changes in the receptor protein may not be expected to cause anything but a hyperplastic response of otherwise phenotypically normal cells (cf. Johnsson et al., 1986); it may be a necessary but not sufficient event in tumorigenesis. In terminally differentiating systems, such as in hematopoiesis, such an event must be complemented by a differentiation block in order to cause a malignancy, and this is probably also true for the lymphoid system. It is notable, for instance, that v-*erb*B transformation of erythroid cells requires the cooperativity of v-*erb*A, the role of which probably is to block differentiation (Kahn et al., 1986). In other systems, an aberrant growth signal probably has to be complemented by an immortalizing event.

Data taken from various experimental systems indicate that an autocrine response may be an early as well as a late phenomenon in multistep tumorigenesis. Thus, in SSV-induced sarcomas and gliomas (Deinhardt, 1980), and perhaps also in spontaneous tumors of the same kind, autocrine growth is the first event, which is conceived to be complemented by secondary events in the proliferating population. An analogous situation may prevail in HTLV-associated acute T-cell lymphoma, via transactivation of the IL-2 pathway (Greene et al., 1986). Autocrine growth stimulation can also occur as a late step in tumorigenesis, as inferred from experiments of introducing growth factor cDNA expression vectors into immortalized cells of hematopoietic or fibroblastic origin (Lang et al., 1985; Rosenthal et al., 1986; Stern et al., 1987; Watanabe et al., 1987).

In several systems, an autocrine growth response seems to be only a transient rate-limiting event in tumorigenesis. Several examples have been cited above, in which cells progress from an autocrine response to a nonautocrine stimulation of growth. If we also take points 1) and 2) of page 158 into consideration, we can tentatively define two steps that bring the cell to growth factor independence:

1. Maintenance of a physiological autocrine stimulation (through a differentiation block) or generation of an unscheduled autocrine loop.
2. Complete abolition of the growth factor requirement by a nonautocrine mechanism.

These two events often may occur in sequence, i.e., along a progressional line, as exemplified by the studies of Lang et al. (1985) and Laker et al. (1987), showing the emergence of growth factor–independent clones in cultures of autocrine hematopoietic cells. Similarly, progression from an autocrine to a nonautocrine stimulation of growth has been shown to occur in HTLV-I–transformed cells (Arya et al., 1984) and in human small cell lung carcinoma (Cuttitta et al., 1985), and has been proposed to occur in B-cell–derived tumors (Gordon et al., 1985). It is conceivable that many of the cell lines which have been shown to coexpress a growth factor and the cognate receptor, but which are not growth arrested by growth factor antibodies or by receptor-blocking antibodies, have evolved from autocrine parental cells. This may for instance be true for glioma and sarcoma cells, which express PDGF receptors and produce PDGF-like growth factors, but are refractory to PDGF antibodies (see above).

It is important to point out that steps 1 and 2 above may be taken independently in transformation and tumorigenesis. Thus, step 1 may never be followed by step 2. As discussed by Metcalf, (1984), this may be the case in most instances of myeloid leukemia. Moreover, step 2 may not be preceded by step 1. Although we do not know whether this may occur in the development of spontaneous tumors, there are several examples of oncogenes that subvert the mitogenic pathway by a nonautocrine mechanism, such as those encoding mutated versions of growth factor receptors. Other examples are found among oncogenes whose products have an intracellular site of action. Thus, the v-*myc* and v-*abl* oncogenes cause a bypass of the need for hematopoietic growth factors (Cook et al., 1985; Pierce et al., 1985) and expression of a transfected c-*myc* cDNA reduces the PDGF requirement of Balb/c 3T3 cells (Armelin et al., 1984).

REFERENCES

Adkins, B., Leutz, A., and Graf, T. (1984). Autocrine growth induced by src-related oncogenes in transformed chicken myeloid cells. *Cell 39*: 439–445.

Anzano, M. A., Roberts, A. B., Smith, J. M., Sporn, M. B., and DeLarco, J. E. (1983). Sarcoma growth factor from conditioned medium of virally transformed cells is composed of both type a and type b transforming growth factors. *Proc. Natl. Acad. Sci. U.S.A. 80*: 6264–6268.

Arima, N., Daitoku, Y., Oghaki, S., Fukumori, J., Tanaka, H., Yamamoto, Y., Fujimoto, K., and Onoue, K. (1986). Autocrine growth of interleukin 2-producing leukemic cells in a patient with adult T cell leukemia. *Blood 68*: 779–782.

Armelin, H. A., Armelin, M. C. S., Kelly, K., Stewart, T. A., Leder, P., Cochran, B. H., and Stiles, C. D. (1984). A functional role for c-*myc* in the mitogenic response to platelet-derived growth factor. *Nature 310*: 655–660.

Arya, S. L., Wong-Staal, F., and Gallo, R. C. (1984). T-cell growth factor gene: Lack of expression in human T-cell leukemia-lymphoma virus-infected cells. *Science 223*: 1086–1087.

Balduzzi, P. C., Notter, M. D. F., Morgan, H. R., and Shibuya, M. (1981). Some biological properties of two new avian sarcoma viruses. *J. Virol. 40*: 268–275.

Bargmann, C. I., Hung, M.-C., and Weinberg, R. A. (1986a). The *neu* oncogene encodes an epidermal growth factor-related protein. *Nature 319*: 226–230.

Bargmann, C. I., Hung, M.-C., and Weinberg, R. A. (1986b). Multiple independent activations of the *neu* oncogene by a point mutation altering the transmembrane domain of p185. *Cell 45*: 649–657.

Barrett, T. B., Gajdusek, C. M., Schwartz, S. M., McDougall, J. K., and Benditt, E. P. (1985). Expression of the *sis* gene by endothelial cells in culture and *in vivo*. *Proc. Natl. Acad. Sci. U.S.A. 81*: 6772–6774.

Besmer, P., Snyder, H. W., Jr., Murphy, J. E., Hardy, W. D., Jr., and Parodi, A. (1983). The Parodi-Irgens feline sarcoma virus and simian sarcoma virus have homologous oncogenes, but in different contexts of the viral genomes. *J. Virol 46*: 606–613.

Besmer, P., Murphy, J. E., George, P. C., Qui, F., Bergold, P. J., Lederman, L., Snyder, H. W., Jr., Brodeur, D., Zuckerman, E. E., and Hardy, W. D. (1986). A new acute transforming feline retrovirus and relationship of its oncogene v-*kit* with the protein kinase gene family. *Nature 320*: 415–421.

Betsholtz, C., Heldin, C.-H., Nistér, M., Ek, B., Wasteson, Å., and Westermark, B. (1983). Synthesis of a PDGF-like growth factor in human glioma and sarcoma cells suggests the expression of the cellular homologue of the transforming protein of simian sarcoma virus. *Biochem. Biophys. Res. Commun. 117*: 176–182.

Betsholtz, C., Westermark, B., Ek, B., and Heldin, C.-H. (1984). Coexpression of a PDGF-like growth factor and PDGF receptors in a human osteosarcoma cell line. Implications for autocrine receptor activation. *Cell 39*: 447–457.

Betsholtz, C., Johnsson, A., Heldin, C.-H., Westermark, B., Lind, P., Urdea, M. S., Eddy, R., Shows, T. B., Philpott, K., Mellor, A. L., Knott, T. J., and Scott, J. (1986a). cDNA sequence and chromosomal localization of human platelet-derived growth factor A-chain and its expression in tumor cell lines. *Nature 320*: 695–699.

Betsholtz, C., Johnsson, A., Heldin, C.-H., and Westermark, B. (1986b). Efficient reversion of SSV-transformation and inhibition of growth factor-induced mitogenesis by suramin. *Proc. Natl. Acad. Sci. U.S.A. 83*: 6440–6444.

Betsholtz, C., Bergh, J., Bywater-Ekegärd, M., Pettersson, M., Johnsson, A., Ohlsson, R., Scott, J., Bell, G., Heldin, C.-H., and Westermark, B. (1987). PDGF production in human lung cancer cells suggests a role in tumor stroma formation. *Int. J. Cancer 39*: 502–507.

Beug, H., Hayman, M. J., Raines, M. B., Kung H.-J., and Vennström, B. (1986). Rous-associated virus 1-induced erythroleukemic cells exhibit a c-*erb*B-containing retrovirus unable to transform fibroblasts. *J. Virol. 57*: 1127–1138.

Bigner, S. H., Wong, A. J., Mark, J., Kinzler, K. W., Vogelstein, B., and Bigner, D. D. (1987). Relationships between gene amplification and chromosomal deviations in malignant human gliomas. *Cancer Genet. Cytogenet. 29*: 165–170.

Blazar, B. A., Sutton, L. M., and Strome, M. (1983). Self-stimulating growth factor production by B-cell lines derived from Burkitt's lymphoma and other cell lines transformed *in vitro* by Epstein-Barr virus. *Cancer Res. 43*: 4562–4569.

Browning, P. J., Bunn, H. F., Cline, A., Shuman, M., and Nienhius, A. W. (1986). "Replacement" of COOH-terminal truncation of v-*fms* with c-*fms* sequences markedly reduces transformation potential. *Proc. Natl. Acad. Sci. U.S.A. 83*, 7800–7804.

Cantrell, D. A., and Smith, K. A. (1984). The interleukin-2 T-cell system: A new cell growth model. *Science 224*: 1312–1316.

Carpenter, G., Stoscheck, C. M., Preston, Y. A., and DeLarco, J. E. (1983). Antibodies to the epidermal growth factor receptor block the biological activities of sarcoma growth factor. *Proc. Natl. Acad. Sci. U.S.A. 80*, 5627–5630.

Chen, S. J., Holbrook, N. J., Mitchell, K. F., Vallone, C. A., Freegard, J. S., Crabtree, G., and Lin, Y. (1985). A viral long terminal repeat in the interleukin 2 gene of a cell line that constitutively products interleukin 2. *Proc. Natl. Acad. Sci. U.S.A. 82*: 7284–7288.

Chiu, I.-M., Reddy, E. P., Givol, D., Robbins, K. C., Tronick, S. R., and Aaronson, S. A. (1984). Nucleotide sequence analysis identifies the human c-*sis* proto-oncogene as a structural gene for platelet-derived growth factor. *Cell 37*: 123–129.

Clarke, M. F., Westin, E., Schmidt, D., Josephs, S. F., Ratner, L., Wong-Staal, F., Gallo, R. C., and Reitz, M. S. (1984). Transformation of NIH 3T3 cells by a human c-*sis* cDNA clone. *Nature 308*: 464–467.

Coffey, R. J., Derynck, R., Wilcox, J. N., Bringman, T. S., Goustin, A. S., Moses, H. L., and Pihelkow, M. R. (1987). Production and autoinduction of transforming growth factor-α in human keratinocytes. *Nature 328*: 817–820.

Collins, T., and Pober, J. S. (1986). The 5′ non-coding region of c-*sis* mRNA reduces translational efficiency. *Fed. Proc. 45*: 1073.

Collins, T., Ginsburg, D., Boss, J. M., Orkin, S. H., and Pober, J. S. (1985). Cultured human endothelial cells express platelet-derived growth factor B-chain: cDNA cloning and structural analysis. *Nature 316*: 748–758.

Collins, T., Pober, J. S., Gimbrone, Jr., M. A., Hammacher, A., Betsholtz, C., Westermark, B., and Heldin, C.-H. (1987). Cultured human endothelial cells express platelet-derived growth factor A chain. *Am. J. Pathol. 126*: 7–12.

Cook, W. D., Metcalf, D., Nicola, N. A., Burgess, A. W., and Walker, F. (1985). Malignant transformation of a growth factor-dependent myeloid cell line by Abelson virus without evidence of an autocrine mechanism. *Cell 41*: 677–683.

Cooper, C. S., Park, M., Blair, D. G., Tainsky, M. A., Huebner, K., Croce, C. M., and Vande Woude, G. F. (1984). Molecular cloning of a new transforming gene from a chemically transformed human cell line *Nature. 311*: 29–33.

Cooper, C. S., Tempest, P. R., Beckmann, M. P., Heldin, C.-H., and Brookes, P. (1986). Amplification and overexpression of the *met* gene in spontaneously transformed NIH3T3 mouse fibroblasts. *EMBO J. 5*: 2623–2628.

Cotton, P. C., and Brugge, J. S. (1983). Neural tissues express high levels of the cellular *src* gene product, $pp60^{c\text{-}src}$. *Mol. Cell. Biol. 3*: 1157–1162.

Coussens, L., Yang-Feng, T. L., Liao, Y.-C., Chen, E., Gray, A., McGrath, J., Seeburg, P. H., Libermann, T. A., Schlessinger, J., Francke, U., Levinson, A., and Ullrich, A. (1985). Tyrosine kinase receptor with extensive homology to EGF receptor shares chromosomal location with *neu* oncogene. *Science 230*: 1132–1139.

Coussens, L., Van Beveren, C., Smith, D., Chen, E., Mitchell, R. L., Isacke, C. M., Verma, I. M., and Ullrich, A. (1986). Structural alteration of viral homologue of receptor proto-oncogene *fms* at carboxyl terminus. *Nature 320*: 277–280.

Cuttitta, F., Carney, D. N., Mulshine, J., Moody, T. W., Fedorko, J., Fischler, A., and Minna, J. N. D. (1985). Bombesin-like peptides can function as autocrine growth factors in human small-cell lung cancer. *Nature 316*: 823–826.

Deinhardt, F. (1980). The Biology of primate retrovirus. In *Viral Oncology*. (Klein, G., ed.). New York, Raven Press, pp. 359–398.

DeLarco, J. E., and Todaro, G. J. (1978). Growth factors from murine sarcoma virus-transformed cells. *Proc. Natl. Acad. Sci. U.S.A. 75*: 4001–4005.

Derynck, R., Roberts, A. B., Winkler, M. E., Chen, E. Y., and Goeddel, D. V. (1984). Human transforming growth factor-α: Precursor structure and expression in E. coli. *Cell 38*: 287–297.

Deuel, T. F., Huang, J. S., Huang, S. S., Stroobant, P., and Waterfield, M. (1983). Expression of a platelet-derived growth factor-like protein in simian sarcoma virus transformed cells. *Science 221*: 1348–1350.

Devare, S. G., Reddy, E. P., Law, J. D., Robbins, K. C., and Aaronson, S. A. (1983). Nucleotide sequence of the simian sarcoma virus genome: Demonstration that its acquired cellular sequences encode the transforming gene product $p28^{sis}$. *Proc. Natl. Acad. Sci. U.S.A. 80*: 731–735.

Dickson, C., and Peters, G. (1987). Potential oncogene product related to growth factors. *Nature 326*: 833.

Doolittle, R. F., Hunkapiller, M. W., Hood, L. E., Devare, S. G., Robbins, K. C., Aaronson, S. A., and Antoniades, H. N. (1983). Simian sarcoma virus oncogene, v-*sis*, is derived from the gene (or genes) encoding a platelet-derived growth factor. *Science 221*: 275–277.

Downward, J., Yarden, Y., Mayes, E., Scrace, G., Totty, N., Stockwell, P., Ullrich, A., Schlessinger, J., and Waterfield, M. D. (1984). Close similarity of epidermal growth factor receptor and v-*erb*-B oncogene protein sequences. *Nature 307*: 521–527.

Duprez, V., Lenoir, G., and Dautry-Varsat, A. (1985). Autocrine growth stimulation of a human T-cell lymphoma line by interleukin 2. *Proc. Natl. Acad. Sci. U.S.A. 82*: 6932–6936.

Ek, B., and Heldin, C.-H. (1984). Use of an antiserum against phosphotyrosine for the identification of phosphorylated components in human fibroblasts stimulated by platelet derived growth factor. *Biol.-Chem. 259*: 11145–11152.

Ek, B., Westermark, B., Wasteson, Å., and Heldin, C.-H. (1982). Stimulation of tyrosine-specific phosphorylation by platelet-derived growth factor. *Nature 295*: 419–420.

Folkman, J., and Klagsbrun, M. (1987). Angiogenic factors. *Science 235*: 442–447.

Frykberg, L., Palmieri, S., Beug, H., Graf, T., Hayman, M. J., and Vennström, B. (1983). Transforming capacities of avian erythroblastosis virus mutants deleted in the v-*erb*A or v-*erb*B oncogenes. *Cell 32*: 227–238.

Gazit, A., Igarashi, H., Chiu, I.-M., Srinivasan, A., Yaniv, A., Tronick, S. R., Robbins, K. C., and Aaronson, S. A. (1984). Expression of the normal human *sis*/PDGF-2 coding sequence induces cellular transformation. *Cell 39*: 80–97.

Gilmore, T., DeClue, J. E., and Martin, G. S. (1985). Protein phosphorylation at tyrosine is induced by the v-*erb*B gene product in vivo and in vitro. *Cell 40*: 609–618.

Golden, A., Nemeth, S. P., and Brugge, J. S. (1986). Blood platelets express high levels of the pp60$^{c\text{-}src}$-specific tyrosine kinase activity *Proc. Natl. Acad. Sci. U.S.A. 83*: 852–856.

Gootenberg, J. E., Ruscetti, F. W., Mier, J. W., Gazdar, A., and Gallo, R. C. (1981). T-cell lymphoma and leukemia cell lines produce and respond to T-cell growth factor. *J. Exp. Med. 154*: 1403–1418.

Gordon, J., Ley, S. C., Melamed, M. D., Aman, P., and Hughes-Jones, N. C. (1984a). Soluble factor requirements for the autostimulatory growth of B lymphomas immortalized by Epstein-Barr virus. *J. Exp. Med. 159*: 1554–1559.

Gordon, J., Ley, S. C., Melamed, M. D., English, L. S., and Hughes-Jones, N. C. (1984b). Immortalized B lymphocytes produce B-cell growth factor. *Nature 310*: 145–147.

Gordon, J., Åman, P., Rosén, A., Ernberg, I., Ehlin-Henriksson, B., and Klein, G. (1985). Capacity of B-lymphocytic lines of diverse tumor origin to produce and respond to B-cell growth factors: A progression model for B-cell lymphomagenesis. *Int. J. Cancer 35*: 251–256.

Gospodarowicz, D., Neufeld, G., and Schweigerer, L. (1986). Fibroblast growth factor. *Mol. Cell. Endocrinol. 46*: 187–203.

Gough, N. M. (1986). The granulocyte-macrophage colony-stimulating factors. In *Oncogenes and Growth Control.* (Kahn, P., and Graf, T., eds.). New York, Springer Verlag, pp. 35–42.

Goustin, A. S., Betsholtz, C., Pfeifer-Ohlsson, S., Persson, H., Rydnert, J., Bywater, M., Holmgren, G., Heldin, C.-H., Westermark, B., and Ohlsson, R. (1985). Co-expression of the *sis* and *myc* proto-oncogenes in human placenta suggest autocrine control of trophoblast growth. *Cell 41*: 301–312.

Graf, T., v. Weizsaecker, F., Grieser, S., Coll, J., Stehelin, D., Patschinsky, T., Bister, K., Bechade, C., Calothy, G., and Leutz, A. (1986). v-*mil* induces autocrine growth and enhanced tumorigenicity in v-*myc* transformed avian macrophages. *Cell 45*: 357–364.

Graves, D. T., Owen, A. J., and Antoniades, H. N. (1985). Demonstration of receptors for a PDGF-like mitogen on human osteosarcoma cells. *Biochem. Biophys. Res. Commun. 129*: 56–64.

Greene, W., Leonard, W., Wano, Y., Svetlik, P., Pfeffer, N., Sodroski, J., Rosen, C. A., Goh, W. C., and Haseltine, W. A. (1986). Transactivator gene of HTLV-II induces IL-2 receptor and IL-2 cellular gene expression. *Science 232*: 877–880.

Hammacher, A., Hellman, U., Johnson, A., Östman, A., Gunnarsson, K., Westermark, B., Wasteson, Å and Heldin, C. H. (1988). PDGF purified from human platelets in a heterodimer of one A and one B chain. *J. Biol. Chem.* (in press).

Heldin, C.-H., and Westermark, B. (1984). Growth factors: Mechanism of action and relation to oncogenes. *Cell 37*: 9–20.

Heldin, C.-H., Westermark, B., and Wasteson, Å. (1980). Chemical and biological properties of a growth factor from human cultured osteosarcoma cells: Resemblance with platelet-derived growth factor. *J. Cell. Physiol. 105*: 235–246.

Heldin, C.-H., Johnsson, A., Wennergren, S., Wernstedt, C., Betsholtz, C., and Westermark, B. (1986). A human osteosarcoma cell line secretes a growth factor structurally related to a homodimer of PDGF A chains. *Nature 319*: 511–514.

Heldin, C.-H., Betsholtz, C., Claesson-Welsh, L., and Westermark, B. (1987). Subversion of growth regulatory pathways in malignant transformation. *Biochim. Biophys. Acta Cancer Rev. 907*: 219–244.

Huang, J. S., Huang, S. S., and Deuel, T. F. (1984). Transforming protein of simian sarcoma virus stimulates autocrine growth of SSV-transformed cells through PDGF cell-surface receptors. *Cell 39*: 79–87.

Hunter, T., and Cooper, J. A. (1985). Protein tyrosine kinases. *Ann. Rev. Biochem. 54*: 897–930.

Hunter, T., and Sefton, B. M. (1980). Transforming gene product of Rous sarcoma virus phosphorylates tyrosine. *Proc. Natl. Acad. Sci. U.S.A. 77*: 1311–1315.

Johnsson, A., Heldin, C.-H., Westermark, B., and Wasteson, Å. (1982). Platelet-derived growth factor: Identification of constituent polypeptide chains. *Biochem. Biophys. Res. Commun. 104*: 66–74.

Johnsson, A., Heldin, C.-H., Wasteson, Å., Westermark, B., Deuel, T. F., Huang, J. S., Seeburg, P. H., Gray, A., Ullrich, A., Scrace, G., Stroobant, P., and Waterfield, M. D. (1984). The c-*sis* gene encodes a procursor of the B chain of platelet-derived growth factor. *EMBO J. 3*: 921–928.

Johnsson, A., Betsholtz, C., Heldin, C.-H., and Westermark, B. (1985). Antibodies against platelet-derived growth factor inhibit acute transformation by simian sarcoma virus. *Nature 317*: 438–440.

Johnsson, A., Betsholtz, C., Heldin, C.-H., and Westermark, B. (1986). The phenotypic characteristics of simian sarcoma virus-transformed human fibroblasts suggest that the v-*sis* gene product acts solely as a PDGF receptor agonist in cell transformation. *EMBO J. 5*: 1535–1541.

Josephs, S. F., Guo, C., Ratner, L., and Wong-Staal, F. (1984a). Human proto-oncogene nucleotide sequences corresponding to the transforming region of simian sarcoma virus. *Science 223*: 487–491.

Josephs, S. F., Ratner, L., Clarke, M. F., Westin, E. H., Reitz, M. S., and Wong-Staal, F. (1984b). Transforming potential of human c-*sis* nucleotide sequences encoding platelet-derived growth factor. *Science 225*: 636–639.

Kahn, P., Frykberg, L., Brady, C., Stanly, I., Beug, H., Vennström, B., and Graf, T. (1986). v-*erb*A cooperates with sarcoma oncogenes in leukemic cell transformation. *Cell 45*: 349–356.

Kaplan, P. L., and Ozanne, B. (1982). Polyoma virus-transformed cells produce transforming growth factor(s) and grow in serum-free medium. *Virology 123*: 372–380.

Kaplan, P. L., Andersson, M., and Ozanne, B. (1982). Transforming growth factor(s) production enables cells to grow in the absence of serum: An autocrine system. *Proc. Natl. Acad. Sci. U.S.A. 79*: 485–489.

King, C. R., Kraus, M. H., and Aaronson, S. A. (1985). Amplification of a novel v-*erb*B-related gene in a human mammary carcinoma. *Science 229*: 974–976.

Kozak, M. (1986). Bifunctional messenger RNAs in eukaryotes. *Cell 47*: 481–483.

Kris, R. M., Lax, I., Gullick, W., Waterfield, M. D., Ullrich, A., Fridkin, M., and Schlessinger, J. (1985). Antibodies against a synthetic peptide as a probe for the kinase activity of the avian EGF receptor and v-*erb*B proteins. *Cell 40*: 619–625.

Laker, C., Stocking, C., Bergholz, U., Hess, N., De Lamarter, J. F., and Ostertag, W. (1987). Autocrine growth stimulation after viral transfer of the granulocyte-macrophage colony stimulating factor gene and geniune factor independent growth are two distinct but interdependent steps in the oncogenic pathway. *Proc. Natl. Acad. Sci. U.S.A. 84*: 8458–8462.

Lang, R. A., Metcalf, D., Gough, N. M., Dunn, A. R., and Gonda, T. J. (1985) Expression of a hemopoietic growth factor cDNA in a factor-dependent cell line results in autonomous growth and tumorigenicity. *Cell 43*: 531–542.

Lax, I., Kris, R., Sasson, I., Ullrich, A., Hayman, M. J., Beug, H., and Schlessinger, J. (1985) Activation of c-*erb*B in avian leukosis virus-induced erythroblastosis leads to the expression of a truncated EGF receptor kinase. *EMBO J. 4*: 3179–3182.

Leal, F., Williams, L. T., Robbins, K. C., and Aaronson, S. A. (1985). Evidence that the v-*sis* gene product transforms by interaction with the receptor for platelet-derived growth factor. *Science 230*: 327–330.

Lee, D. C., Rochford, R., Todaro, G. J., and Villarreal, L. P. (1985). Developmental expression of transforming growth factor-α mRNA. *Mol. Cell. Biol. 5*: 3644–3646.

Libermann, T. A., Nusbaum, H. R., Razon, N., Kris, R., Lax, I., Soreq, H., Whittle, N., Waterfield, M. D., Ullrich, A., and Schlessinger, J. (1985). Amplification, enhanced expression and possible rearrangement of EGF receptor gene in primary brain tumors of glial origin. *Nature 313*: 144–147.

Libermann, T. A., Friese, R., Jaye, M., Lyall, R. M., Westermark, B., Drohan, W., Schmidt, A., Maciag, T., and Schlessinger, J. (1987). An angiogenic growth factor is expressed in human glioma cells. *EMBO J. 6*: 1627–1632.

Little, C. D., Nau, M. M., Carney, D. N., Gazdar, A. F., and Minna, J. D. (1983). Amplification and expression of the c-*myc* oncogene in human lung cancer cell lines. *Nature 306*: 194–196.

Marquardt, H., Hunkapiller, M. W., Hood, L. E., Twardzik, D. R., De Larco, J. E., Stephensson, J. R., and Torado, G. J. (1983). Transforming growth factors produced by retrovirus transformed rodent fibroblasts and human melanoma cells: Amino acid sequence homology with epidermal growth factor. *Proc. Natl. Acad. Sci. U.S.A. 80*: 4684–4688.

Marquardt, H., Hunkapiller, M. W., Hood, L. E., and Todaro, G. J. (1984). Rat transforming growth factor type 1 structure and relation to epidermal growth factor. *Science 223*: 1079–1082.

Martin-Zanca, D., Hughes, S. H., and Barbacid, M. (1986). A human oncogene formed by the fusion of truncated tropomyosin and protein tyrosine kinase sequences. *Nature 319*: 743–748.

Martinet, Y., Bitterman, P. B., Mornex, J.-F., Grotendorst, G., Martin, G. R., and Crystal, R. G. (1986). Activated human monocytes express the c-*sis* proto-oncogene and release a mediator showing PDGF-like activity. *Nature 319*: 158–160.

McKay, I., Malone, P., Marshall, C. J., and Hall, A. (1986). Malignant transformation of murine fibroblast by a human c-Ha-*ras*-1 oncogene does not require a functional epidermal growth factor receptor. *Mol. Cell. Biol. 6*: 3382–3387.

Metcalf, D. (1985). The granulocyte-macrophage colony-stimulating factors. *Science 229*: 16–22.

Miles, B. D., and Robinson, H. L. (1986). High-frequency transduction of c-*erb*B in avian leukosis virus-induced erythroblastosis. *J. Virol. 54*: 295–303.

Moody, T. W., Pert, C. B., Gazdar, A. F., Carney, D. N., and Minna, J. D. (1981). High levels of intracellular bombesin characterize human small-cell lung carcinoma. *Science 214*: 1246–1248.

Morgan, D. A., Ruscetti, F. W., and Gallo, R. C. (1976). Selective in vitro growth of T lymphocytes form normal human bone marrows. *Science 293*: 11007–1008.

Mueller, P. P., and Hinebusch, A. G. (1986). Multiple upstream AUG codons mediate translational control of GCN4. *Cell 45*: 201–291.

Neckameyer, W. S., Shibuya, M., Hsu, M.-T., and Wang, L.-H. (1986). Proto-oncogene c-*ros* codes for a molecule with structural features common to those of growth factor receptors and displays tissue-specific and developmentally regulated expression. *Mol. Cell. Biol. 6*: 1478–1486.

Nilsen, T. W., Matoney, P. A., Goodwin, R. G., Rottman, F. M., Crittenden, L. B., Raines, M. A., and Kung, H.-J. (1985). c-*erb*B activation in ALV-induced erythroblastosis: Novel RNA processing and promoter insertion result in expression of a amino-truncated EGF receptor. *Cell 41*: 719–726.

Nilsson, J., Sjölund, M., Palmberg, L., Thyberg, J., and Heldin, C.-H. (1985). Arterial smooth muscle cells in primary culture produce a platelet-derived growth factor-like protein. *Proc. Natl. Acad. Sci. U.S.A. 82*: 4418–4307.

Nistér, M., Heldin, C.-H., Wasteson, Å., and Westermark, B. (1984). A glioma-derived analog to platelet-derived growth factor: Demonstration of receptor competing activity and immunological cross-reactivity. *Proc. Natl. Acad. Sci. U.S.A. 81*: 926–930.

Nistér, M., Heldin, C.-H., and Westermark, B. (1986). Clonal variation in the production of a platelet-derived growth factor-like protein and expression of corresponding receptors in a human malignant glioma. *Cancer Res. 46*:332–340.

Nistér, M., Libermann, T., Betsholtz, C., Pettersson, M., Welsh, L., Heldin, C.-H., Schlessinger, J., and Westermark, B. (1988a). Expression of messenger RNAs for platelet-derived growth factor and transforming growth factor-α and their receptors in human malignant glioma cell lines. *Cancer Res.* (submitted).

Nistér, M., Hammacher, A., Mellström, K., Siegbahn, A., Rōnnstrand, L., Westermark, B., and Heldin, C.-H. (1988b). A glioma-derived PDGF A chain homodimer has different functional activities than a PDGF AB heterodimer purified from human platelets. *Cell* (in press).

Nusse, R. (1986). The activation of cellular oncogenes by retroviral insertion. *Trends Genet. 2*: 244–247.

Ozanne, B., Fulton, R. J., and Kaplan, P. L. (1980). Kirsten murine sarcoma virus transformed cell lines and a spontaneously transformed rat cell-line produce transforming factors. *J. of Cell. Physiol. 105*: 163–180.

Pantazis, P., Pelicci, P. G., Dalla-Favera, R., and Antoniades, H. N. (1985). Synthesis and secretion of protein resembling platelet-derived growth factor by human glioblastoma and fibrosarcoma cells in culture. *Proc. Natl. Acad. Sci. U.S.A. 82*: 2404–2408.

Park, M., Dean, M., Cooper, C. S., Schmidt, M., O'Brien, S. J., Blair, D. G., and Vande Woude, G. F. (1986). Mechanism of *met* oncogene activation. *Cell 45*: 895–904.

Paulsson, Y., Hammacher, A., Heldin, C.-H., and Westermark, B. (1987). Possible positive autocrine feed back in the prereplicative phase of human fibroblasts. *Nature 328*: 715–717.

Perez, R., Betsholtz, C., Westermark, B., and Heldin, C.-H. (1987). Frequent expression of growth factors for mesenchymal cells in human mammary carcinoma cell lines. *Cancer Res. 47*: 3425–3429.

Pierce, J. H., Di Fiore, P. P., Aaronson, S. A., Potter, M., Pumphrey, J. Scott, A., and Ihle, J. N. (1985). Neoplastic transformation of mast cells by Abelson-MuLV: Abrogation of IL-3 dependence by a nonautocrine mechanism. *Cell 41*: 685–693.

Pike, L. J., Gallis, B., Casnellie, J. E., Bornstein, P., and Krebs, E. G. (1982). Epidermal growth factor stimulates the phosphorylation of synthetic tyrosine-containing peptides by A431 cell membranes. *Proc. Natl. Acad. Sci. U.S.A. 79*: 1443–1447.

Raines, M. A., Lewis, W. G., Crittenden, L. B., and Kung, H.-J. (1985). c-*erb*B activation in avian leukosis virus-induced erythroblastosis: Clustered integration sites and the arrangement of ALV provirus in the c-*erb*B alleles. *Proc. Natl. Acad. Sci. U.S.A. 82*: 2287–2291.

Rao, C. D., Igarashi, H., Chiu, I.-M., Robbins, K. C., and Aaronson, S. A. (1986). Structure and sequence of the human c-*sis*/platelet-derived growth factor 2 (SIS/PDGF 2) transcriptional unit. *Proc. Natl. Acad. Sci. U.S.A. 83*: 2392–2396.

Reynolds, F. H., Jr., Todaro, G. J., Fryling, C., and Stephenson, J. R. (1981). Human transforming growth factors induce tyrosine phosphorylation of EGF receptors. *Nature 292*: 259–262.

Riedel, H., Schlessinger, J., and Ullrich, A. (1987). A chimeric, ligand-binding v-*erb*B/EGF receptor retains transforming potential. *Science 236*: 197–200.

Robbins, K. C., Antoniades, H. N., Devare, S. G., Hunkapiller, M. W., and Aaronson, S.A. (1983). Structural and immunological similarities between simian sarcoma virus gene product(s) and human platelet-derived growth factor. *Nature 305*: 605–608.

Rosenthal, A., Lindquist, P. B., Bringman, T. S., Goeddel, D. V., and Derynck, R. (1986). Expression in rat fibroblasts of a human transforming growth factor-α cDNA results in transformation. *Cell 46*: 301–309.

Roussel, M. F., Dull, T. J., Rettenmier, C. W., Ralph, P., Ullrich, A., and Sherr, C. J. (1987). Transforming potential of the c-*fms* proto-oncogene (CSF-1 receptor). *Nature 325*: 549–551.

Rozengurt, E. (1986). Early signals in the mitogenic response. *Science 234*: 161–166.

Rozengurt, E., Sinnett-Smith, J., and Taylor-Papadimitriou, J. (1985). Production of PDGF-like growth factor by breast cancer cell lines. *Int. J. Cancer 36*: 247–252.

Sacca, R., Stanley, E. R., Sherr, C. J., and Rettenmier, C. W. (1986). Specific binding of the mononuclear phagocyte colony-stimulating factor CSF-1 to the product of the v-*fms* oncogene. *Proc. Natl. Acad. Sci. U.S.A. 83*: 3331–3335.

Sakamoto, H., Mori, M., Taira, M., Yoshida, T., Matsukawa, S., Shimizu, K., Sekiguchi, M., Terada, M., and Sugimura, T. (1986). Transforming gene from human stomach cancers and a noncancerous portion of stomach mucosa. *Proc. Natl. Acad. Sci. U.S.A. 83*: 3997–4001.

Sap, J., Muñoz, A., Damm, K., Goldberg, Y., Gysdael, J., Leutz, A., Beug, H., and Vennström, B. (1986). The c-*erb*-A protein is a high-affinity receptor for thyroid hormone. *Nature 324*: 635–640.

Sato, M., Yoshida, H., Hayashi, Y., Miyakami, K., Bando, T., Yanagawa, T., Yuna, Y., Azuma, M., and Ueno, A. (1985). Expression of epidermal growth factor and transforming growth factor-β in a human salivary gland adenocarcinoma cell line. *Cancer Res. 45*: 6160–6167.

Schrader, K. W., and Crapper, R. M. (1983). Autogenous production of a hemopoietic growth factor, persisting cell-stimulating factor as a mechanism for transformation of bone marrow-derived cells. *Proc. Natl. Acad. Sci. U.S.A. 80*: 6892–6896.

Schweigerer, L., Neufeld, G., Mergia, A., Abraham, A. J., Fiddes, J. C., and Gospodarowicz, D. (1987). Basic fibroblast growth factor in human rhabdomyosarcoma cells: Implications for the proliferation and neovascularization of myoblast-derived tumors. *Proc. Natl. Acad. Sci. U.S.A. 84*: 842–846.

Semba, K., Kamata, N., Toyoshima, K., and Yamamoto, T. (1985). A v-*erb*B related protooncogene, c-*erb*B-2, is distinct from the c-*erb*B-1/epidermal growth factor-receptor gene and is amplified in a human salivary gland adenocarcinoma. *Proc. Natl. Acad. Sci. U.S.A. 82*: 6497–6501.

Seifert, R. A., Schwartz, S. M., and Bowen-Pope, D. F. (1984). Developmentally regulated production of platelet-derived growth factor-like molecules. *Nature 311*: 669–671.

Sejersen, T., Betsholtz, C., Sjölund, M., Heldin, C.-H., Westermark, B., and Thyberg, J. (1986). Rat skeletal myoblasts and arterial smooth muscle cells express the gene for the A chain but not the B chain (c-*sis*) of the platelet-derived growth factor (PDGF) and produce a PDGF-like protein. *Proc. Natl. Acad. Sci. U.S.A. 83*: 6844–6848.

Sherr, C. J., Rettenmier, C. W., Sacca, R., Roussel, M. F., Look, A. T., and Stanley, E. R. (1985). The c-*fms* proto-oncogene product is related to the receptor for the mononuclear phagocyte growth factor, CSF-1. *Cell 41*: 665–676.

Shibuya, M., Hanafusa, H., and Balduzzi, P. C. (1982). Cellular sequences related to three new *onc* genes of avian sarcoma (*fps, yes,* and *ros*) and their expression in normal and transformed cells. *J. Virol. 42*: 143–152.

Shimokado, K., Raines, E. W., Madtes, D. K., Barrett, T. B., Benditt, E. P., and Ross, R. (1985). A significant part of macrophage-derived growth factor consists of at least two forms of PDGF. *Cell 43*: 277–286.

Slamon, D. J., Clark, G. M., Wong, S. G., Levin, W. J., Ullrich, A., and McGuire, W. L. (1987). Human breast cancer: Correlation of relapse and survival with amplification of the HER-2/*neu* oncogene. *Science 235*: 177–182.

Sporn, M. B., and Todaro, G. J. (1980). Autocrine secretion and malignant transformation of cells. *N. Engl. J. Med. 303*: 878–880.

Stanley, E. R., Guilbert, L. J., Tushinski, R. J., and Bartelmez, S. H. (1983). CSF-1 a mononuclear phagocyte lineage-specific hemopoietic growth factor. *J. Cell. Biochem. 21*: 151–159.

Stern, D. F., Hare, D. L., Cecchini, M. A., and Weinberg, R. A. (1987). Construction of a novel oncogene based on synthetic sequences encoding epidermal growth factor. *Science 235*: 321–324.

Stroobant, P., and Waterfield, M. D. (1984). Purification and properties of porcine, platelet-derived growth factor. *EMBO J. 3*: 2963–2967.

Swan, D. C., McBride, O. W., Robbins, K. C., Keithley, F. A., Reddy, E. P., and Aaronson, S. A. (1982). Chromosonal mapping of the simian sarcoma virus *onc*-gene analogue in human cells. *Proc. Natl. Acad. Sci. U.S.A. 79*: 4691–4695.

Taira, M., Yoshida, T., Miyagawa, K., Sakamoto, H., Terada, M., and Sigimura, T. (1987). cDNA sequence of human transforming gene *hst* and identification of the coding sequence required for transforming activity. *Proc. Natl. Acad. Sci. U.S.A. 84*: 2980–2984.

Takahashi, M., and Cooper, G. M. (1987). *ret* transforming gene encodes a fusion protein homologous to tyrosine kinases. *Mol. Cell. Biol. 7*: 1378–1385.

Taniguchi, T., Matsui, H., Fujita, Y., Hatakeymana, M., Kashima, N., Fuse, A., Hamuro, J., Hishi-Takaoka, C., and Yamada, G. (1986). Molecular analysis of the interleukin-2 system. *Immunol. Rev. 92*: 121–133.

Tempest, P. R., Cooper, C. S., and Major, G. N. (1986). The activated human *met* gene encodes a protein tyrosine kinase. *F.E.B.S. Lett. 209*: 357–360.

Temin, H. M. (1967). Control by factors in serum of multiplication of uninfected cells and cells infected and converted by avian sarcoma viruses. In *Growth Regulating Substances for Animal Cells in Cultures.* The Wistar Symposium Monograph No. 7, pp. 103–116.

Todaro, G. J., De Larco, J. E., Marquardt, H., Bryant, M. L., Sherwin, S. A., and Sliski, A. H. (1979). Polypeptide growth factors produced by tumor cells and virus-transformed cells: A possible growth advantage for the producer cells. In *Hormones and Cell Culture.* Book A, Cold Spring Harbor Conferences on Cell Proliferation, 6. (Sato, G. H., and Ross, R. eds.). Cold Spring Harbor, New York, Cold Spring Harbor Laboratory, pp. 113–127.

Todaro, G. J., Fryling, C., and De Larco, J. E. (1980). Transforming growth factors produced by certain human tumor cells: Polypeptides that interact with epidermal growth factor receptors. *Proc. Natl. Acad. Sci. U.S.A. 77*: 5258–5262.

Twardzik, D. R., Todaro, G. J., Marquardt, H., Reynolds, F. H., Jr., and Stephenson, J. R. (1982). Transformation induced by Abelson murine leukemia virus involves production of a polypeptide growth factor. *Science 216*: 894–896.

Twardzik, D. R., Todaro, G. J., Reynolds, F. H., Jr., and Stephenson, J. R. (1983). Similar transforming growth factors (TGFs) produced by cells transformed by different isolates of feline sarcoma virus. *Virology 124*: 201–207.

Twadzik, D. R. (1985). Differential expression of transforming growth factor-a during prenatal developmental of the mouse. *Cancer Res. 45*: 5413–5416.

Ullrich, A., Bell, J. R., Chen, E. Y., Herrera, R., Pertuzelli, L. M., Dull, T. J., Gray, A., Coussens, L., Liao, Y.-C., Tsubokawa, M., Mason, A., Seeburg, P. H., Grunfeld, C., Rosen, O. M., and Ramachandran, J. (1985). Human insulin receptor and its relationship to the tyrosine kinase family of oncogenes. *Nature 131*: 756–761.

Ullrich, A., Coussens, L., Hayflick, J. S., Dull, T. J., Gray, A., Tam, A. W., Lee, J., Yarden, Y., Libermann, T. A., Schlessinger, J., Downward, J., Mayes, E. L. V., Whittle, N., Waterfield, M. D., and Seeburg, P. H. (1984). Human epidermal growth factor receptor cDNA sequence and aberrant expression of the amplified gene in A 431 epidermoid carcinoma cells. *Nature 309*: 418–725.

Ullrich, A., Gray, A., Tam, A. W., Yang-Feng, T., Tsubokawa, M., Collins, C., Henzel, W., Le Bon, T., Kathuria, S., Chen, E., Jacobs, S., Francke, U., Ramachandran, J., and Fujita-Yamaguchi, Y. (1986). Insulin-like growth factor I receptor primary structure: Comparison with insulin receptor suggests structural determinants that define functional specificity. *EMBO J. 5*: 2503–2512.

Ushiro, H., and Cohen, S. (1980). Identification of phosphotyrosine as a product of epidermal growth factor-activated protein kinase in A-431 cell membranes. *J. Biol. Chem. 255*: 8363–8365.

Verbeek, J. S., dc Ruyter, O., Bloemers, H. P. J., and Van de Ven, W. J. M. (1985). Molecular cloning and characterization of feline cellular genetic sequences homologous to the oncogene of the McDonough strain of feline sarcoma virus. *Virology 141*: 322–327.

von Weizsäcker, F., Beug, H., and Graf, T. (1986). Temperature-sensitive mutants of MH2 avian leukemia virus that map in the v-mil and v-myc genes of the virus. *EMBO J. 5*: 1521–1528.

Watanabe, S., Lazar, E., and Sporn, M. B. (1987). Transformation of normal rat kidney (NRK) cells by an infectious retrovirus carrying a synthetic rat type α transforming growth factor gene. *Proc. Natl. Acad. Sci. U.S.A. 84*: 1258–1262.

Waterfield, M. D., Scrace, G. T., Whittle, N., Stroobant, P., Johnsson, A., Wasteson, Å., Westermark, B., Heldin, C.-H., Huang, J. S., and Deuel, T. F. (1983). Platelet-derived growth factor is structurally related to the putative transforming protein $p28^{sis}$ of simian sarcoma virus. *Nature 304*: 35–39.

Weber, S., Zuckerman, J. E., Bostwick, D. G., Bensch, K. G., Sikic, B. I., and Riffin, T. A. (1985). Gastrin releasing peptide is a selective mitogen for small cell lung carcinoma. *J. Clin. Invest. 75*: 306–309.

Westermark, B., Johnsson, A., Paulsson, Y., Betsholtz, C., Heldin, C.-H., Herlyn, M., Rodeck, U., and Koprowski, H. (1986). Human melanoma cell lines of primary and metastatic origin express the genes encoding the constituent chains of PDGF and produce a PDGF-like growth factor. *Proc. Natl. Acad. Sci. U.S.A. 83*: 7197–7200.

Westermark, B., Betsholtz, C., Johnsson, A., and Heldin, C.-H. (1987). Acute transformation by simian sarcoma virus is mediated by an externalized PDGF-like growth factor. In *Viral Carcinogens.* (Kjelgaard, N. O., and Forchhammer, J.). Munksgaard, Copenhagen, pp. 445–457.

Weinberger, C., Thompson, C. C., Ong, E. S., Lebo, R., Gruol, D. J., and Evans, R. M. (1986). The c-*erb*-A gene encodes a thyroid hormone receptor. *Nature 324*: 641–646.

Wheeler, E. F., Roussel, M. F., Hampe, A., Walker, M. H., Fried, V. A., Look, A. T., Rettenmier, C. W., and Sherr, C. J. (1986a). The aminoterminal domain of the v-fms oncogene includes a functional signal peptide that directs synthesis of a transforming glycoprotein in the absence of FeLV *gag* sequences. *J. Virol. 59*: 224–233.

Wheeler, E. F., Rettenmier, C. W., Look, A. T., and Sherr, C. J. (1986b). The v-*fms* oncogene induces factor independence and tumorigenicity in CSF-1 dependent macrophage cell line. *Nature 324*: 377–380.

Williams, L. T., Tremble, P. M., Lavin, M. F., and Sunday, M. E. (1984). Platelet-derived growth factor receptors form a high affinity state in membrane preparations. *J. Biol. Chem. 259*: 5287–5294.

Wood, S. M., Wood, J. R., Ghatei, M. A., Lee, Y. C., O'Shaugnessy, D., and Bloom, S. R. (1981). Bombesin, somatostatin and neurotensin-like immunoreactivity in bronchial carcinoma. *J. Clin. Endocr. Metab. 53*: 1310–1312.

Yamamoto, T., Nishida, T., Miyajima, N., Kawai, S., Ooi, T., and Toyoshima, K. (1983). The *erb*B gene of avian erythroblastisis virus is a member of the *src* gene family. *Cell 35*: 71–78.

Yamamoto, T., Ikawa, S., Akiyama, T., Semba, K., Nomura, N., Miyajima, N., Saito, T., and Toyoshima, K. (1986). Similarity of protein encoded by the human c-*erb*-B-2 gene to epidermal growth factor receptor. *Nature 319:* 230–234.

Yarden, Y., Escobedo, J. A., Kuang, W.-J., Yang-Feng, T. L., Daniel, T. O., Tremble, P. M., Chen, E. Y., Ando, M. E., Harkins, R. N., Francke, U., Fried, V. A., Ullrich, A., and Williams, L. T. (1986). Structure of the receptor for platelet-derived growth factor helps define a family of closely related growth factor receptors. *Nature 323*:226–232.

Ymer, S., Tucker, W. Q. J., Sanderson, C. J., Hapel, A. J., Campbell, H. D., and Young, I. G. (1985). Constitutive synthesis of interleukin-3 by leukemia cell line WEHI-3B is due to retroviral insertion near the gene. *Nature 317*: 255–258.

Young, D., and Griffin, J. D. (1986). Autocrine secretion of GM-CFS in acute myeloblastic leukemia. *Blood 68*: 1178–1181.

SIX

c-*myc* Oncogene Activation and Chromosomal Translocation in BALB/c Plasmacytomas

J. Frederic Mushinski
National Cancer Institute
National Institutes of Health
Bethesda, Maryland

INDUCTION OF PLASMACYTOMAS BY PARAFFIN OILS

Pristane Alone

Susceptible strains of mice, such as BALB/cAnN, regularly develop intraperitoneal plasma cell tumors in the inflammatory granulomata that arise around intraperitoneal plastic objects and nonmetabolizable paraffin oils (1). The experimental details of this system have been worked out best when tumors were induced by injecting a purified branched-chain alkane called pristane (2,6,10,14-tetramethylpentadecane). The percentage of mice that develops tumors is proportional to the total dose of pristane administered and can approach 80% in immunologically mature female BALB/cAnN mice given 1.5 ml of pristane in single or divided doses. More commonly a single intraperitoneal injection of 0.5 ml pristane is used, which causes approximately 30% of these mice to develop tumors that appear between 6 and 24 months, but occasionally as early as 4 months (Fig. 1) (2).

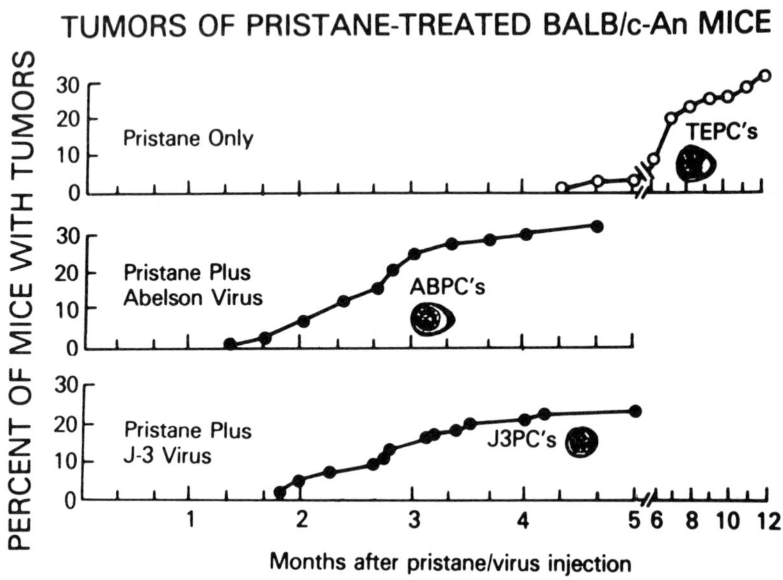

Figure 1 Time of appearance of plasmacytomas after receiving 0.5 ml intraperitoneal pristane at day zero either alone (1), plus Abelson virus (3), or plus J-3 recombinant virus expressing avian v-*myc* (4).

Pristane Plus Retroviruses

The appearance of tumors can be accelerated by administering pristane plus an intraperitoneal injection of oncogene-containing viruses such as Abelson virus (3) or J-3 virus (4). The decrease in mean latent period is shown in Fig. 1, and it can be seen that the incidence remains about the same.

CONSISTENT CHROMOSOMAL ALTERATIONS

G- and Q-banding karyotypic studies of the plasmacytomas that arose following injection of mineral oil (MOPCs) or pristane (TEPCs), alone or in combination with x-irradiation (XRPCs) or Abelson virus infection (ABPCs) permitted identification of one of two specific reciprocal chromosome translocations (rcpt) in nearly all the tumors examined (5–8). The translocations always involved band D2/3 on chromosome 15 (chr. 15), which was later discovered to be the locus of the c-*myc* gene, and the telomeric tip of chr. 12, where the immunoglobulin heavy chain (IgH) locus was found, or the middle of chr. 6, the site for the Ig kappa light chain. Four tumors appeared to have no such rearrangements, but high resolution banding studies revealed internal deletions at the D2/3 area of chr. 15 in three tumors (2). To date only one plasmacytoma, ABPC22, lacks discernible chr. 15 abnormalities. The limitations of this technique, and light microscopy in general, leave plenty of room for molecular rearrangements that are beyond the sensitivity of detection. Analysis of over 40 karyotypes, including those of primary and transplanted plasmacytomas induced with and without Abelson virus in BALB/c and CBB-22 (a BALB/c congenic strain) mice, shows that about 75% have rcpt(12;15), 15% have rcpt(6;15), and 10% have internal chr. 15 deletions (2).

rcpt(12;15)

The upper portion of Fig. 2 depicts a summary of the karyotypic and molecular events that have been shown to occur in the most common form of chromosome translocation in plasmacytomas induced by pristane alone (85% have rcpt[12;15]) and pristane plus Abelson virus (52% have rcpt [12;15]) (2). Some of the plasmacytomas are nearly diploid, but many are nearly tetraploid. Regardless of the ploidy, there are usually equal numbers of normal chr. 12, chr. $12q^+$ (mostly chr. 12 plus the telomeric portion of chr. 15), normal chr. 15 and chr. $15q^-$ (mostly chr. 15 plus a barely perceptible portion from the telomeric tip of chr. 12). The portion of each chromosome involved in the breakage and reciprocal exchange has been expanded, and a sketch of the molecular genetic map of the relevant regions is shown at the side of each chromosome. The normal chromosomes 12 and 15 are shown outside the products of the reciprocal translocation, chr. $12q^+$ and chr. $15q^-$ (9–12). Chr. $12q^+$ retains only a small portion of the IgH locus ($C\alpha$ and a portion of $S\alpha$) which is now apposed to coding $exon_2$ and $exon_3$ of c-*myc*. As shown by the vertical arrows, these genes are oriented in opposite directions relative to ribonucleic acid (RNA) transcription and coding sense. Chr. $12q^+$ is the source of the abundant c-*myc* RNA found in plasmacytomas; chr. 15 has no vertical arrow because it is usually transcriptionally silent in these cells (13–17). The other translocated chromosome ($15q^-$) has so little chromosomal material from chr. 12 that it took molecular genetic studies to prove that the translocation was really reciprocal (18–20). It retains only the 5′ portion of the c-*myc* gene apposed to the bulk of the IgH locus of chr. 12. Since c-*myc* $exon_1$ is filled with translational stop signals, apparently only noncoding c-*myc* sequences are left on chr. $15q^-$. Particularly significant, however, is that many important upstream elements that normally regulate expression of c-*myc* are located in $exon_1$ and its 5′ flanking region, and they have now been separated from the coding exons (2 and 3) of c-*myc*, which have been moved to chr. $12q^+$. In Fig. 2, the IgH gene segments are depicted in a germ-line configuration

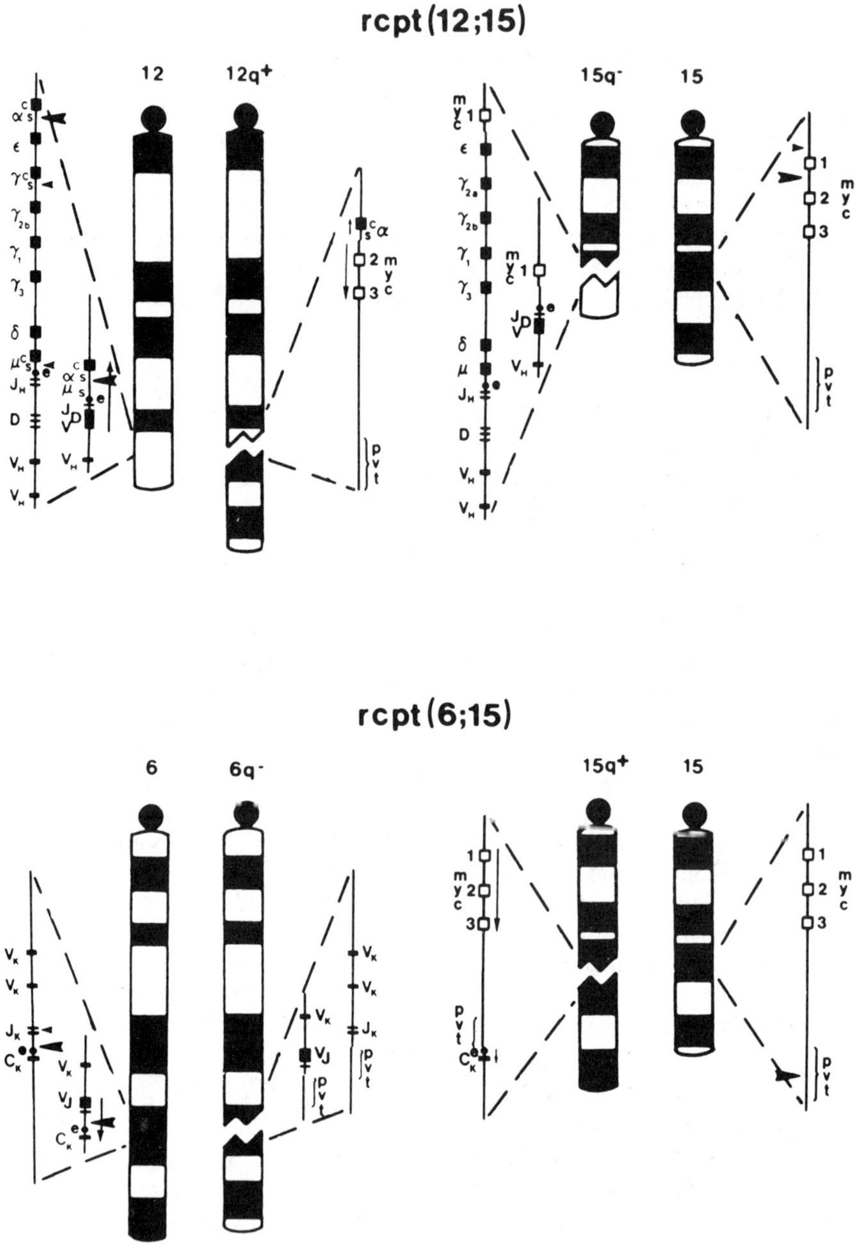

Figure 2 Diagram of mouse chromosomes 6, 12, and 15 plus a sketch of the Ig kappa, Ig heavy chain, and c-*myc* plus *pvt*-1 genes that are the sites of breakage of these chromosomes when they are involved in translocations in plasmacytomas (7,10,12–14, 16, 21, 22). Ig gene segments are shown as filled boxes (V = variable,

and after they have undergone VDJ assembly and C_H switch. Typically, however, any IgH rearrangement on chr. $15q^-$ is nonproductive; hence, there is no vertical arrow to indicate meaningful transcription.

rcpt(6;15)

The lower portion of Fig. 2 depicts the karyotypic and molecular events understood to happen in the less common, so-called variant, form of plasmacytoma translocation. This form has been found in about 10% of plasmacytomas induced by pristane alone and about 20% of those arising after pristane plus Abelson virus (2). The chromosomes and molecular maps are arranged as in the upper panel of Fig. 2, with the normals flanking the translocated chromosomes. Chromosome 6 bears the Ig kappa light chain locus, but its orientation relative to the centromere is opposite from that of IgH on chr. 12, that is, the many V_κ gene segments (of which only two are pictured here) are closer to the centromere than the single C_κ gene segment (21). The outer map is depicted in its germ-line form. The normal chr. 6 in plasmacytomas is generally productively rearranged by bringing one of the V_κ gene segments adjacent to one of the J_κ genes, and this arrangement is depicted between the outer map and the chromosome. The direction of RNA transcription is from top to bottom. The arrowheads show the places where this gene is broken and translocated, the J_κ region or in the intron between J_κ and C_κ (12,22). The most common site, as

---

D = diversity, J = joining, and C = constant region). Each of the seven heavy chain constant region gene segments consists of three to four exons, which are shown here as one filled box designated by a Greek letter, and each is preceded by a 5′ flanking region (introns are shown as lines) designated S (switch sequences). C_δ has no switch region, and only three of the six switch regions ($S\alpha$, $S\gamma_2$, and $S\mu$) are labeled to simplify the figure. In the leftmost heavy chain map the Ig genes are shown in their germ-line configuration. Plasma cells generally have rearranged one or both chromosomes 12 and 6 in assembly of productive V_HDJ_H or $V_\kappa J_\kappa$ variable (antigen-binding) regions. They might also have recombined various heavy chain switch regions to bring the V_HDJ_H next to another C_H gene segment, such as C_α. Examples of such rearranged genes are illustrated closer to the banded chromosomes. Only three of the many D segments, and two of the J_H, J_κ, V_H, and V_κ gene segments are illustrated. The enhancer sequences of the IgH and kappa genes are shown as filled circles labeled e. The direction of RNA transcription is from bottom to top for IgH and top to bottom for kappa. The three c-*myc* exons are shown as open boxes, and the c-*myc* allele actively being transcribed is indicated by the long vertical arrow from top to bottom. The small vertical arrows indicate the direction of transcription of C_κ and C_α genes in the translocated chromosomes. The large horizontal arrowheads point out the usual molecular locations of the chromosome breaks that give rise to the recombinations illustrated here in the middle diagrams; the smaller arrowheads indicate other breakpoints documented by cloning and sequencing. (Reviewed in Ref. 9.)

indicated by the larger arrowhead, is in the latter region, and it may be important to note that all of these translocations occur just 5′ of the C_κ enhancer (the filled circle marked *e* in Fig. 2).

As above, the normal chr. 15 is on the far right, but in these translocations the c-*myc* gene segments are not interrupted. Most, but not all, of the tumors with rcpt(6;15) have been shown to interrupt a region called *pvt*-1 (for plasmacytoma variant translocations) which is at least 94 kb downstream and telomeric from c-*myc* (9,12,21). Similar to the situation with rcpt(12;15), there are tumors with translocations known to involve chromosomes 6 and 15, but at sites that have not yet been mapped.

The reciprocally translocated chromosomes are shown in the center of the lower half of Fig. 2. In this form of translocation, the entire c-*myc* gene remains on chr. $15q^+$, and the C_κ gene segment plus its enhancer and the telomeric portion of chr. 6 are joined to it. This is presumed to be the active c-*myc* allele (9,12,21), as indicated by the vertical arrow. In contrast to the situation with the IgH transcription in rcpt(12;15), in rcpt(6;15) the direction of c-*myc* RNA transcription is the same as that for C_κ. Since the translocated C_κ is devoid of the V_κ promoter and the C_κ enhancer (12), significant transcription of that part of the $15q^+$ chromosome is unlikely. The active transcription of c-*myc* from this chromosome is thought to repress transcription from the normal chr. 15, but this is difficult to establish unambiguously. The $6q^-$ chromosome retains the V_κ and J_κ gene segments apposed to a portion of *pvt*-1 from chr. 15 and the remaining telomeric components of chr. 15. Interestingly, *pvt*-1 has been shown to be the site of proviral integration in about 10% of AKR T-cell lymphomas (23) and in Mo-MuLV–induced rat T-cell lymphomas (24). Molecular studies (24) suggest that breakpoints utilized in translocations and virus integrations, which define *pvt*-1, may occur over a distance of 70 kilobase pairs (kbp) or so. No enhanced transcription has been demonstrated from the *pvt*-1 locus in translocated or untranslocated chromosomes, so it is unlikely that this region contains oncogene elements. It is commonly assumed that deoxyribonucleic acid (DNA) sites of active RNA transcription, such as oncogenes and growth-related genes, are uncovered, have an open configuration of chromatin, and thus are vunerable to chromosome breakage, viral insertion, and recombination (25). Thus it remains mysterious why the *pvt*-1 site is frequently involved in plasmacytoma chromosome translocations, but only when chr. 6 is the reciprocating partner of the exchange of chromosomal material.

Internal Abnormalities Within Chromosome 15

Four (∿10%) of the karyotyped plasmacytomas lack visible chromosome translocations (2,8). High-resolution banding techniques permitted the detection of internal deletions within one chr. 15 in three of these tumors (26). The site of the deletion was the same as where c-*myc* has been localized, qD1qE, and the site usually involved in rcpt(12;15) and rcpt(6;15). Only one of these tumors (ABPC45) had a rearranged c-*myc* gene that enabled it to be cloned and studied at the molecular level. These studies (27) revealed that something more complicated than a simple deletion has occurred inasmuch as an insertion of two fragments from the IgH locus of chr. 12 had occurred upstream of c-*myc* $exon_1$. Because these fragments were found to be in opposite orientations, it appears that at least two chromosomal rearrangements had occurred, one or both of which may have been a rcpt(12;15). Thus, the banding pattern that appears as a deletion in chr. 15 (del. 15 qD1qE) may really be the result of a multistep translocation involving chr. 12. There are other examples of such a complicated multichromosomal rearrangement in ABPC17 (28) and the NZB plasmacytoma PC7183 (29) in which chr. 6 as well as chr. 12 and chr. 15 may have been involved in a concerted translocation.

There remains a single karyotyped plasmacytoma, ABPC22, in which no sign of chr. 15 aberration has been detected. It also has no rearrangement of the c-*myc* gene by Southern analysis of EcoRI digests (8), yet its level of c-*myc* transcript is within the same range as the other plasmacytomas (unreported data). Thus, there is every reason to suspect that ABPC22 has some chromosomal aberration in the vicinity of c-*myc* that leads to a deregulation of c-*myc* expression. The inability of chromosome studies to detect alterations smaller than 100–300 kbp may have prevented the detection of a karyotypic change in chr. 15 in ABPC22.

TIGHT REGULATION OF NORMAL c-*myc* GENE EXPRESSION

Since c-*myc* expression has proved to be germane to tumorigenesis, normal cell division, and differentiation, the molecular mechanisms that regulate c-*myc* expression have come under intensive study. Despite extensive investigations of the problem in chickens, rats, man, and mouse, it must be said that regulation of c-*myc* expression still holds many mysteries (30). The impression one gets from the manifold regulatory mechanisms and sites involved in regulation that have already been elucidated is that c-*myc* is a gene that is essential for eukaryotic life, and that its expression is under very tight control. There are multiple means to up-regulate c-*myc* expression at the transcriptional, RNA processing, translational, and posttranslational levels, and a similar redundancy exists for down-regulatory mechanisms. Thus, there are many ways to ensure a continued production of c-*myc* protein even in the face of genetic accidents such as point mutations or insertional mutations. Other properties such as transcriptional pausing and very short half-lives of c-*myc* messenger RNA (mRNA) and protein seem designed to preclude excessive accumulation of c-*myc* protein product. This may be because excessive levels of c-*myc* protein may adversely affect cell life. These are also particularly appropriate characteristics for a gene with a central role in regulation of cell proliferation. It is suspected that interruptions in this tight control may contribute to neoplastic transformation. With this kind of perspective, this section will summarize what is known about normal regulation of mouse c-*myc* expression. The next section will examine how this regulation is perturbed by the chromosomal translocations characteristic of mouse plasmacytomas, which were described in the previous section. Occasional reference will be made to studies of human c-*myc* and the plasmacytomalike chromosomal translocations seen in Burkitt's lymphomas, but this subject is dealt with in greater detail in chapter 5 of this book. A recent review that also deals with many of these concepts is recommended for another perspective (31).

Transcription of RNA

Fig. 3 presents a molecular map of the three exons of the mouse c-*myc* gene. Ribonucleic acid polymerase II transcribes this gene from left to right to yield mRNA, which can be translated into c-*myc* protein. Transcription normally starts at both of the two well-characterized promoters, P_1 and P_2 (17,19), which define the 5′ boundary of $exon_1$. Generally, P_2 is more active than P_1 in initiating transcripts. Ribonucleic acid transcription off the complementary strand of DNA, so-called antisense transcription, has been detected and proceeds from right to left. Nuclear run-on experiments hybridized to single-stranded DNA probes from small segments of both strands of DNA have shown that there are transcripts that begin upstream of P_1 (32). Discrete start sites of such transcripts have been described 550–650 bp 5′ of P_1 in the human *myc* gene and called P_0 (33). Homologous start site sequences are not found in the mouse and the origin of the upstream transcription has not been determined. Although these studies have shown RNA transcription throughout the c-*myc* gene in both directions, the RNA synthetic activity is not uniform. The rate of nuclear run-on RNA synthesis is indicated by the thickness of the horizontal lines pointed right (mRNA coding sense) and left (antisense) above the c-*myc* exon/intron map in Fig. 3. In several mouse cell lines transcription of $exon_1$ is very active, but an abrupt drop in transcriptional activity occurs near the end of $exon_1$ (*b* in Fig. 3 [32]). A rapid block of c-*myc* transcription elongation occurs at a similar site in the human c-*myc* gene when

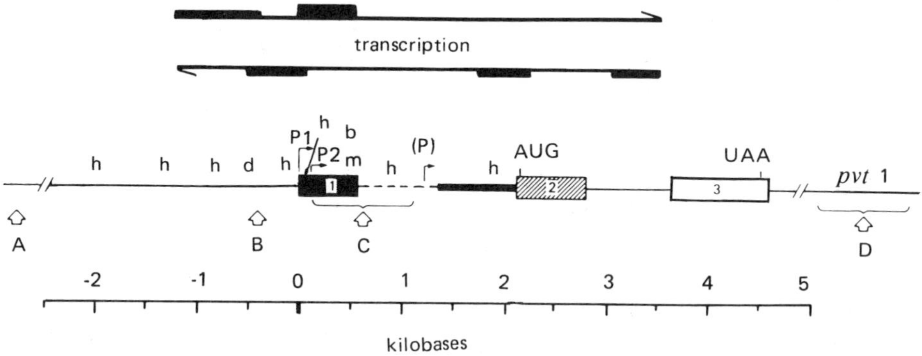

Figure 3 A molecular map of the murine c-*myc* gene is presented as the central line drawing. $Exons_{1-3}$ are indicated by boxes and introns by horizontal lines. Various sites of regulatory regions are indicated by lower case letters above the line: h = DNAase-hypersensitive sites (36); d = dehancer sequences (38); b – site of block or pausing in RNA transcription (32); and m = modulator region with positive effects on transcription (39). P_1 and P_2 are the usual promoters (17,19), and (P) represents one of many possible "cryptic" promoters activated only after loss of P_1 and P_2 (47,93,98,118,119). AUG and UAA indicate the locations of the translation start and stop codons in $exon_2$ and $exon_3$, respectively. *pvt*-1 (12) indicates the region telomeric from c-*myc* that is involved in most rcpt(6;15). The large vertical arrows below the line, labeled A–D, indicate frequent sites of breakage of this gene in chr. 15 translocations and alterations; B indicates the nearby site just 5′ of P_1; C indicates the most common site for breakpoints (it is quite broad, as indicated by the bracket, but the breakpoints of several tumors cluster in a short region just above the C); A and D indicate breaks very far from c-*myc*, most of which have not been localized but some of which fall in the *pvt*-1 region. Above the gene map are thick horizontal arrows representing transcriptional activity (32). The thickness of the top arrow pointing right indicates the activity of nuclear run-on transcription of coding mRNA strands; the line pointing left indicates level of transcription of antisense RNA. (From Ref. 32, used with permission.)

expresion of the amplified c-*myc* gene in the promyelocytic line HL-60 is rapidly down-regulated after differentiation is induced by dimethylsulfoxide or retinoic acid (34,35).

Thus, normal c-*myc* transcription seems to be regulated in or around $exon_1$. The promoters can be up-regulated by exogenous growth factors that stimulate cell division (see below), but a block in transcription toward the end of $exon_1$ greatly attenuates the level of transcription of $intron_1$ and, more significantly, the $exons_2$ and $_3$ which contain the c-*myc* coding regions. The promoter and blocker sequences appear to be negatively regulated by labile proteins. The antiblocker protein seems to act rapidly, presumably by binding directly to the DNA at the *b* site, whereas the promoters seem to be controlled more indirectly by DNA-binding proteins that act at a number of distant sites. Several DNAase-hypersensitive sites (*h*) have been identified upstream of $exon_2$ (36), which are thought to indicate places where an open chromatin structure would make the DNA accessible to controlling protein molecules. A very similar series of DNAase-hypersensitive sites have been reported for the human c-*myc* gene (37). The sites close to P_1 and P_2 are thought to be promoter sites where RNA polymerase binds and initiates mRNA synthesis. Those sites further upstream are felt to be for binding control molecules, mostly positive influences, but the precise effects that these upstream sites exert on c-*myc* transcription are controversial. Particularly close analysis of the effect of some of the sequences around $exon_1$ upon model transcription systems (CAT assays) have revealed down-regulator or "dehancer" sequences (*d*) about 500 bases upstream of P_1 (38), and an up-regulating, positive modulator (*m*) within $exon_1$ itself (39). Studies of the human c-*myc* gene (40) have identified similar positive and negative control elements.

Stabilization of mRNA

The primary effector molecules of c-*myc* expression are the protein products of c-*myc* mRNAs. Tests for levels of c-*myc* protein activity cannot yet be performed, since the principal biological activity of this protein has not yet been deciphered. Quantitative measures of c-*myc* protein have been attempted with various anti-*myc* antibodies, but most attempts at quantitation of c-*myc* expression have focused on levels of c-*myc* mRNA in RNA isolated from cells or tissues of interest. Northern blots of RNAs after electrophoretic separation and S1 nuclease protection assays have been used in conjunction with c-*myc*-specific hybridization probes to determine steady state levels of c-*myc* mRNAs. Although limited in some respects, these methods are the appropriate ones to learn how much c-*myc* message is available for translation at any particular time or under any particular conditions. So far, no stable steady-state mRNAs have been detected with upstream sequences, with short sequences of $exon_1$ alone, or with antisense sequences (32). Thus, these transcripts must be shortlived and in short supply. If they play any role in mouse c-*myc* physiology, they must act intranuclearly and in regulatory, i.e., noncoding, ways that are not yet understood.*

---

*In human cells $exon_1$ mRNAs and translation products have been identified, but their significance remains controversial (41).

It was indeed an observation of considerable importance when the normal half-life of c-*myc* mRNA was found to be very short, i.e., 10–30 min (42,43), but subject to prolongation under certain circumstances (44). As we will discuss below, this mechanism seems to be a very important one in the enhanced c-*myc* expression seen in mouse plasmacytomas and in proliferating normal cells (16,44–47).

Translation of mRNA into Protein

A controversial aspect of c-*myc* metabolism is whether regulation of c-*myc* mRNA translation is important in controlling normal c-*myc* expression. Such a mechanism was proposed when complementary regions about 70 nucleotides long were found in opposite orientations in $exon_1$ and $exon_2$ of a human c-*myc* sequence (48). Since these sequences could allow c-*myc* mRNA to form a stem-loop structure that would render the initiator codon in $exon_2$ inaccessible, it was proposed that normal c-*myc* might be poorly translatable. In contrast, c-*myc* mRNA which lacked $exon_1$ sequences secondary to a decapitating chromosomal translocation would be incapable of forming such a hairpin and, therefore, might be more efficiently translated. The results of in vitro translation of mouse c-*myc* mRNAs (49) were consistent with this hypothesis inasmuch as c-*myc* transcripts with shorter 5′ and 3′ untranslated regions were translated eight- to 10-fold more efficiently without an effect on mRNA stability. Two other studies (50,51) came to the opposite conclusion; namely, that in vitro translation of mouse and human c-*myc* mRNA was unaffected by the presence or absence of 5′ sequences, and that human cell lines contained comparable amounts of ribosome-bound c-*myc* mRNA and synthesized the same amount of immunoprecipitable c-*myc* protein regardless of whether $exon_1$ was present or not. What is more, phytohemagglutinin (PHA)-stimulated human peripheral blood T lymphocytes contained elevated levels of c-*myc* protein comparable to the elevated levels of c-*myc* mRNA (50).

Although its relevance in mammalian systems has not yet been established, translational control of c-*myc* synthesis seems to be important during Xenopus oogenesis. During this process the levels of c-*myc* mRNA remain constant and very high, yet dramatic changes occur in the rate of synthesis of c-*myc* protein (52–54). Dramatic changes in c-*myc* mRNA half-life are also noticed after fertilization and the onset of rapid cell division during embryogenesis. Thus, this system provides many lessons on control of c-*myc* expression. Of particular interest is the conclusion that in this situation, at least, *myc* expression does not completely correlate with cell proliferation.

A very short half-life of about 25 min has also been described for the c-*myc* protein product in the Colo 320 line of neuroectoderm cells from a colon tumor and other cells (55,56). One wonders if still another means of enhancing expression of the c-*myc* gene could be primary structural mutations or posttranslational alterations that could prolong the active half-life of this molecule by rendering it less sensitive to proteolysis. Alternatively, proteins that associate with the c-*myc* protein could stabilize it or enhance its activity, whatever that may be.

Between two and four distinct bands of immunoprecipitable c-*myc* protein have been detected by various *myc*-specific antisera (50,55), generally around 60–67 kd in size. Whether these represent translation products of two or more different c-*myc* mRNAs or result from different posttranslational modifications such as phosphorylation remains to be determined. One of these proteins may have a >6 hr half-life (57), so it is possible that there may be significant functional differences among the different forms of c-*myc* proteins. Another potentially important new observation documents the presence of a cryptic (non-AUG) initiator codon near the 3′ end of $exon_1$ that is used to generate a longer c-*myc* protein. Translation that begins at this upstream site adds ∿20 codons of additional open reading frame in the synthesis of one of the larger forms of c-*myc* protein in mouse, chicken, and man (58). This gives each cell the potential of making two c-*myc* proteins that differ at the aminoterminal and, perhaps, in their functional properties.

Relation to Cell Cycle

Some confusion has developed regarding whether normal c-*myc* expression varies in different parts of the cell cycle. The picture has cleared up recently, since many synthetic and breakdown components that contribute to steady-state levels of c-*myc* mRNA have been dissected. Early reports demonstrated that levels of c-*myc* mRNA were rapidly but temporarily increased 20- to 40-fold when quiescent (G_0) mouse fibroblasts, B, and T lymphocytes were induced to undergo mitotic cycling (44,46,59). This was thought to indicate that c-*myc* expression occurred primarily in the G_1 phase of the cell cycle and functioned as a factor endowing cells with the "competence" to progress through further stages of the mitotic cycle (46). Later studies in chicken embryo fibroblasts and chicken transformed T lymphocytes showed that although c-*myc* mRNAs levels do undergo a transient increase 1–2 hr after mitogenic stimulation of quiescent cells, the level of c-*myc* mRNA and protein synthesis is constant throughout the cell cycle (60,61). Similar results were obtained by these and other authors for murine and human cells, so the phenomenon is thought to be general

(60,62,63). Mitogenic stimuli, such as lectins, peptide growth factors, phorbol esters, calcium ionophores, antireceptor antibodies, lymphokines, and partial hepatectomy, commonly cause marked, transient elevations in c-*myc* mRNA and protein levels in normal cells by a variable combination of increased transcription and decreased breakdown (44,46,50,57,59,63–73). All the agonists that activate the phosphoinositide turnover/protein kinase C cascade also lead to increased c-*myc* expression, so this pathway has been implicated in the transduction of some of these mitogenic stimuli. Another second messenger pathway appears to utilize adenylate cyclase and cAMP instead of protein kinase C to transmit the c-*myc* activation and mitogenic effects of epidermal growth factor on serum-deprived (not confluence-arrested) 3T3 cells (74). These physiological activations of c-*myc* expression apparently do not alter the ratio of $P_2 > P_1$ promoter usage (46). However, under certain circumstances, platelet-derived growth factor can induce cell division in fibroblasts without evidence of c-*myc* activation (69). So although c-*myc* activation is clearly connected with cell division in several systems, it may be only one of several pathways that transduce mitogenic signals (69,71).

Relation to Cell Differentiation and Maturation

As high levels of v-*myc* and c-*myc* expression became associated with normal and neoplastic cell growth, the concept arose that *myc* expression might confer immortality to cells. This has been tested by transfecting cells with expression vectors bearing *myc* sequences, and immortalization was not routinely achieved. Instead, a related phenomenon was observed; namely, high levels of c-*myc* expression were incompatible with many different specialized functions of cells. This has been demonstrated in three different sorts of experiments. First, c-*myc* RNA levels were found to be lower in tumors of B lymphocytes and myelomonocytic cells that expressed more differentiated characteristics (75). The exception here was the plasmacytoma, a nearly end-stage B lymphocyte with high levels of c-*myc* mRNA.

Second, the high levels of c-*myc* mRNA that are present in certain immature cell lines diminished when the cells were induced to become more differentiated. This effect has been repeatedly observed when the HL-60 human promyelocytic leukemia cell line and the WEHI-3B mouse myeloblast line were induced by a variety of agents to develop into mature granulocytic or macrophagic cells (76,77). More recently, the teratocarcinoma cell line F9, myoblast, and Friend erythroleukemia cells have also been shown to exhibit down-regulation of c-*myc* mRNA (frequently biphasic) when induced to differentiate into parietal ectoderm, myotubes, and erythroid cells, respectively (78–83). Whereas the decrease in c-*myc* mRNA levels in the teratocarcinoma system has been shown to be principally a function of posttranscriptional destabilization rather than decreased transcription (79,81), decreased c-*myc* mRNA synthesis (in part operating at the transcription block site at the end of $exon_1$) was the principal cause of its decreased expression in muscle (80) and HL-60 (34,35) differentiation. Both transcriptional and posttranscriptional effects have been detected in erythroleukemia differentiation (83).

Third, expression vectors were used to introduce active recombinant *myc* genes into avian myoblasts or mouse erythroleukemia (Friend) cells. The constitutive *myc* expression from the provirus inhibited the usual differentiation responses seen when these cells are treated with dimethylsulfoxide or similar agents (84–87). Contrariwise, there are reports that expression of c-*myc* increases during differentiation of chronic lymphocytic leukemia (CLL) cells (88) and lens epithelium (89), although the latter increase may be transient.

In summary, the processes involved in terminal differentiation and cell division are multiple, interrelated, and poorly understood. It is clear that c-*myc* expression is closely tied with some of them but uncoupled with others. The protean nature of the stimuli that affect c-*myc* expression and the variety of ways in which that expression can be regulated renders it difficult, at this time, to state with certainty its role in differentiation. Clearly, however, *myc* expression is not totally incompatible with cellular differentiation in certain systems.

DEREGULATION OF c-*myc* GENE EXPRESSION BY CHROMOSOME 15 TRANSLOCATIONS

Evidence for Deregulation of c-*myc* Expression in Plasmacytomas

The earliest observers of the transcriptional characteristics of plasmacytomas were impressed by their prodigious levels of Ig heavy and light chain mRNAs (see Ref. 1 for discussion). The concept of allelic exclusion arose when it was found that usually only one of each pair of chromosomes bearing Ig genes was productively rearranged and being expressed. Later, the c-*myc* locus was found to be involved in translocations with the IgH-bearing chr. 12 or the Ig kappa-bearing chr. 6, in both cases involving the "nonproductively" rearranged Ig alleles or chromosome (90). The c-*myc* transcripts were traced to the translocated allele, and the c-*myc* gene on the nonrearranged chr. 15 was generally found to be transcriptionally silent. Authors varied in the way they viewed the c-*myc* RNA levels. Some regarded the levels as higher than those found in other B-cell neoplasms or in tumors of other cell types that arose in the same induction experiments (16,45), whereas others felt the levels were not substantially elevated (13,14). It was agreed that mRNAs of abnormal size were frequently present. Human Burkitt lymphomas, B-cell neoplasms which sometimes secrete Ig, were found to have similar disruption of their c-*myc* gene due to chromosome translocation (91–94) and similar levels of c-*myc* mRNAs. At least part of the problem in deciding whether these levels were inappropriate was the difficulty of choosing a normal tissue for comparison. There is no good source of nonneoplastic mouse plasma cells or of the normal counterpart of Burkitt lymphoma cells, whatever cell that might be. Mitogen-stimulated B lymphocytes achieve nearly the same high levels of c-*myc* mRNA as plasmacytomas (47), so the absolute levels in these tumor cells cannot be considered completely abnormal. Thus, one must look further to define c-*myc*'s contribution to the transformation process.

Structural studies on normal and translocated c-*myc* mRNAs revealed a few Burkitt lymphomas with mutations, primarily in exon$_1$ and its 5′ and 3′ flanking regions (95–97), but virtually no structural mutations were found in mouse c-*myc* genes (16,17,98,99). The universal association of chromosomal translocations in the vicinity of the c-*myc* locus with mouse plasmacytomas and human Burkitt lymphomas strongly implicated the c-*myc* gene in the pathogenesis of these tumors (100,101). Since structural mutations in the c-*myc* coding regions appeared to be rare, the oncogenic activation of the proto-oncogene c-*myc* was generally agreed to stem not from alteration to the normal protein structure but from an alteration in its expression (102–106). Careful comparison of c-*myc* RNA levels (44,46,47) showed that lipopolysaccharide (LPS)-stimulated splenic B lymphocytes rapidly achieve high levels of c-*myc* RNA transcripts, but these levels usually fall to much more modest levels in the course of a few hours; these modest levels remain as the cells continue through cycles of cell division. Thus, only the initial entry into a proliferative state from a resting state is accompanied by tumorlike levels of c-*myc* mRNA, whereas the high levels characteristic of plasmacytomas appear to be more or less constant. This inappropriately high level of expression, which is constitutive or not regulatable, is felt to constitute c-*myc*'s contribution to neoplasia.

Another way of looking at this situation is to extrapolate from data obtained from B-cell tumors of varying degrees of differentiation (75,102). This predicts that if "normal" plasma cells could be isolated and studied, they would have very low levels of c-*myc* RNA, levels consistent with a highly methylated c-*myc* gene characteristic of a nondividing, terminally differentiated cell stage (107). This is consistent with data from somatic cell hybrids made from human Burkitt cells and mouse plasmacytoma cells (108,109) which indicate that the normal (untranslocated) c-*myc* gene is generally inactive (not generating stable mRNAs). Of course, these data came from cells in which there was abundant transcription of c-*myc* from the translocated chromosomes. Thus, it could also be argued that the normal c-*myc* allele was silenced by feedback from the products of the active allele rather than by stage-specific factors present in nearly end-stage B cells (105).

From our current vantage point it seems important to reexamine the data behind the conclusions that c-*myc* expression is constitutive or deregulated. Fig. 4 is a northern blot analysis of 5 μg of poly(A)$^+$ RNA prepared from 19 BALB/c plasmacytomas, normal mouse spleen, and four other hematopoietic tumors hybridized with a mouse c-*myc* probe. The only tumor negative for c-*myc* RNA is J3PC2093, which harbors an active J-3 provirus that synthesizes large quantities of v-*myc* RNA protein (4). The tumor expresses very little or no c-*myc* mRNA owing to feedback from the J-3 v-*myc* product or a normal plasmacytoma-specific down-regulation or both. Eight of the plasmacytomas (ABPCs) were induced by pristane plus Abelson virus and were chosen because they include examples of all the known types of chromosomal alterations: rcpt(6;15),* rcpt(12;15),† and interstitial chr. 15 deletions.‡ A lymphosarcoma (ABLS109), myeloid lines (ABPL1 and 2), and a mast cell tumor (ABMC20), which also arose in mice given pristane and Abelson virus, are included for comparison. The remaining plasmacytomas were induced with pristane alone in BALB/c mice plus one tumor each from C57BL (BFPC1) and CB20 (CBPC112) mice. Hybridomas (Hy14 and SP2/0) were included as well as plasmacytoma RNA from early transplant generations (TEPC) or from tumors that had been passaged scores of times (LPC1, MOPC104E, SP2/0). All of these plasmacytomas contained steady-state levels of 2.0–2.4 kb c-*myc* RNA that are higher than any normal resting tissue or the other tumors induced by the same regimen. The band of hybridization for ABPC103 is fainter than that of all the other plasmacytomas. This is primarily a result of a lower amount of RNA in this lane as determined by ethidium bromide staining and hybridization of blots to a housekeeping gene (data not shown), but it may also reflect a certain degree of variation in c-*myc* RNA levels among plasmacytomas. On the other end of the scale is TEPC1165, which has an unusually high level of c-*myc* RNA (45). No mitogenically stimulated normal cells are included in this comparison, but LPS-treated splenic B cells only transiently approach the high levels of c-*myc* RNA consistently and continually found in these plasmacytomas (47). What is more, this figure emphasizes that the high steady-state c-*myc* RNA level is found in virtually all plasmacytomas whether they contain a rcpt(12;15), rcpt(6;15), or just a del(15), and regardless of the length of time they have

---

*rcpt(6;15) karyotype: ABPC4, ABPC20, ABPC103 (8).
†rcpt(12;15) karyotype: ABPC24, ABPC60, APBC89 (8); TEPC1017, TEPC1165, J3PC2095 (4,9)
‡del(15) karyotype: ABPC45, ABPC26, CBPC112 (2).

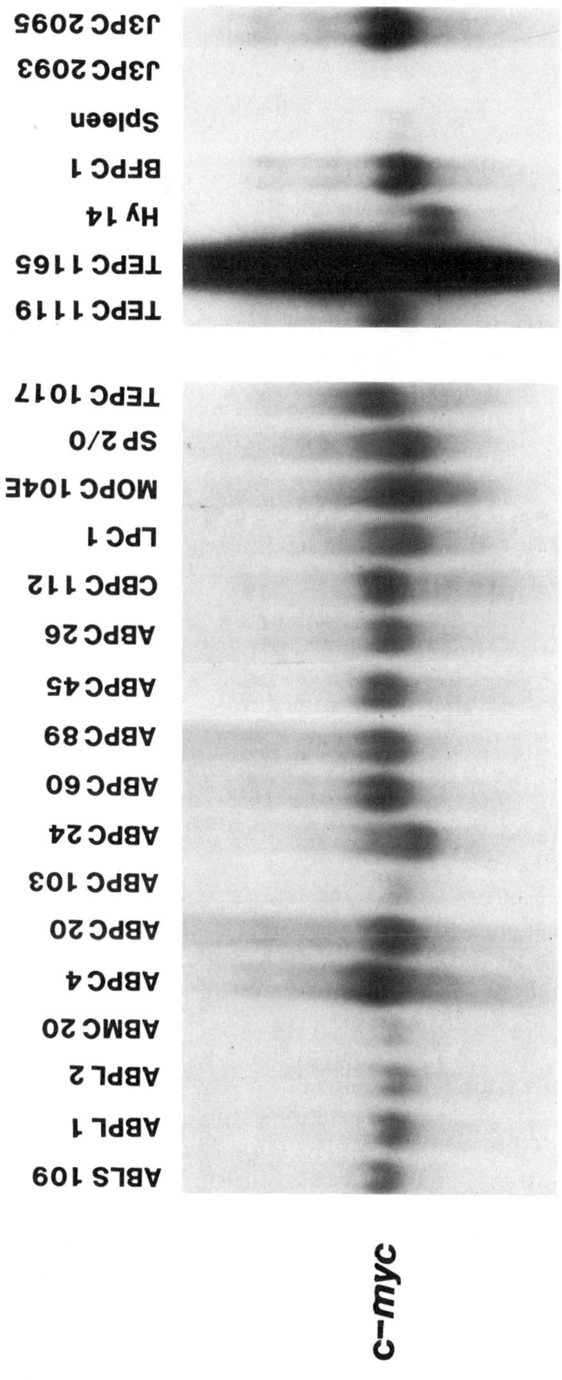

Figure 4 Northern blot of 5 μg of poly(A)$^+$RNA from plasmacytomas (PC) and other tumors and tissues after electrophoresis in 1% agarose containing methyl mercuric hydroxide and blotting onto diazothiophenylether paper (45) The two blots were run simultaneously and probed identically with nick-translated c-*myc* cDNA pMc-*myc* 54 (98) and stringently washed.

been carried in transplant. Since these cells were neither cultured nor synchronized, these high levels cannot be related to stage of cell cycle. Furthermore, studies of c-*myc* levels in plasmacytomas have been found to be invariant in different phases of the cell cycle (110).

What other evidence is there to indicate that expression of one or both c-*myc* alleles is constitutive; i.e., always being expressed, in plasmacytomas (or the very analogous human Burkitt lymphomas)? As mentioned earlier, in plasmacytoma cells, in Burkitt lymphoma cells, and in hybrids of the two cell types, there is usually a difference in the regulation of the c-*myc* locus on the normal and the translocated chromosome. The translocated one is expressed, whereas the normal one is not. This repression of the normal c-*myc* allele may result from a feedback inhibition by the products of the high levels of transcription of the other allele or from other down-regulation signals attendant to final stages of B-cell maturation or both, but the allele on the translocated chromosome no longer responds to these influences. This is also clearly demonstrated in plasmacytomas themselves, at least in those tumors where the normal and (12;15) translocated (decapitated) c-*myc* transcripts can be differentiated by their size. The interrupted c-*myc* transcript is usually small ($\sim$2 kb), whereas the normal transcript is 2.4 kb in size and contains $exon_1$ sequences. In these tumors, no RNA from the normal chromosome is detected (17,93). It also must be true in TEPC1165, which has a rcpt(12;15) that does not interrupt the c-*myc* transcriptional unit, but instead breaks chr. 15 just 198 bases 5′ to P_1 and contains a mutation leading to larger than normal c-*myc* mRNA (111). No 2.4-kb normal mRNA is seen here either. It is not yet clear whether the normal chromosome is inactive in most tumors with rcpt(6;15) or del(15) because the mRNAs from the two chromosomes 15 cannot usually be distinguished (see below).

It is important to bear in mind that these deregulating translocations do not remove all possibilities of regulation from the c-*myc* gene. When the translocated c-*myc* chromosome from a Burkitt lymphoma was put into the cellular context of a quiescent fibroblast or lymphoblastoid cell it became transcriptionally inactive (112,113). Only certain Burkitt lines, such as Daudi, with an IgH enhancer near c-*myc*, retains c-*myc* transcriptional activity in lymphoblastoid cells (114). In a similar vein, c-*myc* expression in the Daudi line of Burkitt's lymphoma cells can be lowered by treatment with interferon α or β (115,116). The interferon effect on Daudi occurs at a posttranscriptional level (116), while it is not yet certain where the tissue-specific regulation of normal and translocated c-*myc* takes place.

Another indication that c-*myc* expression is altered by certain of the translocations in plasmacytomas is the change in usage of the different promoters or start sites for RNA synthesis. Normally, c-*myc* mRNA contains more transcripts beginning at P_2 than at P_1 (cf. Fig. 3) in both human and murine cells (19,117), but translocations that break the c-*myc* locus just 5′ of P_1 alter this promoter usage in favor of P_1 (105,111). Curiously, in the plasmacytoma lines it appeared that the increase in the P_1/P_2 usage ratio may have stemmed more from a decrease in use of P_2 than an increase in P_1 usage. Only three human lines were studied in this way, and the usage of P_1 and P_2 varied too greatly to draw any conclusion concerning the primary change occurring at P_1 and P_2. Of course, in many plasmatomas (and Burkitt's lymphomas) the rcpt(12;15) translocation occurs within $exon_1$ or $intron_1$, removing the usual P_1 and P_2 promoters from their functional position upstream of the coding $exon_2$ and $exon_3$. The majority of the c-*myc* transcripts found in these tumors originate from atypical (lacking TATA boxes) "cryptic" promoters within $intron_1$ (47,93,98,118,119). These may be found at multiple sites within the intron, although only one such (P) is shown in Fig. 3. These cases are even more dramatic evidence that the translocations disrupt the normal transcription of c-*myc*, and we will consider the consequences of this disruption below.

Effects of Interruption 5′ of $Exon_1$

It seems important that all seven of the plasmacytomas with breakpoints upstream of the c-*myc* transcription unit have breaks within a very small area, 200–400 bp 5′ to *myc* $exon_1$ (27,28,111). In fact, two of the three breakpoints that have been precisely located by DNA sequencing, ABPC17 and ABPC45, occur at the very same nucleotide 365 bp upstream of P_1 (27,28). This area is indicated by the large vertical arrow marked B in Fig. 3. The consequences of breakpoints near B are the removal of regions 5′ to this breakpoint, which contain several regions thought to be involved in control of c-*myc* expression: three DNAase-hypersensitive sites (h in Fig. 3 [36]) and the down-regulating anti-enhancer or "dehancer" (d in Fig. 3 [38]). The three h sites have been shown to be associated with active c-*myc* transcription (36), although certain aspects of this interpretation are controversial (37,120,121). This suggests, but does not necessarily mean, that these are sites that bind up-regulating factors. Thus, breakage at B potentially would remove three positive (h) and one negative (d) transcriptional control elements from their normal position upstream of the structural exons. Thus, even ignoring the potential contribution of the 5′ sequences brought in by the translocation, it is not possible to predict a priori what the net effect of these 5′ translocations might have on c-*myc* transcription. It probably is fair to ignore the nature of the new upstream sequences inasmuch as the levels of c-*myc* mRNA seem about the same for five out of the seven plasmacytomas with 5′ interruptions by very different parts of chr. 12.* Three of these five bring in switch regions sequences (ABPC33 [$S\gamma_{2a}$], TEPC1033 [$S\gamma_{2b}$] and TEPC1194 [$S\mu$]; Ref. 111) in head-to-head orientation, whereas two others (ABPC17 and ABPC45 [27,28]) bring $S\mu$ plus the IgH enhancer as an insertion element in head-to-tail orientation. The other effect on transcription, i.e.; a decrease in usage of the P_2 promoter (cf. previous section), occurs equally in each of this group of plasmacytomas regardless of the presence or absence of the IgH enhancer (111). It has been shown that P_1 and P_2 are under independent regulation and that transcription starting at P_2 (not P_1) is turned off when separated from $exon_2$ and $exon_3$ by translocation (118). This may indicate that P_2 is more sensitive that P_1 to down-regulation by excess c-*myc* products, and this difference contributes to the change in ratio of P_1/P_2 usage in this situation. These observations imply that the final common determinant of the constitutively high levels of c-*myc* RNA lies further downstream, such as the regulatable block to continued transcription at the end of $exon_1$ (b) or mRNA stabilization, as discussed in greater detail previously. It may be, then, that the control regions defined upstream are more important in normal fine tuning of c-*myc* transcription or transducing its up-regulation by growth factors. When translocation removes these control regions from the rest of c-*myc*, other influences seem to take over its expression, and these may lack some degree of regulation. This concept is better illustrated in the situation discussed in the following section.

Effects of Interruption Within the Transcription Unit

The majority of plasmacytomas have translocations that break the c-*myc* gene within $exon_1$ or $intron_1$, and all of these appear to be examples of rcpt(12;15), although not all tumors with this molecular finding have been characterized karyotypically. A detailed summary of most of the translocation mapping and chromosome translocation information and breakpoint determinations can be found in Refs. 2 and 9. The area in which these translocations occur is fairly wide, including about 1000 bp, as indicated by a bracket marked C in Fig. 3. This broad region is also the site of most translocations in Burkitt's lymphoma (9), but there is a heavy concentra-

---

*Only TEPC1165 and TEPC2027 have extraordinarily high levels of c-*myc* mRNA owing to a defect in splicing out $intron_1$ due to structural mutations at the $exon_1$-$intron_1$ junction (122).

tion of breakpoints in both forms of malignancies near the C arrow in the 5′ part of intron$_1$. The effect of interruption here (once again ignoring the nature of the new 5′ sequences brought in by the translocation) is to remove all the upstream regulatory sites lost by interruptions at B plus the normal promoters P_1 and P_2 (with their attendant DNAase I-hypersensitive sites, h) and some or all of the other putative control regions indicated as b, m, and h in Fig. 3. As shown in Fig. 4, the levels of *myc* mRNA are elevated to about the same extent after translocation, but frequently the mRNA size is smaller; e.g., 2 kb in ABPC24. The lack of exon$_1$ contributes to the decrease in size of the final mRNA, but it necessitates the usage of alternate, "cryptic" promoters [designated (P) in Fig. 3] within the remaining 3′ part of intron$_1$. The cryptic promoters are not normally used when exon$_1$ and its two typical promoters are present. The cryptic ones are not as well defined as P_1 and P_2, since most lack cannonical TATA box sequences and vary widely in site. Fifteen different RNA start sites have been mapped in this region in a single decapitated plasmacytoma (118) and other different from these 15 have been identified in additional plasmacytomas (47,98,119). What is more, cryptic splice sites, both donor and acceptor, have been utilized in transcripts initiated at these cryptic promoters, but none of these transcripts would generate open reading frames and altered c-*myc* proteins (118). The postulated cryptic translation initiator codon in exon$_1$ (58) would also be removed by most decapitating translocations. Thus, these tumors would have lost the ability to synthesize this larger form of c-*myc* protein, but the contribution this could play in carcinogenesis is still unknown.

One additional effect is achieved by this decapitation of all or part of exon$_1$ and activation of cryptic promoters in intron$_1$. These c-*myc* RNA transcripts start 3′ of exon$_1$ and, therefore, lack the strong, consensus splice donor site at the exon$_1$-intron$_1$ junction. Even though some cryptic splice sites may also be activated (118), at least a portion of intron$_1$ will remain on the mature c-*myc* mRNA after posttranscriptional processing. Most reports have concluded that lack of exon$_1$ sequences leads to longer half-lives of plasmacytoma and Burkitt c-*myc* mRNA (95,123), but recent data indicate that the presence of intron sequences, instead, are responsible in large measure for the increased stability of the c-*myc* mRNAs observed in plasmacytomas (122). Thus, an indirect consequence of typical rcpt(12;15) translocations is an increased level of c-*myc* RNA (and, presumably, protein) due to a prolongation of its normally very short half-life.

Effects of Distant Interruptions of the c-*myc* Chromosome

The maps of the c-*myc* chromosome and exons shown shown in Figs. 2 and 3 indicate that even high-resolution karyotypic studies in themselves cannot determine where (position A, B, C, or D) the c-*myc* locus is interrupted in a particular tumor, because all these chromosome alterations appear as breaks at the same chromosome band. Furthermore, when the alterations occur too far from the c-*myc* exons to cause DNA rearrangements detectable by Southern blot hybridization (i.e., 5′ or 3′ of the EcoRI sites that define the 21-kb EcoRI fragment containing c-*myc*), it is difficult to determine whether the interruptions are centromeric (site A) or telomeric (site D). Although the translocations from two Burkitt's lymphomas have been estimated to be greater than 8 kb 5′ from c-*myc* (97,124), in mouse plasmacytomas none has been mapped between 500 and 8000 bp 5′ of c-*myc*. There are quite a few human and mouse tumors where the breakpoint has not been mapped, so it is possible that some will be found to have occurred at a considerable distance on the 5′ side. Most of the distant translocations that have been successfully mapped have occurred on the 3′ side in the human and mouse tumors. Without exception these distant 3′ translocations have occurred in the rarer "variant" forms of translocation which involve the Ig kappa light chain chromosome in man (124–127) and mouse (21), or the Ig lambda light chain chromosome (128,129), so far found only in Burkitt's lymphomas, not mouse plaasmacytomas. The translocations involving Ig light chain chromosomes are far less common than those with the Ig heavy chain chromosome, and the c-*myc* gene remains on its chromosome rather than translocating to the Ig chromosome (ending up in a head-to-tail transcriptional orientation) unlike the more common form (21,124–129).

Since the variant translocations occur far from the c-*myc* locus on mouse chr. 15, it proved difficult to characterize and map them. The characterization was accomplished using the rearrangement of the Ig kappa locus (generally 5′ of the C_κ gene segment) that usually is involved in the chr. 6 component of the mouse rcpt(6;15) translocation (12,22,29). This procedure isolated clones of an 18-kb portion of chr. 15 that contained the breakpoints involved in six of the nine plasmatomas bearing rcpt(6;15). This region was called *pvt*-1, for plasmacytoma variant translocation (12). The same region (or homologues in other species) was later found to be involved in a number of other alterations: (a) proviral (MCF and Mo-MuLV) integration in about 10% of AKR mouse T lymphomas (23); (b) Mo-MuLV proviral integration in rat thymomas (24); (c) rcpt(2;8) in three variant human Burkitt's lymphomas (130,131);

(d) intrachromosome deletion in a case of HTLV-1–associated human T-cell leukemia (131); and (e) termination of the regions amplified in one mouse tumor (130) and three human tumors bearing c-*myc* amplifications (131). This expansion of the nature of the involvement of the *pvt*-1 area in tumor-and c-*myc*–related genetic alterations has necessitated enlarging the size of the region included in the *pvt*-1 designation to nearly 40 kb, but it has also enabled it to be placed about 300 kb downstream of c-*myc* (131) on the human chromosome. Since the homology between mouse and human sequences is low, cross-hybridization is not detectable. The distance of *pvt*-1 from c-*myc* in mice cannot be determined more precisely than >94 kb (130).

Despite this substantial separation from c-*myc*, it appears that the rcpt(6;15) activates c-*myc* expression. Surely the levels of c-*myc* mRNA in plasmacytomas with this form of translocation are comparable with those of rcpt(12;15) or del(15) as shown in Fig. 4 and Ref. 8. As discussed previously, rcpt(12;15) plasmacytomas generally do not express c-*myc* from the untranslocated "normal" chromosome, either due to the nearly end-stage nature of this cell type or to the presence of excessive transcripts from the other chromosome. In cells bearing rcpt(6;15) with chr. 15 breaks outside of the c-*myc* transcription unit, it is generally impossible to distinguish between transcripts from the normal and the translocated allele. The B-cell line BALTNM17A contains both rcpt(6;15) and rcpt(12;15) translocations and c-*myc* RNAs of 2.4 and 1.9 kb presumably transcribed from these two alleles, respectively (12). Thus, it seems likely that rcpt(6;15) also activates c-*myc* transcription from the involved chromosome and prevents its inactivation by rcpt(12;15) influences which usually inactivate it on normal chromosomes. Data from somatic cell hybrids between plasmacytomas and "variant" Burkitt lymphomas support this concept (125,128). The mechanism of this activation remains unknown, but it offers a fine opportunity for speculation. If *pvt*-1 were another oncogene, as could be anticipated from its frequent involvement in chromosome breaks or provirus integrations, then its product might activate c-*myc* in *cis* or, more likely, in *trans*. Yet no reproducibly detectable transcripts have been detected using probes from this region, even when proviruses or Ig-bearing chromosome regions are integrated within it (12,130). This makes it unlikely that *pvt*-1 is an oncogene. The rather broad stretch of DNA included in the *pvt*-like region (131) makes it unlikely that it represents a single entity or a single gene. Since *pvt*-1 has been shown to be coamplified with c-*myc* in at least four tumors (130,131), it is possible that the c-*myc* unit extends this far and that factors that perturb *pvt*-1 (e.g., open its chromatin) may concomitantly affect c-*myc* at the other end of this unit.

Studies have been carried out on various aspects of c-*myc* expression in tumors with rcpt(6;15). The 5′-most DNAase-hypersensitivity site (cf. Fig. 3) is detected on only one chromosome in these tumors, indicating that the chromatin of only one (presumably the translocated chromosome) is activated and responsive to positive regulating signals (36). Transcriptional activity of the c-*myc* gene in rcpt(6;15) as measured in nuclear run-on studies was determined to be comparable to that of most rcpt(12;15) plasmacytomas and B-cell tumors (123). There is no deviation from the normal ratio of $P_2 > P_1$ promoter usage in rcpt(6;15) plasmacytomas (111), indicating that the breakage and recombination at the distant *pvt*-1 site does not affect this aspect of c-*myc* transcription. It is worthy of mention, however, that several variant human Burkitt's lymphoma lines, both rcpt(2;8) and rcpt(8;22), with breakpoints only 1–5 kbp on the 3′ side of c-*myc*, i.e., much closer than *pvt*-1, did show increased transcription from the normally less utilized P_1 promoter (96,129,132).

Effects on c-*myc* Chromatin Structure

Chromatin structure is an intriguing and controversial aspect of c-*myc* activation and translocation. It may be important not only in regulating c-*myc* expression, but also in determining the sites involved in the nonrandom translocations. It is generally accepted that stretches of DNA are accessible for proviral integration or chromosome translocation only when the local chromatin structure permits (25). Open chromatin structure occurs during DNA replication, but this occurs throughout the entire genome and could not predispose to nonrandom events. Demethylation and opening of chromatin (seen as appearance of DNAase-hypersensitive sites) also are associated with RNA transcription, and this certainly occurs only at certain genes and at certain times or in certain cells due to tissue or differentiation-stage specificity of gene activity. The *myc* gene is active in virtually all cell types to a varying degree, whereas Ig genes are characteristically transcriptionally activated only in B lymphocytes which are the hosts for the c-*myc* translocations presently under discussion. What is more, the Ig genes characteristically undergo breaks and genetic recombination during the $V_L \rightarrow J_L$, $D \rightarrow J_H$, and $V_H \rightarrow DJ_H$ rearrangements required for generation of antigen-binding sites, another process that requires open chromatin configuration. More specifically, Ig switch regions appear to be transcriptionally activated just prior to being involved in isotype switch recombination (133). These switch regions are the most frequent targets of the rcpt(12;15) recombination. The cell factors that lead to the demethylation and opening of the chromatin in these particular genes are very likely to remain present in plasmacytomas after the "nonfunctional" rearrangements of Ig chromosomes with the c-*myc* chromosome (36,107,134,135). The presence of open Ig chromatin atypically close and on the same chromosome as one of the c-*myc* alleles, which normally would be inactive in cells of this stage of maturation, may be sufficient to prevent inactivation of this c-*myc* allele. The specific consequences of the particular breakpoint used in each tumor cell may be less important to causing constitutive c-*myc* expression than the general opening of chromatin structure in the region which may occur secondary to all of the possible chr. 15 alterations common in plasmacytomas. The *myc*-associated region may be very large, as suggested by the frequent involvement of *pvt*-1, perhaps 300 kb distant, in c-*myc* amplification. Thus, activation of *pvt*-1 by virus integration or Ig chromosome integration may affect the chromatin of the whole "amplicon" (including c-*myc* at the other end). Surely, the promoter and enhancer of the requisite LTR of an integrated, active provirus could be a strong chromatin opener. In what may be an analogous situation, every plasmacytoma with rcpt(6;15) that has been cloned and studied contains the Ig kappa enhancer in the *pvt*-1 recombination site. Although the IgH enhancer has only rarely been shown to have been translocated close to the c-*myc* locus, in the two cases where it has been found close to c-*myc* (27,28), it came as an insertional element rather than as part of a simple rcpt(12;15). Thus, there may be additional examples of IgH enhancer insertions that have not been detected because they are so small. Particularly likely candidates would include the other translocation-negative plasmacytomas which cannot easily be studied molecularly.

Very commonly IgH switch regions interrupt c-*myc* in rcpt(12;15), but these regions end up in opposite transcription orientations. Sometimes one can detect transcripts of c-*myc* that originate in these switch regions, but the more important aspect of the proximity of such switch regions may be their influence which keeps the neighboring c-*myc* chromatin accessible for transcriptional machinery. Then, owing to the remarkable redundancy of control regions that can activate the c-*myc* gene, even in the face of point mutations or gross insertions or deletions, it is constitutively transcribed.

Effects of Mutations

Reports of somatic mutations in $exon_1$ of human c-*myc* cloned from Burkitt's lymphomas (95–97) led to enthusiasm for the theory that normal c-*myc* transcription was subject to feedback repression. Mutations could interfere with this feedback and lead to abnormal, constitutive c-*myc* expression (105). The lack of finding such mutations when normal mouse and plasmacytoma c-*myc* sequences were compared led to dissatisfaction with this theory. More recently, there have been additional reports of mutations in DNAs from large numbers of Burkitt's lymphomas (136,137), again involving $exon_1$ and flanking regions. Clusters of these mutations were noted near the 3′ end of $exon_1$, the same region (b in Fig. 3) that recently has been shown to be involved in blocking progression of RNA transcription from $exon_1$ into downstream (coding) regions of the gene (32–35) and the site of the cryptic translation initiation codon (58). It is known that a labile protein is involved in this blockage of transcription progression (32). Since at least in some tumors, the block was gone (34), it is possible that mutations in this site prevent binding of the protein, release the block, and effectively increase the level of c-*myc* RNA. Another possible effect of mutations in this area is to inactivate the cryptic $exon_1$ translation initiator codon (58). This would have an effect similar to those translocations discussed in the preceding section, which decapitate $exon_1$ from the rest of the c-*myc* gene; namely, to preclude synthesis of the larger c-*myc* protein. More examples of analogous mutations in mouse plasmacytomas are being found (122), so this mechanism may prove to play a more widespread and important role in c-*myc* deregulation than expected heretofore. It is worrisome that most Burkitt lines have been maintained in tissue culture for very long periods of time, during which time random point mutations could have occurred that may have nothing to do with the origins of the tumors. This may not be the case for c-*myc*, however, inasmuch as similar mutations were found in primary tumor cells isolated from at least one patient with B-cell acute lymphocytic leukemia (138), and the mutations in mouse plasmacytomas were detected in DNA isolated from early transplant generations of solid tumors (122). It has yet to be determined, however, whether the transcription block at the end of $exon_1$ is a general and normal phenomenon, since so far it has only been reported in neoplastic cells with amplified c-*myc* genes (32–35).

CAUSAL CONNECTION BETWEEN c-*myc* ACTIVATION AND PLASMACYTOMAGENESIS

Chromosome Translocation Can Be Replaced by Retroviruses that Express v-*myc*

The nearly universial association of c-*myc* activation by chromosome alteration with BALB/c plasmacytomas and human Burkitt's lymphomas has begotten considerable confidence that pristane-induced plasmacytomagenesis required these alterations in c-*myc* expression (101). Only recently has evidence accumulated to support this presumption. As shown in the bottom portion of Fig. 1, induction of BALB/c plasmacytomas can be accelerated by infection with the J-3 retrovirus (4), a retroviral construct that contains a hybrid avian v-*myc* gene (and a defective portion of v-*raf*) between the LTRs of the murine sarcoma virus, 3611 (139). As with the Abelson virus induction experiments, helper virus (MoMuLV) is included in the viral inoculum, and pristane must be injected intraperitoneally. Whereas all but one of the Abelson + pristane-induced plasmacytoma contained chr. 15 translocations or alterations, and all had elevated levels of c-*myc* RNAs, most of the J-3 + pristane plasmacytomas had high levels of v-*myc* transcripts from integrated J-3 proviruses and no chromosome translocations or c-*myc* transcripts (4). This indicates that high levels of *myc* expression, either c-*myc* from altered chr. 15 or v-*myc* from integrated viruses, is necessary for the induction of plasmacytomas. Both alterations have never been seen in the same tumor. An important corollary of these experiments is derived from the observation that CDF1 mice which are normally resistant to plasmacytoma induction by pristane do develop plasmacytomas when given J-3 plus pristane (4). This suggests that at least part of the resistance of most inbred mouse strains to this form of carcinogenesis may stem from their inability to develop chr. 15 alterations that activate the c-*myc* gene. When an exogenous virus can supply a *myc* gene actively transcribed owing to the influence of the viral LTR, plasmacytomas can arise in mice that are normally resistant.

Pleomorphic Tumor Induction by *myc* Viruses

The usual form of neoplasm isolated from BALB/c mice after intraperitoneal pristane is the plasmacytoma. When the induction process is accelerated by adding Abelson virus or J-3 virus to the regimen, other forms of tumors arise. As shown in Fig. 5, in addition to the plasmacytomas depicted in Fig. 1, myeloid tumors, B- and T-cell lymphomas also occur. What is more, the v-*raf*- + v-*myc*-expressing J-2 virus causes myeloid tumors and lymphomas, but no plasmacytomas (4). The J-2 virus differs only slightly from J-3 in that the v-*raf* in J-3 has been rendered untranslatable by a 200-bp deletion (139). Other induction studies using different retroviruses that express v-*myc* have shown a wide range of transforming activity (139–141), and transgenic mice with deregulated c-*myc* genes inserted in all cells give rise to a wide spectrum of tumors (142,143). This underscores the pleomorphic potential of c-*myc* activation in tumorigenesis. It is noteworthy that the tumors that arise when the two coding exons of mouse c-*myc* are inserted in retroviruses and injected into pristane-primed BALB/c mice are usually myeloid in character (144,145),

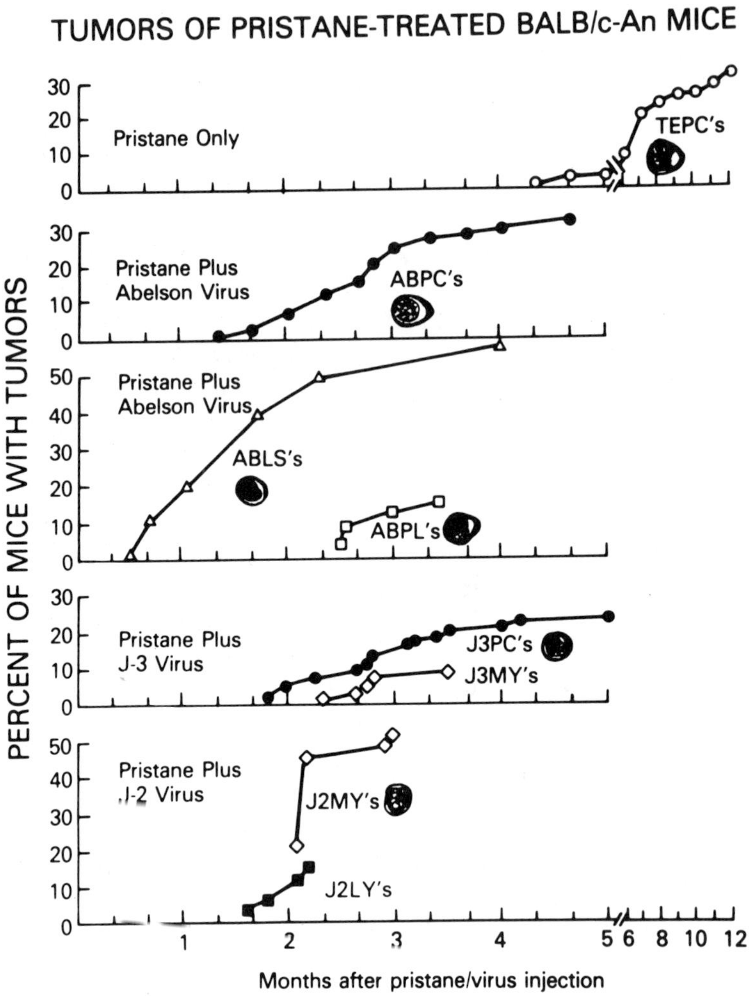

Figure 5 Time course of appearance of plasmacytomas and other hematopoietic neoplasms after BALB/c mice are given intraperitoneal pristane with or without retroviruses, as in the legend of Fig. 1. Besides plasmacytomas (PC), pre-B lymphosarcomas (ABLS [3]) and myeloid lymphomas (ABPL [2]) arise after Abelson virus is added to the regimen. Myeloid tumors (J2MY and J3MY) and T-cell lymphomas (J2LY) arise when J-2 or J-3 recombinant viruses expressing v-*raf* and/or v-*myc* are also administered. (From Ref. 4, used with permission.)

much as were many of the tumors induced by the avian myelocytomatosis viruses from which c-*myc* was originally isolated (146). Only when activated v-Ha-*ras* was coinfected with c-*myc* could plasmacytomas be induced (147). Thus, differences in cell milieu and other influences must play important roles in determining the nature of the tumors that arise when c-*myc* is uncontrollably activated.

EFFECTS OF CHROMOSOMAL TRANSLOCATION AND ACTIVATED c-*myc* EXPRESSION ON OTHER GENES

Activation of Cell Division

Although the normal function of c-*myc* protein product is not yet known, its intranuclear location and its apparent ability to bind DNA suggest that at least one of its functions may be to activate or inactivate other genes involved in cell division. Purified c-*myc* protein has been shown to confer on cells a competence to divide in response to certain growth factors (148), and antibodies to c-*myc* inhibit DNA synthesis and DNA polymerase activity in vitro (149). Inhibition of c-*myc* translation by antisense DNA seems to prevent cells from entering S phase (150). Infection with retroviral vectors that express c-*myc* can decrease various cell lines' requirements for exogenous growth factors (151), thus bypassing certain blocks to cell division. Certainly, this sort of activity could contribute to tumorigenesis. However, primary plasmacytomas have a requirement for a factor in order to grow in culture (151), and this requirement cannot be satisfied by the endogenous c-*myc* levels. Thus, even constitutive c-*myc* expression requires additional growth-related gene activations to achieve normal or neoplastic cell proliferation.

Deactivation of Differentiation-Specific Genes

It has been shown that expression of *myc* can prevent certain kinds of tumor cells from differentiating into more mature forms (see section on effects of mutations above). How this happens is still unknown, but the action of c-*myc* could be to interact with and to interfere with one or more genes essential to various steps involved in cell maturation. This concept is particularly appealing in considering the situation of plasmacytomas. The malignantly dividing cell is an Ig-secreting plasma cell, generally thought to be the end stage of B-lymphocyte differentiation. As such, it is expected to have lost the ability to divide and multiply. It would also be expected to have low c-*myc* RNA levels. Since both these expected characteristics do not obtain in plasmacytomas, it may be that one (the c-*myc* expression) causes the other (failure to stop dividing).

Complementation of Action of Other Genes

Tumorigenesis is felt to be a multistep process, and c-*myc* is thought to be a member of a class of oncogenes (also including c-*fos* and c-*myb*) that act intranuclearly and which can complement or cooperate with members of the cytoplasmic *ras* family in transforming primary rat embryo cells (103). The process of cell division and differentiation mentioned above are also multistep processes. The role that *myc* has been shown to play in these processes must complement other components of these physiological systems. In plasmacytomagenesis the relatively long latent period and the appearance of monoclonal tumors suggests that enhanced expression of *myc*, although necessary for the tumors, may not be sufficient (4). One or more additional genetic alterations, e.g., oncogene mutations, may be required for complete neoplastic transformation. Preliminary evidence suggests that one of the c-*ras* family of oncogenes (frequently Ki-*ras*) may be mutated and/or amplified in most early plasma cell tumors (153). It is not yet known whether the story will stop here, but the complexities of normal and neoplastic cell growth may contain other, still unknown, requirements. A phenomenon that may be related to this process is the recent report that c-*myc* expression may sensitize cells to radiation-induced transformation (154). If the c-*myc* activation occurs early in plasmacytomagenesis, it may serve to predispose the cell to point mutations, e.g., in the *ras* genes or in c-*myc* $exon_1$ itself.

CONCLUSIONS

The c-*myc* gene is a highly conserved gene that is expressed under very tight control befitting a growth-regulating gene. There are multiple factors that up-regulate and down-regulate its expression at the transcriptional and posttranscriptional level and many locations where factors can interact with the c-*myc* gene unit to effect these regulations. Virtually all mouse plasmacytomas have alterations in chr. 15 within the c-*myc* unit, but these alterations may occur far away from, very near to, or even within the three c-*myc* exons. The net effect of all these alterations, be they chromosomal translocations or deletions, is a partial deregulation of the c-*myc* expression. This deregulation may have a critical impact on the progression of B cells through the mitotic cycle. For example, expression of the altered c-*myc* allele in affected plasma cells is not down-regulated by conditions present in that mature form of B cell which do turn off the unaffected c-*myc* allele. Instead, most plasmacytomas contain levels of c-*myc* that are higher than those found in normal resting cells, most tumors of other types of hematopoietic cells, and even mitogenically activated B lymphocytes. In some way, this constitutive expression of c-*myc* contributes an essential component to plasmacytomagenesis, since it can be replaced only by another form of constitutive c-*myc* expression; e.g., under viral promotion or enhancement. Other genetic alterations may also be required for the completion of the neoplastic transformation, such as mutation in other oncogenes or in the c-*myc* gene itself.

ACKNOWLEDGMENTS

I thank my colleagues and collaborators for their inspiration and stimulating discussions, Michael Potter, in particular, for his critical reading of the manuscript, and Susan Brust for her help with the chromosome drawings. I am deeply grateful to Mary Millison for patient and skillful preparation of the manuscript, and to Drs. Robert Eisenman, Konrad Huppi, Kenneth Marcu, Laurent Miribel, and Michael Potter for permission to quote unpublished data.

REFERENCES

1. Potter, M. (1972). Immunoglobulin-producing tumors and myeloma proteins in mice. *Physiol. Rev. 52*: 631–719.
2. Potter, M., Wiener, F., and Mushinski, J. F. (1984). Recent developments in plasmacytomagenesis in mice. *Adv. Viral Oncol. 4*: 139–162.
2. Potter, M., Sklar, M. D., and Rowe, W. P. (1973). Rapid viral induction of plasmacytomas in pristane-primed BALB/c mice. *Science 182*: 592–594.
4. Potter, M., Mushinski, J. F., Mushinski, E. B., Brust, S., Wax, J. S., Wiener, F., Babonits, M., Rapp, U. R., and Morse, H. C., III. (1987). Avian v-*myc* replaces chromosomal translocation in murine plasmacytomagenesis. *Science 235*: 787–789.
5. Yosida, M. C., and Moriwaki, K. (1985). Specific marker chromosomes involving a translocation (12;15) in a mouse myeloma. *Proc. Jpn. Acad. 51*: 588–592.
6. Shepard, J. S., Pettengill, O. S., Wurster-Hill, D. H., and Sorenson, G. D. (1978). A specific chromosome breakpoint associated with mouse plasmacytomas. *J. Natl. Cancer Inst. 61*: 225–258.
7. Ohno, S., Babonits, M., Wiener, F., Spira, J., Klein, G., and Potter, M. (1979). Nonrandom chromosome changes involving the Ig gene-carrying chromosomes 12 and 6 in pristane-induced mouse plasmacytomas. *Cell 18*: 1001–1007.
8. Ohno, S., Migita, S., Wiener, F., Babonits, M., Klein, G., Mushinski, J. F., and Potter, M. (1984). Chromosomal translocations activating *myc* sequences and transduction of v-*abl* are critical events in the rapid induction of plasmacytomas by pristane and Abelson virus. *J. Exp. Med. 159*: 1762–1777.
9. Cory, S. (1986). Activation of cellular oncogenes in hemopoietic cells by chromosome translocation. *Adv. Can. Res. 47*: 189–234.
10. Erikson, J., Miller, D. A., Miller, O. J., Abcarian, P. W., Skurla, R. M., Mushinski, J. F., and Croce, C. M. (1985). The c-*myc* oncogene is

translocated to the involved chromosome 12 in mouse plasmacytoma. *Proc. Natl. Acad. Sci. U.S.A. 82*: 4212–4216.

11. Wirschubsky, Z., Ingvarsson, S., Carstenssen, A., Wiener, F., Klein, G., and Sumegi, J. (1985). Gene localization on sorted chromosomes: Definitive evidence on the relative positioning of genes participating in the mouse plasmacytoma-associated typical translocation. *Proc. Natl. Acad. Sci. U.S.A. 82*: 6975–6979.
12. Cory, S., Graham, M., Webb, E., Corcoran, L., and Adams, J. M. (1985). Variant (6;15) translocations in murine plasmacytomas involve a chromosome 15 locus at least 72 kb from the c-*myc* oncogene. *EMBO J. 4*: 675–681.
13. Adams, J. M., Gerondakis, S., Webb, E., Mitchell, J., Bernard, O., and Cory, S. (1982). Transcriptionally active DNA region that rearranges frequently in murine lymphoid tumors. *Proc. Natl. Acad. Sci. U.S.A. 79*: 6966–6970.
14. Shen-Ong, G. L., Keath, E. J., Piccoli, S. P., and Cole, M. D. (1982). Novel *myc* oncogene RNA from abortive immunoglobulin-gene recombination in mouse plasmacytomas. *Cell 31*: 443–452.
15. Cory, S., Gerondakis, S., and Adams, J. M. (1983). Interchromosomal recombination of the cellular oncogene c-*myc* with the immunoglobulin heavy chain locus in murine plasmacytomas is a reciprocal exchange. *EMBO J. 2*: 697–703.
16. Marcu, K. B., Harris, L. J., Stanton, L. W., Erikson, J., Watt, R., and Croce, C. M. (1983). Transcriptionally active c-*myc* oncogene is contained with NIARD, a DNA sequence associated with chromosome translocations in B-cell neoplasia. *Proc. Natl. Acad. Sci. U.S.A. 80*: 519–523.
17. Bernard, O., Cory, S., Gerondakis, S., Webb, E., and Adams, J. M. (1983). Sequence of the murine and human cellular *myc* oncogenes and two modes of *myc* transcription resulting from chromosome translocation in B lymphoid tumors. *EMBO J. 2*: 2375–2383.
18. Dunnick, W., Shell, B. E., and Dery, C. (1983). DNA sequences near the site of reciprocal recombination between a c-*myc* oncogene and an immunoglobulin switch region. *Proc. Natl. Acad. Sci. U.S.A. 80*: 7269–7273.
19. Stanton, L. W., Yang, J. Q., Eckhardt, L. A., Harris, L. J., Birshtein, B. K., and Marcu, K. B. (1984). Products of a reciprocal chromosome translocation involving the c-*myc* gene in a murine plasmacytoma. *Proc Natl. Acad. Sci. U.S.A. 81*: 829–833.
20. Gerondakis, S., Cory, S., and Adams, J. M. (1984). Translocation of the *myc* cellular oncogene to the immunoglobulin heavy chain locus in murine plasmacytomas is an imprecise reciprocal exchange. *Cell 36*: 973–982.
21. Banerjee, M., Wiener, F., Spira, J., Babonits, M., Nilsson, M.-G., Sumegi, J., and Klein, G. (1985). Mapping of the c-*myc*, *pvt*-1 and immunoglobulin kappa genes in relation to the mouse plasmacytoma-associated variant (6;15) translocation breakpoint. *EMBO J. 4*: 3183–3188.
22. Webb, E., Adams, J. M., and Cory, S. (1984). Variant (6;15) translocation in a murine plasmacytoma occurs near an immunoglobulin κ gene but far from the *myc* oncogene. *Nature 312*: 777–779.

23. Graham, M., Adams, J. M., and Cory, S. (1985). Murine T lymphomas with retroviral inserts in the chromosomal 15 locus for plasmacytoma variant translocations. *Nature 314*: 740–743.
24. Villeneuve, L., Rassart, E., Jolicoeur, P., Graham, M., and Adams, J. M. (1986). Proviral integration site *Mis*-1 in rat thymomas corresponds to the *pvt*-1 translocation breakpoint in murine plasmacytomas. *Mol. Cell. Biol. 6*: 1834–1837.
25. Kirsch, I. R., Brown, J. A., Lawrence, J., Korsmeyer, S. J., and Morton, C. C. (1985). Translocations that highlight chromosomal regions of differentiated activity. *Cancer Genet. Cytogenet. 18*: 159–171.
26. Wiener, F., Ohno, S., Babonits, M., Sumegi, J., Wirschubsky, Z., Klein, G., Mushinski, J. F., and Potter, M. (1984). Hemizygous interstitial deletion of chromosome 15 (band D) in three translocation-negative murine plasmacytomas. *Proc. Natl. Acad. Sci. U.S.A. 81*: 1159–1163.
27. Fahrlander, P. D., Sumegi, J., Yang, J.-Q., Wiener, F., Marcu, K. B., and Klein, G. (1985). Activation of the c-*myc* oncogene by the immunoglobulin heavy-chain gene enhancer after multiple switch region-mediated chromosome rearrangements in a murine plasmacytoma. *Proc. Natl. Acad. Sci. U.S.A. 82*: 3746–3750.
28. Corcoran, L. M., Cory, S., and Adams, J. M. (1985). Transposition of the immunoglobulin heavy chain enhancer to the *myc* oncogene in a murine plasmacytoma. *Cell 40*: 71–79.
29. Van Ness, B. G., Shapiro, M., Kelley, D. E., Perry, R. P., Weigert, M., D'Eustachio, P., and Ruddle, F. (1983). Aberrant rearrangement of the κ-light chain locus involving the heavy chain locus and chromosome 15 in a mouse plasmacytoma. *Nature 301*: 425–427.
30. Piechaczyk, M., Blanchard, J.-M., and Jeanteur, P. (1987). c-*myc* gene regulation still holds its secret. *Trends Genet. 3*: 47–50.
31. Cole, M. D. (1986). The *myc* oncogene: Its role in transformation and differentiation. *Ann. Rev. Genet. 20*: 361–384.
32. Nepveu, A., and Marcu, K. B., (1986). Intragenic pausing and anti-sense transcription within the murine c-*myc* locus. *EMBO J. 5*: 2859–2865.
33. Bentley, D. L., and Groudine, M. (1986). Novel promoter upstream of the human c-*myc* gene and regulation of c-*myc* expression in B-cell lymphomas. *Mol. Cell. Biol. 6*: 3481–3489.
34. Bentley, D. L., Groudine, M. (1986). A block to elongation is largely responsible for decreased transcription of c-*myc* in differentiated HL60 cells. *Nature 321*: 702–706.
35. Eick, D., and Bornkamm, G. W. (1986). Transcriptional arrest within the first exon is a fast control mechanism in c-*myc* gene expression. *Nucleic Acids Res. 14*: 8331–8346.
36. Fahrlander, P. D., Piechaczyk, M., and Marcu, K. B. (1985). Chromatin structure of the murine c-*myc* locus: Implications for the regulation of normal and chromosomally translocated genes. *EMBO J. 4*: 3195–3202.
37. Siebenlist, U., Hennighausen, L., Battey, J., and Leder, P. (1984). Chromatin structure and protein binding in the putative regulatory region of the c-*myc* gene in Burkitt lymphoma. *Cell 37*: 381–391.

38. Remmers, E. F., Yang, J.-Q., and Marcu, K. B. (1986). A negative transcriptional control element located upstream of the murine c-*myc* gene. *EMBO J. 5*: 899–904.
39. Yang, J.-Q., Remmers, E. F., and Marcu, K. B. (1986). The first exon of the c-*myc* proto-oncogene contains a novel positive control element. *EMBO J. 5*: 3553–3562.
40. Chung, J., Sinn, E., Reed, R. R., and Leder, P. (1986). Trans-acting elements modulate expression of the human c-*myc* gene in Burkitt lymphoma cells. *Proc. Natl. Acad. Sci. U.S.A. 83*: 7918–7922.
41. Gazin, C., Rigolet, M., Briand, J. P., Van Regenmortel, M. H. V., and Galibert, F. (1986). Immunochemical detection of proteins related to the human c-*myc* exon 1. *EMBO J 5*: 2241–2250.
42. Dani, C., Blanchard, J.-M., Piechaczyk, M., El Sabouty, El, S., Marty, L., and Jeanteur, P. (1984). Extreme instability of c-*myc* mRNA in normal and transformed cells. *Proc. Natl. Acad. Sci. 81*: 7046–7050.
43. McCormack, J. E., Pepe, V. H., Kent, R. B., Dean, M., Marshak-Rothstein, A., and Sonenshein, G. E. (1984). Specific regulation of c-*myc* oncogene expression in a murine B-cell lymphoma. *Proc. Natl. Acad. Sci. U.S.A. 81*: 5546–5550.
44. Greenberg, M. E., and Ziff, E. B. (1984). Stimulation of mouse 3T3 cells induces transcription of the c-*fos* proto-oncogene. *Nature 311*: 438–442.
45. Mushinski, J. F., Bauer, S. R., Potter, M., and Reddy, E. P. (1983). Increased expression of *myc*-related oncogene mRNA characterizes most BALB/c plasmacytomas induced by pristane or Abelson murine leukemia virus. *Proc. Natl. Acad. Sci. U.S.A. 80*: 1073–1077.
46. Kelly, K., Cochran, B. H., Stiles, C. D., Leder, P. (1983). Cell-specific regulation of the c-*myc* gene by lymphocyte mitogens and platelet-derived growth factor. *Cell 35*: 603–610.
47. Keath, E. J., Kelekar, A., and Cole, M. D. (1984). Transcriptional activation of the translocated c-*myc* oncogene in mouse plasmacytoma: Similar RNA levels in tumor and proliferating normal cells. *Cell 37*: 521–528.
48. Saito, H., Hayday, A. C., Wiman, K., Hayward, W. S., and Tonegawa, S. (1983). Activation of the c-*myc* gene by translocation: A model for translational control. *Proc. Natl. Acad. Sci. U.S.A. 80*: 7476–7480.
49. Darveau, A., Pelletier, J., and Sonenberg, N. (1985). Differential efficiencies of *in vitro* translation of mouse c-*myc* transcripts differing in the 5′ untranslated region. *Proc. Natl. Acad. Sci. U.S.A. 82*: 2315–2319.
50. Persson, H., Hennighausen, L., Taub, R., DeGrado, W., and Leder, P. (1984). Antibodies to human c-*myc* oncogene product: Evidence of an evolutionarily conserved protein induced during cell proliferation. *Science 225*: 687–693.
51. Nilsen, T. W., and Maroney, P. A. (1984). Translational efficiency of c-*myc* mRNA in Burkitt lymphoma cells. *Mol. Cell. Biol. 4*: 2235–2238.
52. Godeau, F., Persson, H., Gray, H. E., and Pardee, A. B. (1986). c-*myc* expression is dissociated from DNA synthesis and cell division in *Xenopus* oocyte and early embryonic development. *EMBO J. 5*: 3571–3577.

53. King, M. W., Roberts, J. M., and Eisenman, R. N. (1986). Expression of the c-*myc* proto-oncogene during development of *Xenopus laevis*. *Mol. Cell. Biol.* *6*: 4499–4508.
54. Taylor, M. V., Gusse, M., Evan, G. I., Dathan, N., and Mechali, M. (1986). *Xenopus myc* proto-oncogene during development: Expression as a stable maternal mRNA uncoupled from cell division. *EMBO J. 5*: 3563–3570.
55. Hann, S. R., and Eisenman, R. N. (1984). Proteins encoded by the human c-*myc* oncogene: Differential expression in neoplastic cells. *Mol. Cell. Biol. 4*: 2486–2497.
56. Beimling, P., Benter, T., Sander, T., and Moelling, K. (1985). Isolation and characterization of the human cellular *myc* gene product. *Biochemistry 24*: 6349–6355.
57. Persson, H., Gray, H. E., and Godeau, F. (1985). Growth-dependent synthesis of c-*myc*-encoded proteins: Early stimulation by serum factors in synchronized mouse 3T3 cells. *Mol. Cell. Biol. 5*: 2903–2912.
58. Hann, S. R., King, M. W., Bentley, D. L., Anderson, C. W., and Eisenman, R. N. (1988). Anon-AUG translational initiation in c-*myc* $exon_1$ generates an N-terminally distinct protein whose synthesis is disrupted in Burkitt's lymphoses. *Cell 52*: 185–189.
59. Campisi, J., Gray, H. E., Pardee, A. B., Dean, M., and Sonenshein, G. (1984). Cell-cycle control of c-*myc* but not c-*ras* expression is lost following chemical transformation. *Cell 36*: 241–247.
60. Thompson, C. B., Challoner, P. B., Neimann, P. E., and Groudine, M. (1985). Levels of c-*myc* oncogene mRNA are invariant throughout the cell cycle. *Nature 314*: 363–366.
61. Hann, S. R., Thompson, C. B., and Eisenman, R. N. (1985). c-*myc* oncogene protein synthesis is independent of the cell cycle in human and avian cells. *Nature 314*: 366–369.
62. Rabbitts, P. H., Watson, J. V., Lamond, A., Forster, A., Stinson, M. A., Evan, G., Fischer, W., Atherton, E., Sheppard, R., and Rabbitts, T. H. (1985). Metabolism of c-*myc* gene products: c-*myc* mRNA and protein expression in the cell cycle. *EMBO J. 4*: 2009–2015.
63. Dean, M., Levine, R. A., Ran, W., Kindy, M. S., Sonenshein, G. E., and Campisi, J. (1986). Regulation of c-*myc* transcription and mRNA abundance by serum growth factors and cell contact. *J. Biol. Chem., 261*: 9161–9166.
64. Reed, J. C., Nowell, P. C. and Hoover, R. G. (1985). Regulation of c-*myc* mRNA levels in normal human lymphocytes by modulators of cell proliferation. *Proc. Natl. Acad. Sci. U.S.A. 82*: 4221–4224.
65. Goyette, M., Petropoulos, C. J., Shank, P. R., and Fausto, N. (1984). Regulated transcription of c-Ki-*ras* and c-*myc* during compensatory growth of rat liver. *Mol. Cell. Biol. 4*: 1493–1498.
66. Armelin, H. A., Armelin, M. C. S., Kelly, K., Stewart, T., Leder, P., Cochran, B. H. and Stiles, C. D. (1984). Functional role for c-*myc* in mitogenic response to platelet-derived growth factor. *Nature 310*: 655–660.
67. Makino, R., Hayashi, K., and Sugimura, T. (1984). c-*myc* transcript is induced in rat liver at a very early stage of regeneration or by cycloheximide treatment. *Nature 310*: 697–698.
68. Blanchard, J. M., Piechaczyk, M., Dani, C., Chambard, J.-C., Franchi, A., Pouyssegur, J., and Jeanteur, P. (1985). c-*myc* gene is transcribed at high rate in G_0-arrested fibroblasts and is post-transcriptionally regulated in response to growth factors. *Nature 317*: 443–445.

69. Coughlin, S. R., Lee, W. M. F., Williams, P. W., Giels, G. M., and Williams, L. T. (1985). c-*myc* gene expression is stimulated by agents that activate protein kinase C and does not account for the mitogenic effect of PDGF. *Cell 43*: 243–251.
70. Reed, J. C., Sabath, D. E., Hoover, R. G., and Prystowsky, M. B. (1985). Recombinant interleukin 2 regulates levels of c-*myc* mRNA in a clonal murine T lymphocyte. *Mol. Cell. Biol. 5*: 3361–3368.
71. Smeland, E., Godal, T., Rund, E., Beiske, K., Funderud, S., Clark, E. A., Pfeifer-Ohlsson, S., and Ohlsson, R. (1985). The specific induction of *myc* proto-oncogene expression in normal human B cells is not a sufficient event for aquisition of competence to proliferate. *Proc. Natl. Acad. Sci. U.S.A. 82*: 6255–6259.
72. Conscience, J.-F., Verrier, B., and Martin, G. (1986). Interleukin-3-dependent expression of the c-*myc* and c-*fos* proto-oncogenes in hemopoietic cell lines. *EMBO J. 5*: 317–323.
73. Lacy, J., Sarkar, S. N., and Summers, W. C. (1986). Induction of c-*myc* expression in human B lymphocytes by B-cell growth factor and anti-immunoglobulin. *Proc. Natl. Acad. Sci. U.S.A. 83*: 1458–1462.
74. Ran, W., Dean, M., Levine, R. A., Henkle, C., and Campisi, J. (1986). Induction of c-*fos* and c-*myc* mRNA by epidermal growth factor or calcium ionophore is cAMP dependent. *Proc. Natl. Acad. Sci. U.S.A. 83*: 8216–8220.
75. Mushinski, J. F., Davidson, W. F., and Morse, H. C., III. (1987). Activation of cellular oncogenes in human and mouse leukemia-lymphomas: Spontaneous and induced oncogene expression in murine B lymphocytic neoplasms. *Cancer Invest. 5*: 345–368.
76. Westin, E. H., Wong-Staal, F., Gelmann, E. P., Dalla Favera, R., Papas, T. S., Lautenberger, J. A., Eva, A., Reddy, E. P., Tronick, S. R., Aaronson, S. A., and Gallo, R. C. (1982). Expression of cellular homologus of retroviral *onc* genes in human hematopoietic cells. *Proc. Natl. Acad. Sci. U.S.A. 79*: 2490–2494.
77. Gonda, T. J., and Metcalf, D. (1984). Expression of *myb, myc,* and *fos* proto-oncogenes during the differentiation of a murine myeloid leukemia. *Nature 310*: 249–251.
78. Lachman, H. M., and Skoultchi, A. I. (1984). Expression of c-*myc* changes during differentiation of mouse erythroleukemia cells. *Nature, 310*: 592–594.
79. Dony, C., Kessel, M., and Gruss, P. (1985). Post-transcriptional control of *myc* and p53 expression during differentiation of the embryonal carcinoma cell line F9. *Nature 317*: 636–639.
80. Endo, T., and Nadal-Ginard, B. (1986). Transcriptional and posttranscriptional control of c-*myc* during myogenesis: Its mRNA remains inducible in differentiated cells and does not suppress the differentiated phenotype. *Mol. Cell. Biol. 6*: 1412–1421.
81. Dean, M., Levine, R. A., and Campisi, J. (1986). c-*myc* regulation during retinoic acid-induced differentiation of F9 cells is posttranscriptional and associated with growth arrest. *Mol. Cell. Biol. 6*: 518–524.
82. Schneider, M. D., Payne, P. A., Ueno, H., Perryman, M. F., and Roberts, R. (1986). Dissociated expression of c-*myc* and a *fos*-related competence gene during cardiac myogenesis. *Mol. Cell. Biol. 6*: 4140–4143.

83. Mechti, N., Piechaczyk, M., Blanchard, J. M., Marty, L., Bonnieu, A., Jeanteur, P., and Lebleu, B. (1986). Transcriptional and post-transcriptional regulation of c-*myc* expression during the differentiation of murine erythroleukemia Friend cells. *Nucleic Acids Res. 14*: 9653–9666.
84. Falcone, G., Tato, F., and Alema, S. (1985). Distinctive effects of the viral oncogenes *myc, erb, fps* and *src* on the differentiation program of quail myogenic cells. *Proc. Natl. Acad. Sci. U.S.A. 82*: 426–430.
85. Coppola, J. A., and Cole, M. D. (1986). Constitutive c-*myc* oncogene expression blocks mouse erythroleukemia cell differentiation but not commitment. *Nature 320*: 760–763.
86. Dmitrovsky, E., Kuehl, W. M., Hollis, G. F., Kirsch, I. R., Bender, T. P., and Segal, S. (1986). Expression of a transfected human c-*myc* oncogene inhibits differentiation of a mouse erythroleukemia cell line. *Nature 322*: 748–750.
87. Lachman, H. M., Cheng, G., and Skoultchi, A. I. (1986). Transfection of mouse erythroleukemic cells with *myc* sequences changes the rate of induced commitment to differentiate. *Proc. Natl. Acad. Sci. U.S.A. 83*: 6480–6484.
88. Larsson, L.-G., Gray, H. E., Totterman, T., Pettersson, U., and Nilsson, K. (1987). Drastically increased expression of *MYC* and *FOS* protooncogenes during *in vitro* differentiation of chronic lymphocytic leukemia cells. *Proc. Natl. Acad. Sci. U.S.A. 84*: 223–227.
89. Nath, P., Getzenberg, R., Beebe, D., Pallansch, L., and Zelenka, P. (1987). c-*myc* mRNA is elevated as differentiating lens cells withdraw from the cell cycle. *Exp. Cell. Res. 169*: 215–222.
90. Calame, K., Kim, S., Lalley, P., Hill, R., Davis, M., and Hood, L. (1982). Molecular cloning of translocations involving chromosome 15 and the immunoglobulin C_{α} from chromosome 12 in two murine plasmacytomas. *Proc. Natl. Acad. Sci. U.S.A. 79*: 6994–6998.
91. Taub, R., Kirsch, I., Morton, C., Lenoir, G., Swan, D., Tronick, S., Aaronson, S., and Leder, P. (1982). Translocation of the c-*myc* gene into the immunoglobulin heavy chain locus in human Burkitt lymphoma and murine plasmacytoma cells. *Proc. Natl. Acad. Sci. U.S.A. 79*: 7837–7841.
92. Dalla-Favera, R., Bregni, M., Erikson, J., Patterson, D., Gallo, R. C., and Croce, C. M. (1982). Human c-*myc* onc gene is located on the region of chromosome 8 that is translocated in Burkitt lymphoma cells. *Proc. Natl. Acad. Sci. U.S.A. 79*: 7824–7827.
93. Adams, J. M., Gerondakis, S., Webb, E., Corcoran, L. M., and Cory, S. (1983). Cellular *myc* oncogene is altered by chromosome translocation to an immunoglobulin locus in murine plasmacytomas and is rearranged similarly in human Burkitt lymphomas. *Proc. Natl. Acad. Sci. U.S.A. 80*: 1982–1986.
94. Erikson, J., ar-Rushdi, A., Drwinga, H. L., Nowell, P. C., and Croce, C. M. (1983). Transcriptional activation of the translocated c-*myc* oncogene in Burkitt lymphoma. *Proc. Natl. Acad. Sci. U.S.A. 80*: 820–824.
95. Rabbitts, T. H., Hamlyn, P. H., and Baer, R. (1983). Altered nucleotide sequences of a translocated c-*myc* gene in Burkitt lymphoma. *Nature 306*: 760–765.

96. Taub, R., Moulding, C., Battey, J., Murphy, W., Vasicek, T., Lenoir, G. M., and Leder, P. (1984). Activation and somatic mutations of the translocated c-*myc* gene in Burkitt lymphoma cells. *Cell 36*: 339–348.
97. Rabbitts, T. H., Forster, A., Hamlyn, P., and Baer, R. (1984). Effect of somatic mutation within translocated c-*myc* genes in Burkitt's lymphoma. *Nature 309*: 592–597.
98. Stanton, L. W., Watt, R., and Marcu, K. B. (1983). Translocation, breakage and truncated transcripts of c-*myc* oncogene in murine plasmacytomas. *Nature 303*: 401–406.
99. Stanton, L. W., Fahrlander, P. D., Tesser, P. M., and Marcu, K. B. (1984). Nucleotide sequence comparison of normal and translocated murine c-*myc* genes. *Nature 310*: 423–425.
100. Klein, G. (1981). The role of gene dosage and genetic transposition in carcinogenesis. *Nature 294*: 314–318.
101. Klein, G. (1983). Specific chromosomal translocations and the genesis of B-cell-derived tumors in mice and man. *Cell 32*: 311–315.
102. Varmus, H. A. (1984). The molecular genetics of cellular oncogenes. *Ann. Rev. Genet. 18*: 553–612.
103. Land, H., Parada, L. F., and Weinberg, R. A. (1983). Tumorigenic conversion of primary embryo fibroblasts requires at least two cooperating oncogenes. *Nature 304*: 596–601.
104. Keath, E. J., Caimi, P. G., and Cole, M. D. (1984). Fibroblast lines expressing activated c-*myc* oncogenes are tumorigenic in nude mice and syngeneic animals. *Cell 39*: 339–348.
105. Leder, P., Battey, J., Lenoir, G., Moulding, C., Murphy, W., Potter, H., Stewart, T., and Taub, R. (1983). Translocations among antibody genes in human cancer. *Science 222*: 765–771.
106. Kelly, K., and Siebenlist, U. (1985). The role of c-*myc* in the proliferation of normal and neoplastic cells. *J. Clin. Immunol. 5*: 65–77.
107. Dunnick, W., Baumgartner, J., Fradkin, L., Schultz, C., and Szurek, P. (1985). Methylation of plasmacytoma c-*myc* genes. *Gene 39*: 287–292.
108. Nishikura, K., ar-Rushdi, A., Erikson, J., Watt, R., Rovera, G., and Croce, C. M. (1983). Differential expression of the normal and of the translocated human c-*myc* oncogenes in B cells. *Proc. Natl. Acad. Sci. U.S.A. 80*: 4822–4826.
109. Feo, S., ar-Rushdi, A., Huebner, K., Finan, J., Nowell, P. C., Clarkson, B., and Croce, C. M. (1985). Suppression of the normal mouse c-*myc* oncogene in human lymphoma cells. *Nature 313*: 493–495.
110. Neckers, L. (1985). Expression of transferrin receptors and c-*myc* in plasmacytoma cells. In *Mechanisms of B Cell Neoplasia 1985*. (Melchers, F., and Potter, M. eds.). Editiones Roche, Basle, Switzerland, pp. 36–47.
111. Yang, J.-Q., Bauer, S. R., Mushinski, J. F., and Marcu, K. B. (1985). Chromosome translocations clustered 5′ of the murine c-*myc* gene qualitatively affect promoter usage: Implications for the site of normal c-*myc* regulation. *EMBO J. 4*: 1441–1447.

112. Nishikura, K., ar-Rushdi, A., Erikson, J., DeJesus, E., Dugan, D., and Croce, C. M. (1984). Repression of rearranged μ gene and translocated c-*myc* in mouse 3T3 cells X Burkitt lymphoma cell hybrids. *Science 224*: 399–402.
113. Croce, C. M., Erikson, J., ar-Rushdi, A., Aden, D., and Nishikura, K. (1984). Translocated c-*myc* oncogene of Burkitt lymphoma is transcribed in plasma cells and repressed in lymphoblastoid cells. *Proc. Natl. Acad. Sci. U.S.A. 81*: 3170–3174.
114. Croce, C. M., Erikson, J., Huebner, K., and Nishikura, K. (1985). Coexpression of translocated and normal c-*myc* oncogenes in hybrids between Daudi and lymphoblastoid cells. *Science 227*: 1235–1238.
115. Einat, M., Resnitzky, D., and Kimchi, A. (1985). Close link between reduction of c-*myc* expression by interferon and G_0/G_1 arrest. *Nature 313*: 597–600.
116. Knight, E., Jr., Anton, E. D., Fahey, D., Friedland, B. K., and Jonak, G. J. (1985). Interferon regulates c-*myc* expression in Daudi cells at the post-transcriptional level. *Proc. Natl. Acad. Sci. U.S.A. 82*: 1151–1154.
117. Battey, J., Moulding, C., Taub, R., Murphy, W., Stewart, T., Potter, H., Lenoir, G., and Leder, P. (1983). The human c-*myc* oncogene: Structural consequences of translocation into the IgH locus in Burkitt lymphoma. *Cell 34*: 779–787.
118. Prehn, J., Mercola, M., and Calame, K. (1984). Translocation affects normal c-*myc* promoter usage and activates fifteen cryptic c-*myc* transcription starts in plasmacytoma M603. *Nucleic Acids Res. 12*: 8987–9007.
119. Calabi, F., and Neuberger, M. S. (1985). Chromosome translocation activates heterogeneously initiated, bipolar transcription of a mouse c-*myc*. *EMBO J. 4*: 667–674.
120. Dyson, P. J., and Rabbitts, T. H. (1985). Chromatin structure around the c-*myc* gene in Burkitt lymphomas with upstream and downstream translocation points. *Proc. Natl. Acad. Sci. U.S.A. 82*: 1984–1988.
121. Dyson, P. J., Littlewood, T. D., Forster, A., and Rabbitts, T. H. (1985). Chromatin structure of transcriptionally active and inactive human c-*myc* alleles. *EMBO J. 4*: 2885–2891.
122. Bauer, S. R., Piechaczyk, M., Marcu, K. B., Nordan, R. P., Potter, M., and Mushinski, J. F. (1986). Mutations which stabilize *myc* transcripts and enhance *myc* transcription in two mouse plasmacytomas. *Curr. Top. Microbiol. Immunol. 132*: 339–344.
123. Piechaczyk, M., Yang, J.-Q., Blanchard, J.-M., Jeanteur, P., and Marcu, K. B. (1985). Posttranscriptional mechanisms are responsible for accumulation of truncated c-*myc* RNAs in murine plasma cell tumors. *Cell 42*: 589–597.
124. Davis, M., Malcolm, S., and Rabbitts, T. H. (1984). Chromosome translocation can occur on either side of the c-*myc* oncogene in Burkitt lymphoma cells. *Nature 308*: 286–288.

125. Erikson, J., Nishikura, K., ar-Rushdi, A., Finan, J., Emanuel, B., Lenoir, G., Nowell, P. C., and Croce, C. M. (1983). Translocation of an immunoglobulin k locus to a region 3′ of an unrearranged c-*myc* oncogene enhances c-*myc* transcription. *Proc. Natl. Acad. Sci. U.S.A. 80*: 7581–7585.
126. Rappold, G. A., Hameister, H., Cremer, T., Adolph, S., Henglein, B., Freese, U. K., Lenoir, G. M., and Bornkamm, G. W. (1984). c-*myc* and immunoglobulin kappa light chain constant genes are on the 8q+ chromosome of three Burkitt lymphoma lines with t(2;8) translocations. *EMBO J. 3*: 2951–2955.
127. Taub, R., Kelly, K., Battey, J., Latt, S., Lenoir, G. M., Tantravahi, U., Tu, Z., and Leder, P. (1984). A novel alteration in the structure of an activated c-*myc* gene in a variant t(2;8) Burkitt lymphoma. *Cell 37*: 511–520.
128. Croce, C. M., Thierfelder, W., Erikson, J., Nishikura, K., Finan, J., Lenoir, G. M., and Nowell, P. C. (1983). Transcriptional activation of an rearranged and untranslocated c-*myc* oncogene by translocation of a C_l locus in Burkitt lymphoma cells. *Proc. Natl. Acad. Sci. U.S.A. 80*: 6922–6926.
129. Hollis, G. F., Mitchell, K. F., Battey, J., Potter, H., Taub, R., Lenoir, G. M., and Leder, P. (1984). A variant translocation places the l immunoglobulin genes 3′ to the c-*myc* oncogene in Burkitt's lymphoma. *Nature 307*: 752–755.
130. Graham, M., and Adams, J. M. (1986). Chromosome 8 breakpoint far 3′ of the c-*myc* oncogene in a Burkitt's lymphoma 2;8 variant translocation is equivalent to the murine *pvt*-1 locus. *EMBO J. 5*: 2845–2851.
131. Mengle-Gaw, L., and Rabbitts, T. H. (1987). A human chromosome 8 region with abnormalities in B cell, HTLV-I$^+$ T cell and c-*myc* amplified tumors. *EMBO J. 6*: 1959–1965.
132. Denny, C. T., Hollis, G. F., Magrath, I. T., and Kirsch, I. R. (1985). Burkitt lymphoma cell line carrying a variant translocation creates new DNA at the breakpoint and violates the hierarchy of immunoglobulin gene rearrangement. *Mol. Cell. Biol. 5*: 3199–3207.
133. Stavezer-Nordgren, J., and Sirlin, S. (1986). Specificity of immunoglobulin heavy chain switch correlates with activity of germline heavy chain genes prior to switching. *EMBO J. 5*: 95–102.
134. Dean, M., Kent, R. B., and Sonenshein, G. E. (1983). Transcriptional activation of immunoglobulin alpha heavy-chain genes by translocation of the c-*myc* oncogene. *Nature 305*: 443–446.
135. Kakkis, E., Prehn, J., and Calame, K. (1986). An active chromatin structure acquired by translocated c-*myc* genes. *Mol. Cell. Biol. 6*: 1357–1361.
136. Pelicci, P.-G., Knowles, D. M., Magrath, I., and Dalla-Favera, R. (1986). Chromosomal breakpoints and structured alterations of the c-*myc* locus differ in endemic and sporadic forms of Burkitt lymphoma. *Proc. Natl. Acad. Sci. U.S.A. 83*: 2984–2988.
137. Szajnert, M.-F., Saule, S., Bornkamm, G. W., Wajcman, H., Lenoir, G. M., and Kaplan, J.-C. (1987). Clustered somatic mutations in and around first exon of non-rearranged c-*myc* in Burkitt lymphoma with t(8;22) translocation. *Nucl. Acids. Res. 15*: 4553–4565.

138. Care, A., Cianetti, L., Giampaolo, A., Sposi, N. M., Zappavigna, V., Mavilio, F., Alimena, G., Amadori, S., Mandelli, F., and Peschle, C. (1986). Translocation of c-*myc* into the immunoglobulin heavy-chain locus in human acute B-cell leukemia. A molecular analysis. *EMBO J. 5*: 905–911.
139. Rapp, U. R., Cleveland, J. L., Fredrickson, T. N., Holmes, K. L., Morse, H. C., III, Patschinsky, T., and Bister, K. (1985). Rapid induction of hematopoietic neoplasms in newborn mice by a *raf* (*mil*)/*myc* recombinant murine retrovirus. *J. Virol. 55*: 23–33.
140. Vennstrom, B., Kahn, P., Adkins, B., Enrietto, P., Hayman, M. J., Graf, T., and Luciw, P. (1984). Transformation of mammalian fibroblasts and macrophages *in vitro* by a murine retrovirus encoding an avian v-*myc* oncogene. *EMBO J. 3*: 3223–3229.
141. Morse, H. C., III, Hartley, J. W., Fredrickson, T. N., Yetter, R. A., Majumdar, C., Cleveland, J. L., and Rapp, U. R. (1986). Recombinant murine retroviruses containing avian v-*myc* induce a wide spectrum of neoplasms in newborn mice. *Proc. Natl. Acad. Sci. U.S.A. 83*: 6868–6872.
142. Adams, J. M., Harris, A. W., Pinkert, C. A., Corcoran, L. M., Alexander, W. S., Cory, S., Palmiter, R. D., and Brinster, R. L. (1985). The c-*myc* oncogene driven by immunoglobulin enhancers induces lymphoid malignancy in transgenic mice. *Nature 318*: 533–538.
143. Leder, A., Pattengale, P. K., Kuo, A., Stewart, T. A., and Leder, P. (1986). Consequences of widespread deregulation of the c-*myc* gene in transgenic mice: Multiple neoplasms and normal development. *Cell 45*: 485–495.
144. Baumbach, W. R., Keath, E. J., and Cole, M. D. (1986). A mouse c-*myc* retrovirus transforms established fibroblast lines *in vitro* and induces monocyte-macrophage tumors *in vivo*. *J. Virol. 59*: 276–283.
145. Wolff, L., Mushinski, J. F., Gilboa, E., and Morse, H. C., III. (1986). Induction of hematopoietic tumors using a viral construct containing c-*myc* cDNA from normal mouse spleen. *Curr. Top. Microbiol. Immunol. 132*: 33–39.
146. Graf, T., and Beug, H. (1978). Avian leukosis viruses: Interaction with their target cells *in vivo* and *in vitro*. *Biochim. Biophys. Acta 516*: 269–299.
147. Marcu, K., and Potter, M. personal communication.
148. Kaczmarek, L., Hyland, J. K., Watt, R., Rosenberg, M., and Baserga, R. (1985). Microinjected c-*myc* as a competence factor. *Science 228*: 1313–1315.
149. Studzinski, G. P., Brelvi, Z. S., Feldman, S. C., and Watt, R. A. (1986). Participation of c-*myc* protein in DNA synthesis of human cells. *Science 234*: 467–470.
150. Heikkila, R., Schwab, G., Wickstrom, E., Loke, S. L., Pluznik, D. H., Watt, R., and Neckers, L. M. (1987). A c-*myc* antisense oligodeoxynucleotide inhibits entry into S phase but not progress from G_0 to G_1. *Nature 328*: 445–449.
151. Rapp, U. R., Cleveland, J. L., Brightman, K., Scott, A., and Ihle, J. N. (1985). Abrogation of IL-3 and IL-2 dependence by recombinant murine retroviruses expressing v-*myc* oncogenes. *Nature 317*: 434–438.

152. Nordan, R., and Potter, M. (1986). A macrophage-derived factor required by plasmacytomas for survival and proliferation *in vitro*. *Science 233*: 566–569.
153. Huppi, K., and Miribel, L. personal communication.
154. Sorrentino, V., Drozdoff, V., Zeitz, L., and Fleissner, E. (1987). Increased radiation-induced transformation in C3H/10T-1/2 cells after transfer of an exogenous c-*myc* gene. *Proc. Natl. Acad. Sci. U.S.A. 84*: 4131–4134.

SEVEN

c-*myc* Deregulation by Chromosomal Translocation in Burkitt's Lymphoma

Georg W. Bornkamm,
Axel Polack, and
Dirk Eick
Institut für Medizinische Mikrobiologie und Hygiene der Universität Freiburg, Freiburg, Federal Republic of Germany

INTRODUCTION

Regulated cell growth is the result of a complex interplay between signals acting from outside the cell and the cellular response to these environmental signals. A first step in the chain of events is the interaction of a receptor on the cell surface with molecules which either stimulate or inhibit cell growth. As a second step, the signal has to be transmitted from the receptor into the cytoplasm and nucleus, and has finally to be converted into a pleiotropic response which includes a change in the pattern of gene expression. Cellular proto-oncogenes are coding for proteins which are involved physiologically in this complex regulation. These genes, when transduced by oncogenic retroviruses, apparently cause cancer by interfering with the normal signal

---

This chapter is dedicated to the memory of Werner Henle.

transduction pathway at one or the other level in a cell. Constitutive production of a growth factor may, for instance, continuously stimulate the own receptor, thus leading to autocrine growth. Experimental support for such a receptor stimulation model was provided by the observation that the cellular homologue of the v-*sis* oncogene is coding for a growth factor; i.e., the B chain of platelet-derived growth factor (PDGF) [1,2]. As a second possibility, alteration of the growth factor receptor may excite the receptor constitutively, thus switching-on the intracellular cascade leading to cell proliferation (receptor mimicking model). Evidence for such a model stems from the fact that the cellular homologues of some oncogenes are genes for growth factor receptors; i.e., c-*erb*B1 for the epidermal growth factor (EGF) receptor and c-*fms* for the mononuclear phagocyte growth factor (CSF-1) receptor [3,4].

Third, perturbation at any step of the signal transduction pathway between growth factor receptor and nucleus may switch on cellular proliferation (receptor circuiting model). Oncogenes coding for cytoplasmic and nuclear proteins are thought to belong in this last category.

An important implication of these models is that unregulated cell proliferation may be induced not only by transduction of an oncogene through a retrovirus, but also by altering either the structure or the regulation of a cellular proto-oncogene. This is strongly supported by the fact that cellular proto-oncogenes are targets for mutations, gene amplification, or chromosomal translocations in naturally occurring tumors in which there is no evidence for involvement of oncogenic retroviruses.

The first tumors in which a cellular proto-oncogene could be assigned to the site of the chromosomal translocation are Burkitt's lymphoma and mouse plasmacytoma. In both types of tumors, the locus carrying the cellular proto-oncogene c-*myc* is fused to an immunoglobulin locus. According to the receptor circuiting model, juxtaposition of c-*myc* to an immunoglobulin (Ig) locus may render the c-*myc* gene unregulatable to signals from outside the cell, thus making expression constitutive.

In this chapter, we shall summarize our current knowledge in support of this hypothesis. We shall first give an introduction into the biology of Burkitt's lymphoma. We shall then describe the structural features of the chromosomal translocations and the consequences of the translocation for c-*myc* expression. Some aspects which evolved from the analysis of mouse plasmacytomas will also be included because of the biological similarity of both types of tumors. Finally, we shall discuss models and new experimental approaches which may help to provide a better understanding of c-*myc* regulation and deregulation at a molecular level.

BURKITT'S LYMPHOMA

Definition of the Tumor

Burkitt's lymphoma (BL), a highly malignant human B-cell tumor, was first recognized by Denis Burkitt in 1958 as a pathoclinical entity with particular epidemiological peculiarities [5]. In some parts of Africa and New Guinea, the tumor is the predominant childhood malignancy, with an incidence of about five to 15 children per 100,000/year, whereas in all other parts of the world the tumor occurs with a 20- to 100-fold lower frequency. In the high incidence areas, the tumor is preferentially localized at the jaws and abdomen, abdominal presentation being the predominant clinical feature of the tumor in low-incidence areas. Burkitt's lymphoma is predominantly a childhood tumor with a peak incidence at the age of 4–12 years, and a sex preference of males over females of 2:1 to 3:1, but it is also observed less commonly in adolescents and young adults. The definition of Burkitt's lymphoma is based exclusively on histopathological and cytological grounds: BL is a malignant lymphoma comprising a monomorphic picture of undifferentiated lymphoid cells with little variation in size and shape, an amphophilic cytoplasm with clear vacuoles, and a noncleaved nucleus with several basophilic nucleoli [6]. At low magnification, a "starry sky" pattern is observed, caused by macrophage infiltration into this rapidly growing tumor. In the new working formulation of non-Hodkin's lymphomas, BL belongs to the group of high-grade malignant small cell lymphomas with noncleaved nuclei [7]. Burkitt's lymphoma consists of a clonal proliferation of lymphocytes of the B-cell type, all of which synthesize heavy chain immunoglobulins, predominantly μ chains. Immunoglobulin light chain expression is observed in most but not all tumors.

Factors Associated with High Incidence of Burkitt's Lymphoma

The distribution of BL in Africa and New Guinea is highly dependent on geographical and climatic factors, such as temperature, rainfall, and altitude [8]. This initiated the search for an arthropodborne virus, and finally led to the discovery of the Epstein-Barr virus (EBV) in cell lines established from BL biopsies. This virus, however, turned out to be an ubiquitous virus, which infects more than 95% of the population in all parts of the world and whose transmission is not related to climatic factors. The epidemiological characteristics of BL can best be explained by its relation to hyper- and holoendemic malaria [9]. The high incidence of BL is restricted to areas where *Plasmodium falciparum* is transmitted to the vast majority of the population at a high rate all during the year. In children which have not yet developed antimalarial immunity, the high rate of transmission is associated with a heavy parasitemia leading to polyclonal B-cell activation [10]. While the B-cell system is unspecifically stimulated, the immune response against individual antigens is impaired [11,12].

Despite its ubiquitous distribution, EBV is apparently associated with the high incidence of BL in Africa and New Guinea. This is documented on one hand by high antiviral antibody titers in BL patients, and on the other by the presence of viral genomes and viral antigens in the tumor cells [13]. The virus is, however, not an indespensible factor for the development of BL, since it is only associated with a minority of cases (10–20%) in the low-incidence areas. Remarkably, the EBV-positive and -negative tumors are histologically and, with respect to surface markers, phenotypically identical. Neither of both express the activation antigens (CD23, K:24, K:1) expressed on cells immortilized by EBV in vitro [14,15], suggesting that the role of the virus in BL is different from that during in vitro immortalization of normal cells.

Another condition which predisposes to the development of BL is the acquired immune deficiency syndrome (AIDS), in which undifferentiated Burkitt-type lymphomas as well as large cellular lymphomas are frequently observed [16,17].

The involvement of several defined parameters such as EBV, malaria, and specific chromosomal translocations as well as immunostimulation and immunosuppression in the setting of AIDS make BL an attractive model for the study of multistep carcinogenesis. The role of EBV and malaria is not precisely understood. Different models have been proposed, as to the interaction of the various parameters in the pathogenesis of Burkitt's lymphoma. The opposing views have recently been the subject of a detailed controversial discussion [18,19] and therefore not treated here.

This chapter focuses only on one particular aspect in the multistep process of Burkitt's lymphoma development; i.e., the deregulation of the c-*myc* gene brought about by chromosomal translocation.

Specific Chromosomal Translocations are a Consistent Feature of BL

Since it became apparent during the 1970s that EBV is not regularly associated with BL in low-incidence areas, and is thus not an indispensible factor for the development of the disease, the interest of many researchers focused on features which are common to BL in low- as well as high-incidence areas. The cytogenetic abnormalities observed in BL cells fulfilled this criterion.

Before the introduction of banding techniques cytogenetic studies on BL gave conflicting results and did not reveal specific chromosomal abnormalities. In 1972, however, at a time when most research on BL was devoted to the etiological role of EBV, Manolov and Manolova [20], using the newly developed banding technique, demonstrated that BL cells carry a specific marker chromosome, $14q^+$, which carries extra material at the extremity of the long arm of chr. 14. This observation was soon confirmed and expanded. It was shown that the extra material on chromosome 14 was derived from chr. 8, and that the exchange of material from both chromosomes was reciprocal and balanced [21–23]. Most importantly, the chromosomal translocations were observed in EBV-positive as well as EBV-negative BL cases and were independent of the geographical origin of the tumor.

In 1979 and 1980, a number of single case reports from different countries with low incidence of BL revealed another important fact: the presence of either of two variant translocations, t(2;8) and t(8;22), in Burkitt's lymphoma cells instead of the well-known t(8;14) translocation [24–27]. The important feature was that in all three cases—t(8;14), t(2;8), and t(8;22)—the breakpoint was localized on the same band of the long arm of chr. 8: band 8q24. Variant translocations were soon later also reported for cases from high-incidence areas [28], indicating that chromosomal translocations involving band q24 of chr. 8 and one of three loci on chr. 14 (14q32), chr. 2 (2p12), and chr. 22 (22q11) are a consistent feature of BL, regardless of the geographical origin of the tumor and its association with EBV (Fig. 1).

The t(8;14) translocations are by far most common and represent about 75% of all tumors. The remainder comprise the variant translocations, the t(8;22) translocations being about twice as frequent as the t(2;8) translocations [29].

Are there exceptions to the rule that BL cases have a translocation involving 8q24? Far more than 100 cell lines and fresh tumor biopsies have been studied, in which one of the three characteristic translocations has been found. One EBV-negative African B-cell line, BJAB, was initially described to be of BL origin and has no abnormality on chr. 8 [21,30]. However, the diagnosis has remained uncertain and is still considered doubtful (G. Klein, personal communication). In two cases of Burkitt-type leukemia, a $6q^-$ marker without detectable abnormality of chr. 8 was reported [31]. Unfortunately, no cell lines could be established from these cases to allow for a more detailed cytogenetic and molecular analysis of clonally proliferating tumor cells.

Are the t(8;14), t(2;8), and t(8;22) translocations specific for BL? Mitelman [32] and Sigaux and coworkers [33] have pointed out that a

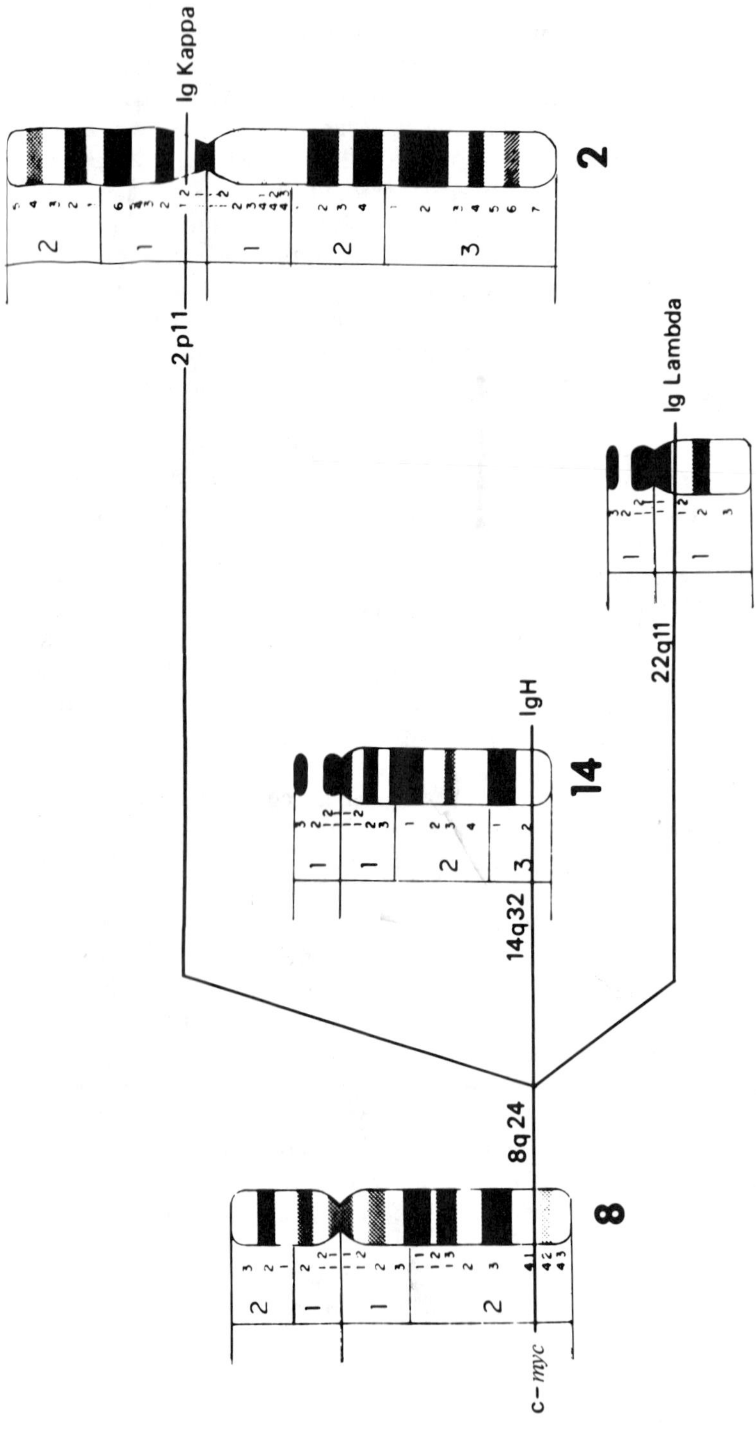

Figure 1 The chromosomal translocations in Burkitt's lymphoma.

translocation involving 8q24 is not strictly confined to BL, but is also found in non-Burkitt malignant lymphoproliferations of the B-cell lineage, such as immunoblastic lymphomas.

EBV does not appear to be capable of inducing specific chromosomal translocations. Epstein-Barr virus–transformed cells in vitro maintain their normal phenotype when established in culture. Upon prolonged cultivation these cells acquire chromosomal changes, but preferentially numerical aberrations and never the specific translocations observed in BL [34,35].

In BL patients, the translocation has only been observed in the malignant cells and never in other hemopoetic cells. This is different from the situation in chronic myelocytic leukemia where the Philadelphia chromosome (Ph^1) is present also in non-leukemic cells of other lineages, indicating that a precursor is the target for the chromosomal translocation generating the Ph^1 marker [36].

Taken together, with the above cited reservations in mind, the specific chromosomal translocations may be regarded as a specific and characteristic feature of Burkitt's lymphoma.

The Link Between Classic and Molecular Cytogenetics

The genes located at both sides of the chromosomal translocations in BL served as a tool for the molecular analysis of the breakpoints. This was possible because the genes involved, the immunoglobulin genes and c-*myc*, were in fact already known and waited to be brought into context with the chromosomal translocations. Translocation breakpoints of mouse plasmacytomas had even been cloned and characterized as aberrantly rearranged immunoglobulin genes [37]. The link was achieved on the one hand by assignment of the immunoglobulin genes to chr. 14 (IgH), chr. 2 (Igκ), and 22 (Igλ) (for review see Refs. [38 and 39]), and on the other hand by assignment of the proto-oncogene c-*myc* to band q24 on the long arm of chr. 8 [40,41,42].

Another hallmark was the finding that during B lymphomagenesis in chicken the cellular proto-oncogene c-*myc* is activated by insertion of avian leukosis virus into the vicinity of the gene [43]. This finding provided for the first time evidence for involvement of a cellular proto-oncogene in the development of cancer and initiated the search for an activated oncogene in Burkitt's lymphoma and mouse plasmacytoma [38,44].

Thus, by the demonstration of fused c-*myc* and immunoglobulin loci in Burkitt's lymphoma and mouse plasmacytoma, in 1982 for the first time the gap was bridged between classic and molecular cytogenetics.

THE c-*myc* GENE

The c-*myc* Gene and Its Gene Product

The Gene

The c-*myc* gene was originally described as the cellular homologue of a gene transduced by avian oncogenic retroviruses (reviewed in Ref. 45). It is a member of a family of related genes, including N-*myc* and L-*myc*, which have been implicated in oncogenesis in various species in association with retrovirus insertion, gene amplification, and chromosomal translocations. c-*myc* is transcribed into a messenger ribonucleic acid (mRNA) of 2.4 kb, consisting of one noncoding exon of about 550 b and two exons of 778, and about 900 b coding for the 439 aminoacid c-*myc* protein. The N-terminal coding $exon_2$ is acidic, whereas the C-terminal $exon_3$ is basic and may account for the deoxyribonucleic acid (DNA) binding property of the protein [46].

The c-*myc* protein is highly conserved in evolution. The homology between the mouse and human c-*myc* proteins is 93% [47], and between the avian and mammalian proteins 73% [48]. The sequence conservation is highest for the third exon. The untranslated first exon, and the untranslated 3′ region are also conserved between mouse and man to 76 and 78%, respectively [47]. There is, however, no conservation between $exon_1$ in avians and mammals [49].

Transcription

In mouse and man, the c-*myc* RNA is transcribed from two promoters, P_1 and P_2, about 160 bp apart from each other. In normal cells, P_2 transcripts are three to five times more abundant then transcripts initiated at P_1. The c-*myc* RNA is terminated at one of two polyadenylation sites located 300 and 440 bp downstream of the end of the c-*myc* reading frame (reviewed in Refs. 50 and 51). The 3′ region of the message carries a signal which seems to be required to confer rapid mRNA degradability [52,53].

The first exon is rich in guanine and cytosine, and carries partly homologous sequences to $exon_2$ in opposite orientation. The c-*myc* RNA has probably a high degree of secondary structure which may have important implications for posttranscriptional c-*myc* regulation [54]. A third promoter (P_0) is located about 600 bp upstream of P_1, and gives rise to a 3.1-kb transcript which is present at a 20- to 100-fold lower abundancy than P_1 and P_2 transcripts [55]. Ribonucleic acid initiated at P_0 comprises two additional open reading frames which may potentially code for proteins of 114 and 188 amino acids, respecitively [55,56]. These two open reading frames are not conserved in evolution [47], which questions their biological importance. The transcriptional situation in the c-*myc* locus is further complicated by the finding of antisense transcription in the region upstream of P_2, a phenomenon whose biological significance is again unclear [57,58].

Chromatin

Six DNAase-hypersensitive sites have been identified in the human as well as in the murine c-*myc* locus. Two of the sites (III1 and III2) are located immediately upstream of P_1 and P_2, respectively, suggesting that they represent sites where transcription factors bind to the promoter region. Site II is located immediately upstream of P_0 and may play a similar role for P_0 transcription. Site II was found to be closed on the transcriptionally silent c-*myc* allele in one Burkitt's lymphoma line [59] and in HL60 cells 4 days after induction of differentiation [60]. Site I is located 1100 bp further upstream. The biological role of site I is not clear, since it has been implicated with both repression [59] and activation [61]. The 2-kb region upstream of P_1 containing DNAase-hypersensitive sites I, II, and III is conserved to about 70% between mouse and man with four clusters of 80–85% homology [47,56,62]. The evolutionary conservation of the upstream region suggests that it contains target sequences for transcriptional regulation. Several attempts to identify *cis*-acting target sequences for transcriptional regulation have revealed a complex interaction between positively and negatively acting elements [63–66]. Another DNAase-hypersensitive site is located in front of $exon_2$ [60,61]. In primary human tonsil lymphocytes, two additional sites were found in $exon_2$ whose function is unknown [67].

The Protein

The c-*myc* RNAs initiated at P_1 and P_2 have the same coding capacity and code for two closely related proteins with an apparent size of 60–67 kd [68–70]. The size heterogeneity of the c-*myc* protein is still not understood. It may reflect conformational variations [69,71], or heterogeneity in initiation of translation with alternative starts in the first exon (S. R. Hann and R. N. Eisenman, personal communication). As its viral counterpart, the c-*myc* protein is phosphorylated, resides in the nucleus, and has DNA-binding capacity in vitro [68–75]. A discrepancy between calculated (48 kd) and apparent molecular weight (60–67 kd) has also been observed for other proteins and may reflect a peculiar secondary structure of the *myc* protein, probably due to its high proline content. The c-*myc* protein is labile with a half-life of 30 min [68,70,76]. The rapid turnover of the protein as well as of the c-*myc* mRNA [52] may be regarded as mechanisms allowing rapid adjustment of the c-*myc* protein level in the cell to changes in the environmental conditions. A metabolically more stable variant of the c-*myc* protein has recently been described [77]. The biochemical and physiological function of the c-*myc* protein has remained largely unknown until recently, but may soon start to be elucidated. The *myc* protein has been found associated with small nuclear ribonucleoproteins (RNPs), suggesting a possible role in RNA processing or transport [78]. It has furthermore been implicated in DNA synthesis [79]. Recently the c-*myc* protein was reported to bind specifically to *ori*-containing sequences, and was shown to promote eucaryotic DNA replication [80,81].

The Role of c-*myc* in Cellular Proliferation and Differentiation

In many different types of cells, c-*myc* expression correlates with proliferation. c-*myc* is turned off in quiescent cells and highly expressed in rapidly proliferating cells [82].

The analysis of c-*myc* expression in embryonic development has suggested, however, that this correlation is not absolute and that other pathways, possibly by involving other members of the *myc* family, may also induce proliferation [83]. The correlation between c-*myc* expression and growth state is an indication that c-*myc* is somehow involved in growth control. How this is achieved is largely unknown.

Most of our knowledge about the role of c-*myc* in growth control comes from systems in which the transition from quiescence to proliferation and eventually back to growth arrest can easily be manipulated. Addition of serum to serum-deprived fibroblasts, antigenic or mitogenic stimulation of lymphocytes [84], and partial hepatectomy [85,86] lead to a 50- to 100-fold increase in c-*myc* RNA with a maximum after 1–2 hr, well before the cell enter into S phase. The induction of c-*myc* is preceded by an induction of c-*fos*, which is expressed at maximal level already after 15–30 min [87].

Induction of c-*fos* and c-*myc* is preceded by intracellular ionic changes, including an increase in intracellular free Ca^{2+} and a rise in intracellular pH by about 0.4–0.5 pH units [88]. These ionic changes appear to be essential steps in the pathway converting a signal from outside the cell into a cellular proliferation response which includes an altered program of gene expression.

Induction of c-*myc* is associated with the transition from G_0 to G_1, but is not sufficient to induce proliferation [89,90]. This indicates that induction of cell growth involves at least two signals, a first, which induces the transition from G_0 to G_1 (competence signal), and makes the cell susceptible to respond to a second signal which drives the cell to proliferation (progression signal) [91]. In lymphocytes mitogen or antigen may be regarded as competence factors which drive the cell into G_1 and induce expression of c-*myc* and growth factor receptors, thus rendering the cell responsive to the action of growth actors. A role of c-*myc* as a competence factor was suggested by experiments in which introduction of c-*myc* into mouse fibroblasts, by DNA transfection or microinjection of the protein, reduced the requirement for PDGF (competence signal) [92,93].

c-*myc* expression appears to be required, however, not only for the transition form G_0 to G_1, but also for progression through the G_1 phase, as indicated by the analysis of T lymphocytes arrested in G_1 by withdrawal of interleukin 2 [94,95].

Taken together, c-*myc* may be regarded as an intracellular amplifier of growth-promoting signals which renders the cell more susceptible to growth factors and/or less sensitive to growth-inhibiting factors. This could be achieved in several ways: by changing the number of receptor molecules (which has been studied and not observed [96]), by modulating the affinity of receptors, or by a postreceptor mechanism, possibly by regulating transcription of other genes [97]. *myc* reduces the requirement for growth factors, but does not abrogate it [96,98–102]. This is also supported from the analysis of tumors associated with an activated viral or cellular c-*myc* gene. Myelomonocytic cells transformed by *myc* containing retroviruses usually remain dependent on the respective colony-stimulating factors [103,104,197]. Likewise, primary mouse plasmacytomas with Ig-*myc* translocations, when placed into culture, require a specific growth factor which is provided by the pristane-induced granuloma in vivo [105–107].

However, abrogation from a specific growth factor requirement has been observed in myeloid and T cells infected with a *myc*-containing retrovirus [108], and may be a secondary event occurring with a considerable frequency in cells with an active *myc* gene. This is supported by the fact that Burkitt's lymphoma cells can be established as cell lines quite successfully in vitro, and that mouse plasmacytoma cells lose their specific growth factor requirement upon serial passage in vivo [109,110].

The induction of c-*myc* during transition from G_0 to G_1 had initially suggested that c-*myc* expression is specific for and restricted to G_1 phase of the cell cycle [84,111]. It was, however, shown that in proliferating cells c-*myc* expression and the rate of c-*myc* protein turnover is invariant throughout the cell cycle [76,112,113]. In light of the possible role of c-*myc* in DNA replication, it will be interesting to see whether c-*myc* expression is required for progression through the cell cycle beyond the restriction point in G_1 after which serum can be withdrawn without affecting the progression of the cell through the rest of the cycle [114]. Once the cell cycle is completed, the level of *myc* expression appears to determine whether a cell is entering another cell cycle or is going into G_0. Thus, decreased expression may be required for a cell to escape the cell cycle, whereas constitutive high expression forces the cells to keep cycling [115].

In a number of cell systems, cycling of the cells and induction of differentiation appear to be mutually exclusive. In the best studied systems of in vitro differentiation, mouse erythroleukemia cells (MEL), and the human promyelocyhic leukemia cell line HL60, c-*myc* RNA decreases rapidly after addition of inducers of differentiation [116,117]. At least in MEL cells, the c-*myc* decrease is biphasic with an intermittent increase after about 8 hr [118]. Enforced *myc* expression from an exogeneously introduced gene carrying a constitutive promoter is able to inhibit induction of differentiation by various inducers, indicating that induction of differentiation in these cells is critically dependent on decreased c-*myc* expression [119–121].

It should be emphasized, however, that a mutually exclusive relationship between c-*myc* expression and differentiation may only exist for terminally differentiating cells. *myc*-containing retroviruses cause tumors with a differentiated phenotype such as myelomonocytic leukemias and carcinomas [122]. Likewise, mouse tumors associated with c-*myc* translocations are tumors of highly differentiated, immunoglobulin-secreting B cells (plasmacytomas). It thus appears that *myc* expression is not necessarily interfering with the differentiation program of a cell as long as the cell is kept proliferating.

c-*myc* Regulation

Systems in which the level of c-*myc* RNA can be modulated from outside the cell provided not only information about the role of c-*myc* in cell proliferation and differentiation, but served also as tools to study the mechanism of c-*myc* regulation. In all of these systems, it became apparent that c-*myc* RNA levels are rapidly increased or decreased by one of two, or a combination of the two mechanisms: regulation of RNA elongation and of RNA stability. Regulation at the level of transcription initiation does, however, not seem to play an important role for rapid adjustment of c-*myc* RNA levels. Regulation at the level of RNA stability has been reported for serum-stimulated fibroblasts [123] for differentiating mouse teratocarcinoma [124] and erythroleukemia (MEL) cells [125], and for Daudi cells treated with interferon [126,127].

Transcriptional regulation was observed in diferentiating HL60 and MEL cells [125,128], and in interferon-treated Daudi cells [129]. A more detailed description of the c-*myc* transcription pattern in nuclei of differentiating HL60 cells by nuclear run-on analysis revealed that the observed transcriptional regulation is largely due to a block of RNA elongation [57,130]. This was concluded from the fact that the density of RNA polymerases was almost unchanged on c-*myc* $exon_1$, whereas it was dramatically reduced on the distal part of the gene upon addition of differentiation-inducing agents.

For differentiating MEL cells, it was shown that two mechanisms cooperate to reduce the c-*myc* RNA level in the cell, a block of RNA elongation and decreased stability of c-*myc* RNA [125]. This is likely to be true also in other systems.

The observed regulation at the level of RNA elongation is reminiscent to regulation by attenuation in the trp operon of *Escherichia coli* [131]. A similar attenuation type control has been described by Hay and Aloni [132] for the regulation of late SV40 gene expression.

Based on these model systems, Eick and Bornkamm [130] proposed that two conformations may be formed at the end of $exon_1$, a read-through conformation with one stem and loop, and an alternative conformation with two stems and loops followed by a polyU stretch, which might serve as a transcription termination signal. Regulation by attenuation, in *E. coli* as well as in SV40, involves a small protein encoded by the RNA leader that stabilizes one of both RNA conformations. The analogy between the different systems has reemphasized the search for proteins which may eventually be encoded by the reading frame in $exon_1$ [56,133], and by the upstream reading frame present in c-*myc* RNA initiated at P_0 [55].

Most importantly, regulation at the level of RNA elongation appears to be the dominant mechanism to regulate the c-*myc* RNA level in lymphocytes before and after mitogenic stimulation [67,134]. The distribution of RNA polymerases on the c-*myc* gene in resting tonsil lymphocytes mirrors that in differentiating HL60 cells. Transcription is apparently going on from P_1/P_2 and P_0 without generating a full transcript, since RNA elongation is blocked. This transcriptional activity of the c-*myc* gene in resting lymphocytes is also reflected by the c-*myc* chromatin conformation. The pattern of DNAase-hypersensitive sites is indistinguishable in resting and proliferating cells, indicating that the c-*myc* gene is in a transcriptionally active configuration already before mitogenic stimulation. The resting tonsil lymphocytes may therefore be regarded as preactivated cells, in which the c-*myc* RNA level can easily and rapidly be increased by releasing the RNA elongation block upon mitogenic stimulation [67].

This type of regulation appears to be particularly well suited for cells whose biological function involves an immediate response to growth-promoting signals. Whether this type of regulation is realized in cells not belonging to the hemopoetic lineage is not yet known.

THE IMMUNOGLOBULIN LOCI AND THE TARGETS OF IMMUNOGLOBULIN GENE REGULATION

The immunoglobulin genes are composed of various genetic elements which are localized distantly apart from each other in germ-line configuration, and are assembled to a functional gene during B-cell differentiation. Two different types of recombinations are involved in the formation of immunoglobulin genes: VDJ and switch recombinations. VDJ rearrangements in the heavy and VJ rearrangements in the light chain loci are sequence-specific recombinations which lead to the formation of functional Ig genes. The sequence specificity is mediated by inverted heptamer-spacer-nonamer signals with 12- and 23-bp spacers, respectively, adjacent to both targets of recombination. The activity of the VDJ and VJ recombinase is believed to be turned down once a functional immunoglobulin heavy and light chain is made [135].

The second type of recombination is the switch recombination. Switch recombination is mediated by repeated sequence elements located upstream of heavy chain constant genes, and gives rise to the production of a new immunoglobulin isotype with the same antigenic specificity. The isotype or class switch is usually occurring in a cell with a reassembled functional immunoglobulin gene during the secondary immune response. However, class switching does not necessarily require a functional immunoglobulin gene rearrangement, as shown by switching in Abelson virus–transformed mouse pre–B-cell lines [135]. Furthermore, the class switching machinery is incapable of discriminate between a functionally and nonfunctionally rearranged immunoglobulin gene, and is operating at both alleles [136].

The expression of immunoglobulin genes is highly regulated in a differentiation-specific fashion. A functional immunoglobulin gene is expressed in B cells, and not in cells of other lineages [137]. Fusion of B cells with fibroblasts leads to extinction of Ig gene expression [138,139]. A shut-off of cell-specific functions is also observed in somatic hybrids between fibroblasts and hepatocytes, suggesting that extinction is a more general biological phenomenon not restricted to B cells [140,141]. The mechanism of extinction in somatic hybrids is not understood at a molecular level.

Different elements in the immunoglobulin locus are involved in conferring tissue specificity of transcription. The elements first identified were enhancers in the heavy chain and κ light chain loci [142–145]. The heavy chain enhancer is located between the joining region and the switch site, and thus remains within a functional heavy chain gene after isotype switch. The κ enhancer is located between the κ joining and constant region. The enhancer appears to be required for initiation of transcription, possibly by opening the chromatin, but not for continued immunoglobulin gene expression [146–148]. In the λ light chain locus, an enhancer has not been identified so far.

A second element conferring tissue specificity of transcription is located in the immunoglobulin gene promoter region [149–151]. This element involves an octamer (ATTTGCAT) in κ light chain promoters and its inversed complementary version (ATGCAAAT) in heavy chain promoters 70 bp 5′ of the cap site [149,150]. The octamer was shown to mediate binding of a protein which may be involved in tissue-specific transcription [152].

Less well defined is the role of sequences for tissue-specific expression which are located either in the body of an Ig constant gene or 3′ thereof. Grosschedl and Baltimore [151] demonstrated that the constant μ gene contributes significantly to B-cell-specific expression when cloned behind a tissue-unspecific promoter and enhancer. Whether the contribution of the μ constant region to tissue specific expression stemmed from transcriptional or posttranscriptional regulation, had not been studied.

Evidence for a regulatory element in the 3′ part of immunoglobulin genes was also reported by Gregor and Morrison [153]. These authors described that expression of the α heavy chain in a myeloma is substantially decreased at the level of transcription by a 4-kb deletion downstream of Cα which involves the membrane domain.

With regard to the potential importance of elements located located in the 3′ part of the Ig locus for c-*myc* deregulation in Burkitt's lymphoma and mouse plasmacytoma, more work is apparently needed to define such an element(s) in more detail.

THE BREAKPOINTS OF THE CHROMOSOMAL TRANSLOCATIONS

When the juxtaposition of c-*myc* and immunoglobulin genes was recognized in Burkitt's lymphoma and mouse plasmacytoma, it became immediately apparent that the breakpoints are heterogeneous with regard to c-*myc* as well as to the immunoglobulin genes. The orientation of c-*myc* and immunoglobulin genes on their respective chromosomes and the position of the genes relative to each other after the chromosomal translocation are shown in Figs. 2 and 3. In all cases, one chromosome 8 and one of the immunoglobulin loci carrying chromosomes participate in the translocation. Significantly, c-*myc* RNA is always derived from the gene on the affected chromosome, whereas the normal allele is silent. Oppositely, the immunoglobulin is usually derived from the normal chromosome. A consistent difference between t(8;14) and variant translocations is that the breakpoints are always located 5′ of the c-*myc*-coding region in t(8;14), and downstream thereof in t(2;8) and t(8;22) translocations (Fig. 3). Accordingly, the coding part of c-*myc* always moves onto chr. 14 in t(8;14) translocations (14q+), whereas it remains on chr. 8 in the variants (8q+) (Fig. 2). As a common denominator, in all cases the coding part of c-*myc*, regardless of distance and orientation, is brought to a position 5′ of an immunoglobulin-constant gene. Most importantly, the open reading frame coding for the c-*myc* protein is in no case violated.

The t(8;14) Translocation

The orientation of the heavy-chain locus on chr. 14 toward the centromer and of c-*myc* on chr. 8 toward the telomer implies that c-*myc* and heavy chain genes are always fused to each other in opposite orientation in t(8;14) translocation. There is considerable heterogeneity of the breakpoints on chr. 8 (Figs. 3 and 4). They are located either in the first exon or intron of the c-*myc* gene (class I according to Cory [51]), within a few kb upstream of P_1 in the presumed regulatory region (class II), or further upstream in an unknown distance (class III). As pointed out by Lanfrancone and coworkers [154], in the majority of cases from low-incidence areas the breakpoints are located within the 12.5-kb c-*myc*-carrying EcoRI fragment (classes I and II), whereas in a large number of cases from Africa and New Guinea, the breakpoint is distant from c-*myc*. This difference is not related to the presence or absence of EBV (M. Falk, G. M. Lenoir, and G. W. Bornkamm, unpublished data). It was proposed to reflect differences in the developmental stage of the B cell when the cell was hit by the translocation [154,155]. In three cell lines with class II t(8;14) translocation which have been studied in detail (P3HR1, 380, Daudi), the breakpoints were found clustered within a small distance on chr. 8 [155]. It remains to be seen whether this will hold true also for other cases.

In the heavy chain locus the breakpoints are also variable; however, to a lesser extent than on chr. 8 (Fig. 5). In the majority of cases of t(8;14), in

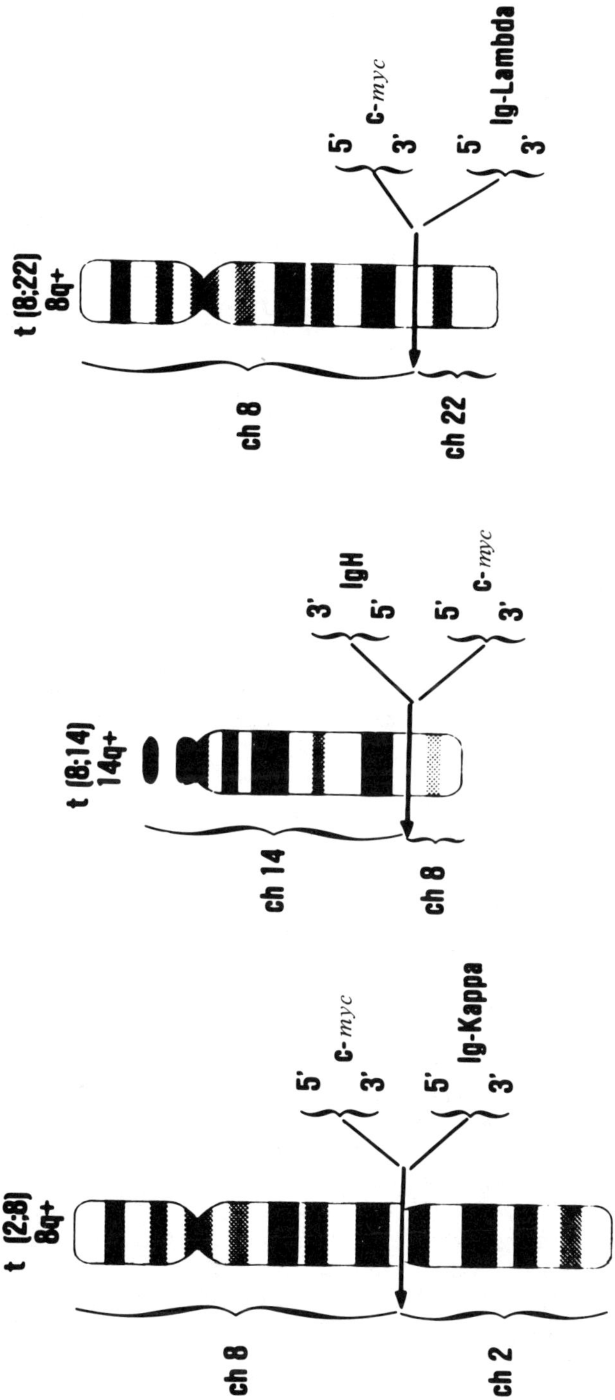

Figure 2 Orientation of the c-*myc* and immunoglobulin genes on the 8q + and 14q + marker chromosomes in Burkitt's lymphoma.

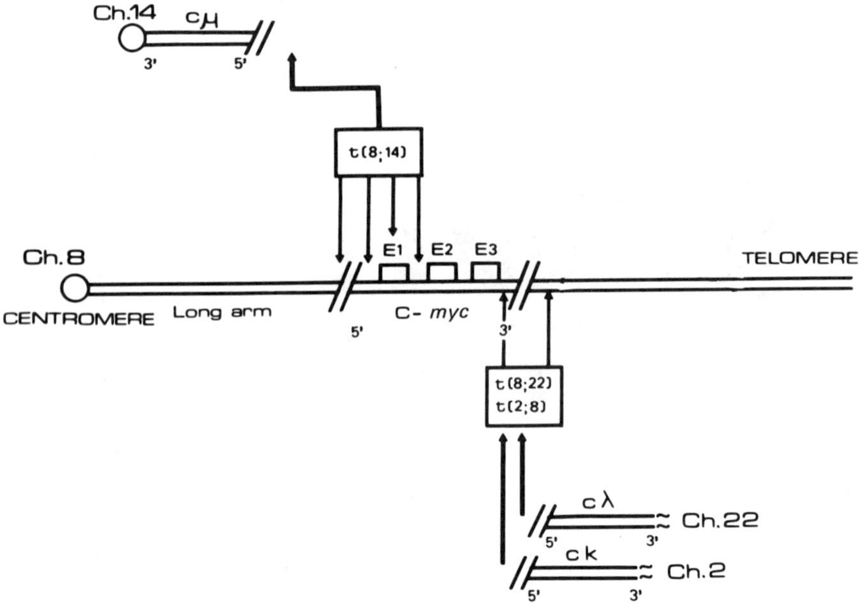

Figure 3 Location of chromosomal breakpoints of t(8;14), t(2;8), and t(8;22) translocations relative to the c-*myc* gene with exon$_1$, exon$_2$, and exon$_3$ (E_1, E_2, E_3) and the immunoglobulin heavy and light chain genes.

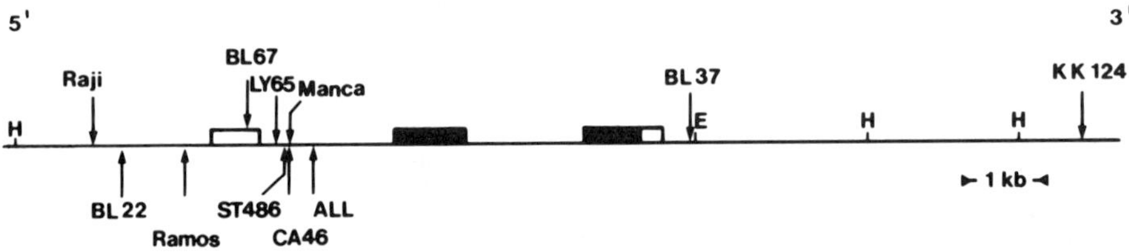

Figure 4 Location of chromosomal breakpoints which were sequenced and of which the distance to the c-*myc* gene is known. The noncoding region of c-*myc* is represented by open boxes, the coding region by filled boxes. Raji [156;218], BL22 [219], Ramos [186], BL67 [162], LY65 [184], ST 486 [220], CA46 [157], Manca [159], and a case of B-cell leukemia (ALL) [158] have t(8;14) translocations, BL37 [169] and KK124 [170] t(8;22) translocations. In two cases with t(8;22) translocations (BL2 [189] and JI [172]) sequenced breakpoints lie 10 and 28 kb downstream of c-*myc*. In two cell lines with t(8;14) translocation (P3HR1 and 380 [155]) and three lines with t(2;8) translocations (JBL2 [174], BL64 [171], and LY91 [179]) the sequenced breakpoints are located at unknown distance upstream and downstream of c-*myc*, respectively.

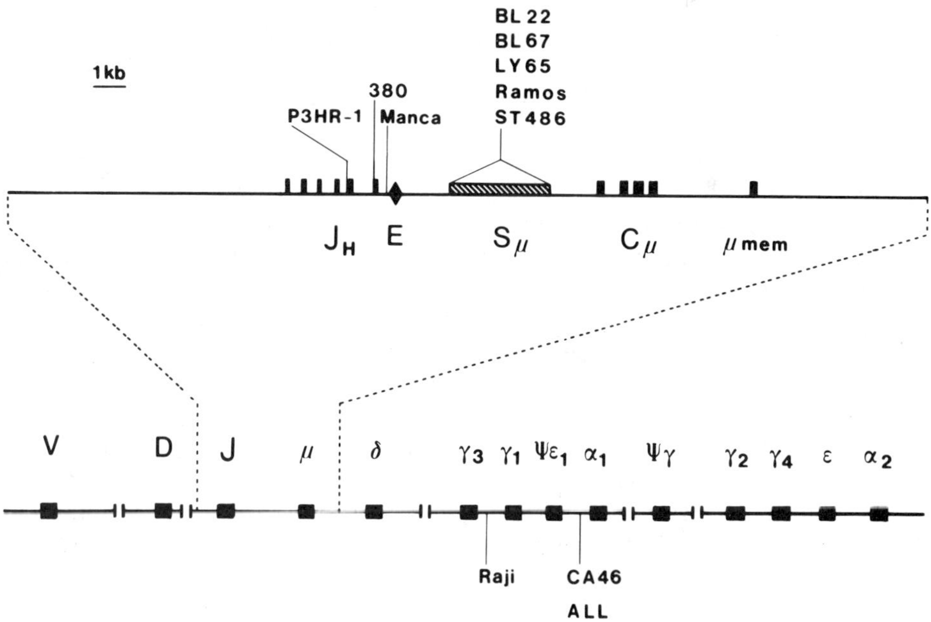

Figure 5 Location of sequenced chromosomal breakpoints of cases with t(8;14) translocations within the immunoglobulin heavy chain locus. Filled boxes represent the coding parts of immunoglobulin genes. The filled rhombus shows the IgH enhancer, the dashed region the μ switch region.

classes I and II translocations the breaks are located in switch sites, usually in front of the μ constant gene and less frequently in front of Cγ [156] or Cα [157,158]. This is in contrast to mouse plasmacytomas that affect in most cases the Cα locus. The translocation is an imprecise reciprocal event involving nonhomologous recombination and usually leads to loss or acquisition of a few base pairs at the recombination sites (reviewed in Ref. 51).

The head-to-head rearrangement of c-*myc* and immunoglobulin heavy chain genes has ruled out the model that the c-*myc* gene comes under the control of a strong and constitutive immunoglobulin promoter, and has rather favored an enhancer insertion model for the deregulation of the c-*myc* gene. It was therefore surprising to note that the IgH enhancer located in the heavy chain locus between the joining and switch region is only in few cases juxtaposed to the c-*myc* gene [59,159]. The enhancer usually moves to the reciprocal fragment of the translocation and is thus unavailable for the c-*myc* gene.

The situation may, however, be quite different for t(8;14) class III translocations. In two of the three cases mentioned above, the breakpoints are located within the heavy chain joining region (P3HR1, 380) [155]. In all three cases, the IgH enhancer is fused to that piece of chr. 8, although at considerable distance, which carries the c-*myc* gene. Whether this is a general feature of t(8;14) translocations remains to be determined.

The consequences of the translocation for c-*myc* expression are much more evident in cases with a truncated versus a nontruncated c-*myc* gene. The translocation into $intron_1$ or $exon_1$ disrupts the c-*myc* gene and separates the coding part from its physiological promoters and the presumed regulatory upstream region. In these cases, transcription is initiated at multiple cryptic promoters in the first intron and proceeds into the coding part of the gene without splicing, thus providing the c-*myc* RNA with a new leader of about similar size (reviewed in Ref. 51). As documented in mouse plasmacytoma and also observed in the Burkitt lymphoma line BL67 (D. Eick, unpublished), initiation of transcription in the first intron is bidirectional and gives rise to aberrant c-*myc* as well as truncated immunoglobulin heavy chain RNA transcribed across the breakpoint of the translocation into the immunoglobulin locus [160, 161]. Calabi and Neuberger [161] cloned and sequenced complementary DNAs (cDNAs) of such truncated heavy chain RNAs, and showed that multiple stop codons are present in front of the constant coding region, thus making expression of a truncated protein unlikely.

In BL67, BL18, and possibly also in a number of other lines [47], the high transcriptional activity around the breakpoint of the translocation is underlined by the finding that transcription is additionally initiated within the immunoglobulin locus in antisense orientation with respect to the constant μ gene and proceeds across the breakpoint of the translocation into the c-*myc* gene, giving rise to a second large c-*myc* RNA of about 3.5 kb [162]. Small transcripts initiated at P_1 and P_2 on the reciprocal fragment of the translocation are present in some and absent in other lines [162,163], whereas the normal c-*myc* allele is usually silent. Structurally aberrant c-*myc* RNAs transcribed from truncated c-*myc* genes are more stable than their normal counterparts [162,164,165]. The increased stability can not be ascribed solely to the absence of $exon_1$ and is rather the consequence of an altered secondary structure of the aberrant c-*myc* RNA [162,166].

The Variant t(2;8) and t(8;22) Translocations

In about 25% of the Burkitt's lymphoma cases, variant translocations have been observed which affect chr. 8 and chromosomes 2 or 22, carrying the immunoglobulin $\varkappa$ and λ light chain loci. Remarkably, in the first series of BL cells with variant translocations, a perfect correlation was observed between the type of translocation and the type of light chain expressed by the respective cells. Thus cells with t(2;8) translocations expressed $\varkappa$ and cells with t(8;22) translocations λ light chains [167]. By now, five exceptions have been observed from this rule, four of which are cell lines with t(8;22) translocation expressing $\varkappa$ light chains [168–170, 221]. The opposite a cell line with t(2;8) translocation expressing λ light chains, has been observed once [221].

In all cases, the breakpoints are downstream of c-*myc* and upstream of an immunoglobulin light chain constant gene. In contrast to the t(8;14) translocations, both loci are thus arranged in head-to-tail orientation. With regard to the light chain locus, the breakpoints are in most cases in or around the joining region. The hepta- and nonamer structures used for VJ joining have been implicated in two cases with t(2;8) translocation [171,172], but do not seem to be generally involved.

On chr. 8, the breakpoints of variant translocations seem to be scattered throughout a large distance of probably several hundred kb downstream of c-*myc*. No apparent cluster of breakpoints has been identified within 47 kb [173]. The only small cluster so far identified contains the breakpoints of three cell lines with t(2;8) translocation and is located >60 kb downstream of c-*myc* (B. Henglein and M. Lipp, personal communication). At an unknown distance further downstream of this small breakpoint cluster is another interesting region at the site of the t(2;8) breakpoint of the Burkitt's lymphoma line JBL2 [174]. This latter region has been defined by its partial sequence homology to the mouse *pvt*-1 locus [175]. The mouse *pvt*-1 locus was initially identified as a region in which five out of 17 breakpoints of mouse plasmacytoma variant translocations were clustered [176]. Mouse *pvt*-1 is not only a chromosomal breakpoint cluster but also a site of preferential provirus integration in Moloney murine leukemia virus (MoMuLV), induced T-cell lymphomas in mice [177] and rats [178] as well as in primary tumors of AKR mice [177].

Even though the human *pvt*-1 like region does not seem to contain a breakpoint cluster, it appears to be a particularly interesting locus for a number of reasons [179]: (a) it contains the 3′ end of the c-*myc* amplification unit of the human tumor line COLO 320, (b) it shows sequence homology to the Moloney proviral integration site in rat T-cell lymphomas, and (c) contains, in a human T-cell leukemia line, the 3′ end of an interstitial deletion of chr. 8, which may have been caused by proviral integration and excision during the course of this HTLV1-associated malignancy. Thus, a structural alteration of the *pvt*-1–like region may have contributed to the development of the leukemic T-cell clone [179].

As suggested by Manolov and coauthors [180], another interesting locus may be located on chr. 8 still further downstream containing the breakpoints of many of the t(8;22) translocations.

The biological role of loci like *pvt*-1 for the development of Burkitt's lymphoma and mouse plasmacytoma is not at all understood. Until now, no gene has yet been assigned to the *pvt*-1 locus [176]. It therefore seems that loci far distant from c-*myc* like *pvt*-1 may exert their effect on c-*myc* regulation over a large distance in *cis*, possibly by altering the high-order chromatin structure in a fashion still to be defined.

Structural Alterations of the c-*myc* Gene in Cell Lines With the Breakpoint Distant From c-*myc*

Duplications

The c-*myc* gene has been studied in detail in several Burkitt's lymphoma lines with variant translocations. In two cases with t(2;8) translocation from Japan (JBL2) and Algeria (IARC-BL64), an additional band was detected on Southern blots with a c-*myc* probe. Remarkably, in these two cases the additional c-*myc* band turned out not to contain the breakpoints of the translocations as expected, but rather duplications of the first exon (JBL2) [174] and the coding part of c-*myc* (IARC-BL64) [171], both derived from the respective 8q+ chromosomes. While in JBL2 the normal tissue of the patient was not available for analysis, the duplication in IARC-BL64 turned out to be constitutional. An identical constitutional duplication has furthermore been observed in a child with Ewing's sarcoma derived from another area in Algeria [181]. Family studies did not provide evidence for a generally increased risk of cancer for the carriers of this abnormal c-*myc* allele [181].

Mutations

The great emphasis on the point mutations in the ras gene during the last few years has also led to an extensive search for mutations in the c-*myc* gene. Mutations in the coding part of c-*myc* have in fact been found in several Burkitt's lymphomas [157,182–184], including one case of Burkitt-type leukemia in which fresh clinical material could be studied [158]. In other cases, however, no change in the coding sequence of the translocated c-*myc* gene was detected [182,185,186].

Despite the lack of changes in $exon_2$ and $exon_3$ of c-*myc* in some cell lines, mutations have been frequently observed in and around the first exon. Thus, all BL lines studied in detail which have the breakpoint distant of the c-*myc* gene, regardless of whether they represent t(8;14) or variant translocations, have either multiple or at least one mutation in the first exon [170,171,183,186–190]. The biological role of these mutations will be discussed in detail below.

The Generation of the Translocations

For our understanding of the pathogenesis of BL, it is an important question at which stage of B-cell development the chromosomal translocations are acquired. Is the translocation an accident of immunoglobulin rearrangement? This is indeed suggested by the fact that the breakpoints of the chromosomal translocations are usually located at or close to sites that are also used for one or the other type of physiological Ig rearrangement; i.e., VDJ/VJ joining or isotype switch. In most cases with t(8;14) translocation the breakpoints are situated in the μ switch region, in variant translocations, and in some t(8;14) cases within or close to the joining region. In some cases, sequences were identified at the breakpoints which closely resemble the nonamer-spacer-heptamer signals used for physiological VJ and VDJ joining. This suggests that in those cases, the translocation has occurred at an early stage of B-cell differentiation as an accident of VJ/VDJ rearrangement [155,171, 172,189]. Differences in the location of breakpoints in cases from high-and low-incidence areas have been interpreted to indicate that the translocations were acquired at different stages of B-cell differentiation in both types of tumors [154,155].

However, involvement of the μ switch site in many t(8;14) translocations does not necessarily imply that the translocation occurred in a mature B cell which is induced to switch to another isotype. It is also conceivable that in cases involving the μ switch site, the translocation occurred before a functional heavy chain gene is formed, the μ switch region just being a favored site of illegitime recombination. Two essential requirements for recombinaton at the μ switch site are also fulfilled in pre–B cells: (a) the site is accessible to the switch recombinase by transcriptional activation (apparently also required for VDJ joining [135], and (b) the switch recombinase is active also in pre–B cells as shown by the possibility of class switching in Abelson virus–transformed pre–B cell lines [135]. Thus, the vast majority of BL cells does in fact produce IgM and not another isotype whose expression requires class switch. It is furthermore interesting that a t(6;14) translocation acquired in a human EBV-immortalized pre–B-cell line in vitro has also targeted the μ switch site in the heavy chain locus [191].

Taken together, the structural analysis of the breakpoints does not provide us a definite answer as to the time when the translocation occurred during B-cell differentiation.

c-*myc* DEREGULATION IN BURKITT'S LYMPHOMA

c-*myc* Plays a Decisive Role in the Development of B-Cell Neoplasias

The structural analysis of the c-*myc* locus in avian bursal lymphoma, mouse plasmacytoma, and Burkitt's lymphoma had provided circumstantial evidence for a role of the c-*myc* gene in the development of these tumors. Direct evidence for a decisive role of *myc* in the development of mouse neoplasias has recently been obtained in two experimental systems. Introduction of *myc* into the germ line of mice leads to a high rate of spontaneous tumors in the animals [192–194]. A transgenic c-*myc* gene fused to an immunoglobulin heavy chain enhancer specifically induces B-cell neoplasias in almost 100% of the offspring [193]. Most importantly, the tumors are monoclonal in origin surrounded by apparently normal tissue, indicating that additional events must have occurred in the tumor cell clone to make the *myc*-expressing cells fully malignant.

In the second experimental system, conclusive evidence for a decisive role of *myc* in the development of B-cell neoplasias was provided by demonstrating that infection of mice with a *myc*-containing retrovirus can substitute for the chromosomal translocation juxtaposing c-*myc* and Ig loci in the development of pristane-induced mouse plasmacytoma [195].

Quantitative Versus Qualitative Changes in c-*myc* Expression

As mentioned above, mutations in the coding part of c-*myc* have been observed in a number of Burkitt's lymphomas. Qualitative changes in the c-*myc* protein may therefore contribute to the development of a malignant cell; e.g., by changing the stability of the protein and/or its interaction with other molecules.

In other cases, the coding sequence of the translocated allele is, however, identical to the germ-line c-*myc* gene, indicating that alteration of the *myc* protein is not a necessary feature of Burkitt's lymphoma. This is consistent with the fact that a normal c-*myc* gene when transfected [196] or inserted into a retrovirus [197,198] exerts transforming activity in vitro and oncogenic potential in vivo [197]. It stresses the importance of quantitative rather than qualitative changes in c-*myc* expression.

Is thus c-*myc* overexpressed in Burkitt's lymphoma cells? A higher c-*myc* expression was in fact reported in cells with the translocation versus cells without the translocation [199,200]. However, the amount of c-*myc* RNA in Burkitt's lymphoma cells as well as mouse plasmacytoma cells is quite variable and does not exceed that in lymphocytes after induction of proliferation with mitogens [201]. Similarly, in transgenic mice c-*myc* expression is not exceedingly high in the premalignant stage as well as in B-cell tumors [202]. This indicates that the failure to downregulate c-*myc* is critical rather than the absolute level of expression.

One reservation should be kept in mind, however, concerning the conclusion that qualitative changes of the c-*myc* protein(s) are irrelevant. We still do not have a definite answer as to the molecular basis for the heterogeneity of the c-*myc* protein. If, as proposed by Hann and Eisenman, an alternative initiation codon in the first exon is used to generate the large c-*myc* protein, truncation of the gene as well as mutations in $exon_1$ could eventually contribute to qualitative changes in the c-*myc* protein(s). Likewise, the small proteins encoded by the open reading frames in P_0 RNA, if they exist, could also serve as targets for mutations in and around $exon_1$.

The possibility that qualitative changes in c-*myc* expression are also important in addition to perturbated regulation has, therefore, not been definitely ruled out.

The Various Models of c-*myc* Deregulation

The structural analysis of the breakpoints in various cases of Burkitt's lymphoma has revealed a remarkable heterogeneity with regard to c-*myc* as well as to the Ig loci. The consequences of the translocation may therefore be quite different in cases with a truncated versus a nontruncated c-*myc* gene and in cases with or without an Ig enhancer juxtaposed to c-*myc*. The c-*myc* gene is a gene which is apparently tightly regulated at many different levels within the cell. This implies as many possibilities to perturbate c-*myc* regulation. We shall discuss first the various models of c-*myc* regulation and deregulation which reflect this diversity and shall then try to evaluate features of deregulation which are common in the different types of translocations.

Transcriptional Deregulation

The separation of the c-*myc* gene from its dual promoter in many cases of Burkitt's lymphomas, and as a result, its transcription from nonphysiological cryptic promoters has immediately suggested that the translocation has deprived the c-*myc* gene of its transcriptional control. Strong support for such a model came from the observation that the c-*myc* RNA in Burkitt's lymphoma cells is always derived from the c-*myc* allele on the translocation chromosome while the normal allele is silent. Shut-off of the normal c-*myc* allele appears to occur at the transcriptional level [55,61].

Another indicator of perturbated c-*myc* transcription in Burkitt's lymphoma and plasmacytoma cells is the shift in promoter usage in cell lines with a nontruncated c-*myc* in favor of P_1 [187,203]. In these cells, the ratio of P_1 to P_2 usage is $\geqslant 1$ compared to a P_1/P_2 ratio of 0.2–0.3 in normal cells. The molecular basis of this promoter shift is still not understood.

Differences in the transcriptional activity of the c-*myc* gene could be correlated with differences in DNAase I–hypersensitive sites in c-*myc* chromatin [59,60], supporting the importance of transcriptional regulation.

The model of transcriptional regulation and deregulation proposed by Leder [50], Dunnick [204], Rabbitts [183], and their coworkers implies that the normal c-*myc* gene would be negatively regulated at a transcriptional level by binding of a repressor. A DNAase-hypersensitive site 2 kb upstream of the two promoters, which is also present on the transcriptionally silent allele [59] and the sequences around the first exon [183], were proposed as putative repressor binding sites. Truncation of the c-*myc* gene or mutations in or around the first exon would abolish repressor binding, thus leading to unregulated c-*myc* expression.

This model does not account for the fact that in some cases with t(8;14), translocations which have their breakpoints in the first intron, $exon_1$ remains continuously transcribed from P_1 and P_2 on the reciprocal fragment of the translocation, giving rise to small RNAs of about 700–900 bp [162,163], whereas the normal c-*myc* allele is turned off. This can, however, be explained by assuming that the Ig heavy chain enhancer which is now juxtaposed to c-*myc* $exon_1$ on chr. 8q−, is overriding the negative transcriptional regulation.

The transcriptional regulation model implies that the c-*myc* gene product exerts a negative control on the normal c-*myc* gene either directly, being its own repressor, or by an in direct mechanism (autoregulation).

The most compelling evidence for an autoregulatory model was provided by the demonstration that expression of an exogeneous constitutively expressed *myc* gene leads to down-regulation of the endogeneous normal *myc* gene in myeloid cells and lymphocytes [102,108,193,205,206]. There is, however, also a considerable amount of data which is in variance with the feedback regulation model.

Thus, in mouse and rat fibroblasts [99,207,208], in mouse erythroleukemia cells [119,120,209], and in tissue of transgenic mice harboring a mouse mammary tumor virus long-terminal repeat c-*myc* fusion gene in their germ line [192], transcription of the endogeneous c-*myc* gene is retained while the exogeneous gene is abundantly transcribed. At least in some of these cases, the endogeneous c-*myc* gene is shown to respond normally to a change in environmental conditions [207], or to the addition of inducers of differentiation [119,120], thus excluding the possibility that the endogeneous c-*myc* gene became spontaneously constitutive.

It still remains to be definitely settled whether the observed differences in c-*myc* autoregulation reflect different thresholds for suppression in different types of cells. Alternatively, it is also conceivable that absence of expression from the normal c-*myc* allele is, for still unknown reasons, an important factor in the evolution of a tumor which is being selected for in vivo [99,193,205,208].

Enhancer Insertion

As mentioned above, in most cases with t(8;14) classes I and II translocation, the IgH enhancer is on the reciprocal fragment of the translocation unavailable for the c-*myc* gene. It is thus possible that the IgH enhancer does play a role only in those cases where it is juxtaposed to c-*myc*. In the t(8;14) class III translocations, the IgH enhancer may always be on the same fragment as c-*myc*, and may exert its effect over a large distance.

Another possibility is that activation of the c-*myc* gene is an indirect rather than a direct effect of the Ig enhancer. The Ig enhancer appears to be required for initiation of transcription, possibly by opening the chromatin conformation, but not for maintainance of transcription. Once the Ig locus is transcriptionally active, removal of the enhancer should have no major effect on transcription. This assumption is based on the observation that Ig genes remain active in vivo even if the enhancer was lost by deletion [146,147]. Such a gene with a deleted enhancer, when cloned and reintroduced into B cells, is however inactive unless the enhancer is present [148].

Based on the analysis of c-*myc* expression in somatic hybrids between Burkitt's lymphoma cells and various lymphoid and fibroblastic cells [138,210,211], Croce and coworkers have postulated an as yet unidentified enhancer element in the 3′ part of immunoglobulin heavy and light chain genes required also for maintenance of transcription, which is supposed to operate over a large distance in certain stages of B-cell differentiation (long-range enhancer).

Mutations May Destroy the Transcription Terminator in $Exon_1$

The discovery that c-*myc* expression in differentiating HL60 cells is regulated mainly at the level of RNA elongation has provided an alternative attractive hypothesis for the role of mutations in and around $exon_1$. Such mutations may alter the secondary structure of DNA or RNA in such a way that the transcription termination signal can no longer be formed and c-*myc* transcription becomes constitutive.

Stabilization of c-*myc* RNA

The effect of the chromosomal translocation on c-*myc* RNA stability in mouse plasmacytoma and Burkitt's lymphoma cells has been analyzed by several groups. In all cases studied, truncation of the c-*myc* gene resulted in an increased stability of the c-*myc* mRNA [162,164,165]. However, mutations in $exon_1$ have no stabilizing effect on c-*myc* RNA [52,171].

Altered Translation Efficiency?

Sequences in the first and second exon are partly homologous in inverted orientation. These sequences allow the formation of a hairpin loop carrying the initiation codon for translation. If the hairpin loop is formed, the initiation codon should not be available for translation. According to the model of Saito and coworkers [54], truncation of the c-*myc* gene might abolish the capacity of the cell to regulate c-*myc* translation via the formation of RNA secondary structure, and would presumably lead to enhanced c-*myc* protein synthesis. Studying the in vitro translation efficiency of c-*myc* RNAs with and without the first exon, data in favor of such a model have been presented [212]. However, Hann and Eisenman [68] did not find a correlation between truncation of the c-*myc* gene and amount of c-*myc* protein in Burkitt's lymphoma lines. By studying transfected *myc* constructs with and without the first exon, it was furthermore impossible to lend direct experimental support for this model [213].

Susceptibility of Burkitt's Lymphoma Cells to Negative c-*myc* Regulation

Under certain experimental conditions, a c-*myc* gene located on a translocation chromosome is still susceptible to negative regulation. This is an important point which might question the concept that the c-*myc* gene is constitutively expressed in Burkitt's lymphoma cells. However, this susceptibility does, of course, not imply that the gene is also capable of responding to negative regulation under physiological conditions. It may, therefore, be more appropriate to talk of deregulated rather than of constitutive c-*myc* expression in Burkitt's lymphoma cells.

The susceptibility of the c-*myc* gene in Burkitt's lymphoma cells to some kind of negative regulation may be instrumental in defining at which level in the cell c-*myc* regulation is working and at which level it is perturbated. Such systems are, therefore, powerful experimental tools to define targets of c-*myc* regulation and to test at least some of the models of c-*myc* deregulation in Burkitt's lymphoma cells which have been discussed above.

The first system in which the c-*myc* gene of a Burkitt's lymphoma cell can be down-regulated is the system of Daudi cells responding to interferon, in which c-*myc* appears to be down-regulated at a transcriptional [129] as well as at a posttranscriptional level [126,127]. Since most Burkitt's lymphoma cell lines do not respond to interferon, this system has the disadvantage of being a special case which can not be generalized.

The second system, the system of somatic cell fusion between Burkitt's lymphoma cells and various other types of cells, has been widely exploited by Croce and coworkers and has unraveled a number of important features of c-*myc* regulation. Most importantly, this system has provided the only direct experimental evidence so far for a role of the Ig locus for c-*myc* deregulation in Burkitt's lymphoma cells. Fusion of Burkitt's lymphoma cells carrying t(8;14) translocations with mouse fibroblasts has been shown to lead to extinction of immunoglobulin gene expression as well as of the human c-*myc* gene derived from the translocation chromosome which had been transcriptionally active before cell fusion [138]. Remarkably, fusion with fibroblasts caused down-regulation also of a truncated c-*myc* gene which had been transcribed from cryptic promoters in Burkitt's lymphoma cells.

This finding has important implications. First of all, it demonstrates that c-*myc* activation in Burkitt's lymphoma cells is not mediated exclusively by deprivation of a repressor binding site [214], as suggested by the transcriptional deregulation model. Loss of a repressor binding site could not account for the fact that c-*myc* transcription from the translocated allele is switched off, whereas the c-*myc* gene derived from the fibroblastic fusion partner is continuously expressed.

The second important implication of these experiments is that the translocated c-*myc* gene must have come under the control of an as yet unidentified *cis*-acting element within the Ig locus in the Burkitt's lymphoma cell. The concominant extinction of Ig and c-*myc* genes in the hybrid cells indicates that c-*myc* expression from the translocated allele is dependent on factors which are active in B cells and inactive or absent in fibroblasts and the respective hybrids. Such factors should interact with target sequences within the immunoglobulin locus and should mediate their effect on c-*myc* expression in *cis* across the breakpoint of the translocation.

A third system in which c-*myc* down-regulation in Burkitt's lymphoma cells can be assessed experimentally, has recently been described by Polack and coworkers [215]. They showed that c-*myc* expression is turned down in Burkitt's lymphoma cells by addition of sodium butyrate. The rational behind these experiments had been provided by the fact that sodium butyrate induces c-*myc* down-regulation and differentiation in HL60 and mouse erythroleukemia cells, linked to the observation of Anisimova and coworkers [216] that sodium butyrate induces morphological, plasmablastlike changes in Raji cells. As shown in Fig. 6, sodium butyrate is capable of down-regulating a nontruncated as well as a truncated c-*myc* gene. It exerts its effect at a transcriptional level on RNA initiated at cryptic promoters in intron$_1$ as well as on the 3.5-kb c-*myc* RNA of BL67 which is initiated as Ig-antisense RNA and transcribed across the breakpoint of the translocation. Notably, transcription of the immunoglobulin constant m gene is also turned off, whereas other genes are either not affected (bcr, b-actin) or are induced (2–5 A synthetase, EBV genes) [215].

There are two possibilities to explain the effect of sodium butyrate on c-*myc* transcription. First, the effect of sodium butyrate may be mediated by target sequences which are located either in the body of the c-*myc* gene or 3′ thereof. Alternatively, sodium butyrate may act on two different targets in a nontruncated and a truncated c-*myc* gene. In a nontruncated gene, it may act on transcription initiation or elongation in the 5′ part of the c-*myc* gene. In cases with a truncated gene, it may have its target within the immunoglobulin locus and may act bidirectionally on immunoglobulin as well as c-*myc* transcription. This hypothesis is supported by the fact that sodium butyrate switches off immunoglobulin transcription concomitantly with c-*myc*, and that at least in some cases of Burkitt's lymphoma (BL18 and BL67), there is direct evidence for transcription initiation within the immunoglobulin locus in antisense orientiation [162].

A butyrate-responsive element in the immunoglobulin locus, if it exists, might be identical with the B cell-specific long-range enhancer postulated by Croce [217] from the fusion experiments just described between Burkitt's lymphoma cells and fibroblasts.

Most importantly, the susceptibility of the c-*myc* gene in Burkitt's lymphoma cells to sodium butyrate may provide an experimental system for the identification of target sequences which mediate this regulation and of the factors which may interact at the respective sites.

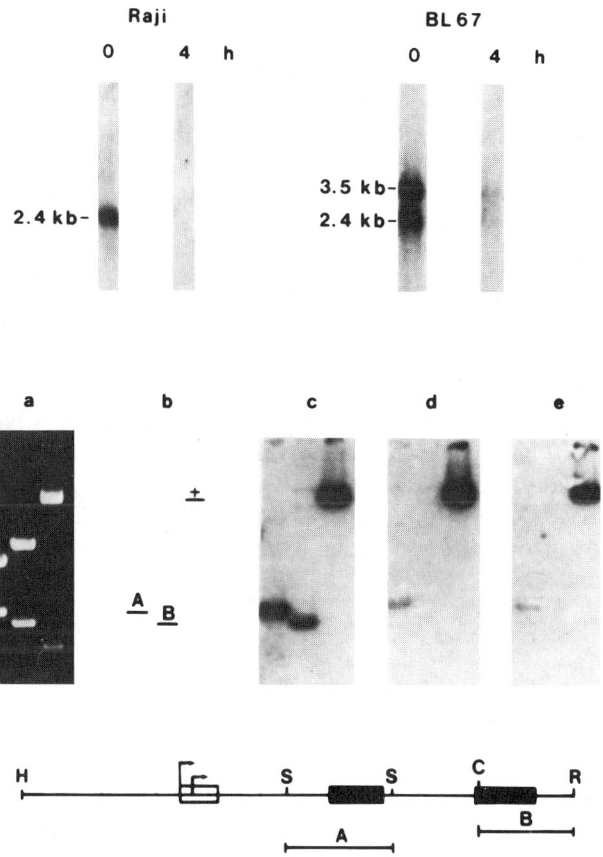

Figure 6 Transcriptional down-regulation of the c-*myc* gene in Burkitt's lymphoma cells by sodium butyrate. The upper part shows Northern blots of c-*myc* RNA in Raji and BL67 cells before and 4 hr after addition of sodium butyrate. The 3.5-kb RNA in BL67 cells is an aberrant c-*myc* RNA transcribed from the immunoglobulin locus across the breakpoint of the translocation into the c-*myc* gene [162]. The lower part demonstrates that the c-*myc* RNA decrease is due to down-regulation at the transcriptional level. ^{32}P-labeled RNA synthesized in isolated BL67 nuclei before (c) and 1 hr (d) and 4 hrs (e) after sodium butyrate treatment was hybridized to small Southern blots containing separated fragments with c-*myc* $exon_2$ (A) and $exon_3$ (B). Transcription of the β-actin gene (+) is unchanged in the presence of sodium butyrate. Bands in the gel (a) without designation in the schematic drawing (b) represent plasmid vector DNA.

Common Features of c-*myc* Deregulation in Burkitt's Lymphoma Cells

We have discussed above various modes of c-*myc* deregulation in Burkitt's lymphoma cells. These various modes reflect on one hand the complex regulation of the c-*myc* gene which may be perturbated at many different levels, and on the other hand the structural diversity of the translocations.

In individual tumors, different modes of c-*myc* deregulation may be realized which reflect particular features of the respective tumors (e.g., stabilization of c-*myc* RNA, juxtaposition of an Ig enhancer, abolished transcription termination). Alternatively, some features of c-*myc* deregulation may be common to all cases of Burkitt's lymphoma, whereas other features, related to particular types of translocations, may be additionally superimposed.

To discuss this second possibility, we classify Burkitt's lymphoma in two groups: one group with the breakpoint within c-*myc* or in its immediate vicinity, and a second, with the breakpoint at a long distance from c-*myc*. These two groups, for which a common mechanism or c-*myc* deregulation is least evident, have nevertheless important features in common:

1. c-*myc* is always located 5′ of an immunoglobulin constant gene.
2. in all cases studied in detail, mutations were found in and around $exon_1$ of the c-*myc* gene.
3. c-*myc* RNA is derived from the allele on the translocation chromosome, whereas the normal allele is silent.

Models of c-*myc* deregulation which may account for both groups of tumors with the breakpoint distant and close to c-*myc*, have to be based either on the juxtaposition of the c-*myc* locus to an immunoglobulin-constant gene (a), or on the mutations in c-*myc* $exon_1$ (b), or on both. Following the autoregulation model, the transcription exclusion of the normal c-*myc* allele may be regarded as a consequence rather than the cause of unregulated c-*myc* expression.

Model 1

As yet unidentified enhancer elements, located within or close to immunoglobulin-constant genes may activate c-*myc* expression over a large distance. Such long-range enhancers should operate only in B cells, and should be dominant over other types of c-*myc* regulation, such as regulation at the level of RNA elongation. Mutations in and around $exon_1$ would be epiphenomena which are not causally related to the development of the tumor. The mutations might therefore not necessarily be present in the tumor cells in vivo.

As a modification of this model, c-*myc* activation might be mediated either directly or indirectly by the known Ig enhancers (the λ light chain enhancer still being to be identified). The Ig enhancer would function in initiation of transcription, but would not be required for maintenance of transcription once the locus is activated. An additional element located in the 3′ part of immunoglobulin genes should be required for maintenance of transcription and should operate over a large distance in a B cell–specific fashion.

Model 2

In the second model, $exon_1$ is the crucial site of c-*myc* regulation. If $exon_1$ and its neighborhood would be mutated, c-*myc* down-regulation by termination of transcription would be abolished, thus making the cell unresponsive to negative signals. According to this model, mutations have necessarily to be present also within the tumor cells in vivo. By exposing c-*myc* to the mechanism which induces somatic mutations, the Ig locus would only have to induce mutations in and around c-*myc* $exon_1$, notably over a considerable distance.

As an implication of this model, it should be possible in rare instances to find typical Burkitt's lymphoma without chromosomal translocations. These cases should have acquired mutations in the first exon of c-*myc* spontaneously. It is unfortunate that of the two cases described by Berger and coworkers, which did not show the typical chromosomal translocations [31], no material is left to test this hypothesis experimentally.

Model 3

Models 1 and 2 may be combined with each other in two different ways, either in an alternative or in an additive fashion. In the alternative model, one of the mechanisms would be dominant, depending on the distance of the Ig locus to c-*myc*. In cases where the breakpoint is close to c-*myc*, the Ig element might override the elongation block in $exon_1$. However, with increasing distance, the importance of regulation at the level of RNA elongation might be dominant. In such an alternative model, mutations in $exon_1$ would be required only if the breakpoint is distant from the c-*myc* gene.

Model 4

In the additive model (models 1 and 2 combined), perturbation of c-*myc* regulation may require the cooperation of both mechanisms, transcriptional activation by an Ig element as well as abrogation of regulation at the level of RNA elongation, whereas neither of both mechanisms would be sufficient to fully deregulate the c-*myc* gene. Transcriptional activation of c-*myc* by an Ig element according to model 1 might be efficiently compensated by blocking RNA elongation unless $exon_1$ is mutated. Likewise, mutations in $exon_1$ without transcriptional activation of c-*myc* by an Ig element might be compensated by other regulatory mechanisms.

PERSPECTIVES

The validity of models is dependent of the possibility to test them experimentally. Therefore, we want to close by discussing the experimental tools which may allow discrimination between the various models. Experimental systems are required for both, transcriptional control elements in the Ig locus as well as for the role of mutations in $exon_1$. Two approaches appear most promising: the technique of somatic cell fusion between Burkitt's lymphoma cells and cells of other origin, which has been already widely used by Croce and coworkers [217]; and, the analysis of c-*myc* regulation by drugs in normal B cells and in Burkitt's lymphoma cells.

The power of the technique of somatic cell fusion for the analysis of c-*myc* regulation in Burkitt's lymphoma cells has already been stressed above. Only in this system, evidence has been provided for the existence of an as yet unidentified element within the Ig locus which drives c-*myc* transcription in Burkitt's lymphoma cells in a cell-specific fashion. With increasing knowledge about the distance of c-*myc* from the translocation breakpoint in various Burkitt's lymphoma lines, it will be interesting to repeat the experiments with selected lines which have the breakpoint at a defined distance far away from c-*myc*. It should thus be possible to test whether c-*myc* expression in Burkitt's lymphoma cells is invariably under the control of the Ig locus regardless of the distance of the breakpoint from c-*myc* (which would rule out model 2). Preliminary evidence for such a role of the Ig locus has come from fusion between P3HR1 cells and mouse fibroblasts [138]. However, in P3HR1 cells nothing is known about the distance of the breakpoint to c-*myc*, so that it is not possible to draw generalizing conclusions.

The system of somatic cell fusion may furthermore be most useful to identify *trans*-acting functions involved in expression or extinction of immunoglobulins and other B cell-specific functions in hybrid cells.

The second experimental system which seems promising to us makes use of drugs to study c-myc regulation.

We have described experiments which demonstrate that even truncated c-*myc* genes respond to transcriptional down-regulation by sodium butyrate. This system may allow us to define a butyrate responsive element in the Ig locus which may eventually be identical with the long-range enhancer of Croce [217].

To evaluate the various models, it will be essential to study not only transcriptional control elements in the Ig locus, but also the role of mutations in and around $exon_1$. It will, first of all, be interesting to see whether the same mutations will also be present in the primary tumor in cases where the primary tumor is still available. Still more important will be the availbility of a functional assay for the role of mutations in c-*myc* $exon_1$.

For this purpose, it may be possible to identify drugs which, similarly to the action of retinoic acid and dimethysulfoxide (DMSO) in HL60 cells, block RNA elongation in normal proliferating B cells. With the aid of such substances it should be possible to see whether mutations in $exon_1$ will prevent transcription termination, thus making transcriptional readthrough constitutive.

With the experimental systems designed here it may be possible to gain deeper insight at a molecular level in the problem of c-*myc* regulation and deregulation.

ACKNOWLEDGMENTS

We are grateful to Gilbert M. Lenoir for helpful discussions, for critically reading the manuscript, and for the permission to reproduce figures. Work from our laboratory described in this chapter was supported by the Deutsche Forschungsgemeinschaft (SFB 31 and Schwerpunktprogramm: Molekulare und klassische Tumorzytogenetik).

REFERENCES

1. Waterfield, M. D., Scrace, G. T., Whittle, N., Stroobant, P., Johnsson, A., Wasteson, A., Westermark, B., Heldin, C. H., Huang, J. S., and Deuel, T. F. (1983). Platelet-derived growth factor is structurally related to the putative transforming protein p28sis of simian sarcoma virus. *Nature 304*: 35–39.
2. Doolittle, R. F., Hunkapiller, M. W., Hood, L. E., Devare, S. G., Robbins, K. C., Aaronson, S. A., and Antoniades, H. N. (1983). Simian sarcoma virus oncogene, v-sis, is derived from the gene (or genes) encoding a platelet-derived growth factor. *Science 221*: 275–277.
3. Downward, J., Yarden, Y., Mayes, E., Scrace, G., Totty, N., Stockwell, P., Ullrich, A., Schlessinger, J., and Waterfield, M. D. (1984). Close similarity of

epidermal growth factor receptor and v-erb B oncogene protein sequences. *Nature 307*: 521–527.

4. Sherr, C. J., Rettenmier, C. W., Sacca, R., Roussel, M. F., Look, A. T., and Stanley, E. R. (1985). The c-fms proto-oncogene product is related to the receptor for the mononuclear phagocyte growth factor, CSF-1. *Cell 41*: 665–676.
5. Burkitt, D. P. (1958). A sarcoma involving the jaws in African children. *Br. J. Surg. 46*: 218–223.
6. Berard, C. W., O'Conor, G. T., Thomas, L. B., and Torloni, H. (1969). Histopathological definition of Burkitt's tumour. *Bull. W. H. O. 40*: 601–607.
7. Rosenberg, S. A. (chairman). (1982). National cancer institute sponsored study of classifications of non-Hodgkin's lymphomas. Summary and description of a working formulation for clinical usage. *Cancer 49*: 2112–2135.
8. Burkitt, D. P. (1962). A children's cancer dependent on climatic factors. *Nature 194*: 232–234.
9. Kafuko, G. W., and Burkitt, D. P. (1970). Burkitt's lymphoma and malaria. *Int. J. Cancer 6*: 1–9.
10. O'Conor, G. T. (1970). Persistent immunologic stimulation as a factor in oncogenesis with special reference to Burkitt's tumour. *Am. J. Med. 48*: 279–285.
11. Morrow, R. H., Jr. (1985). Epidemiological evidence for the role of falciparum malaria in the pathogenesis of Burkitt's lymphoma. In: *Burkitt's lymphoma: A Human Cancer Model.* Lenoir, G. M., O'Conor, G. T., and Olweny, C. L. M. (eds.) IARC Scientific Publication No. 60, Lyon, pp. 177–186.
12. Greenwood, B. M. (1985). The immunology of malaria — A view from the bush. *Parasite Immunol. 7*: 191–199.
13. Henle, W., and Henle, G. (1985). Epstein-Barr virus and human malignancies. *Adv. Viral Oncol. 5*: 201–238.
14. Rooney, C. M., Gregory, C. D., Rowe, M., Finerty, S., Edwards, C., Rupani, H., and Rickinson, A. B. (1986). Endemic Burkitt's lymphoma: Phenotypic analysis of tumor biopsy cells and of derived tumor cell lines. *J. Natl. Cancer Inst. 77*: 681–687.
15. Rowe, M., Rowe, D. T., Gregory, C. D., Young, L. S., Farrell, P. J., Rupani, H., and Rickinson, A. B. (1987). Differences in B cell growth phenotype reflect novel patterns of Epstein-Barr virus latent gene expression in Burkitt's lymphoma cells. *EMBO J. 6*: 2743–2751.
16. Ziegler, J. L., Miner, R. C., Rosenbaum, E., Lennette, E. T., Shillitoe, E., Casavant, C., Drew, W. L., Mintz, L., Gershow, J., Greenspan, J., Beckstead, J., and Yamamoto, K. (1982). Outbreak of Burkitt's lymphoma in homosexual men. *Lancet 2*: 631–633.
17. Kalter, S. P., Riggs, S. A., Cabanillas, F., Butler, J. J., Hagemeister, F. B., Mansell, P. W., Newell, G. R., Velasquez, W. S., Salvador, P., Barlogie, B., Rios, A., and Hersh, E. M. (1985). Aggressive non-Hodgkin's lymphomas in immunocompromised homosexual males. *Blood 66*: 655–659.

18. Lenoir, G. M., and Bornkamm, G. W. (1987). Burkitt's lymphoma, a human cancer model for the study of the multistep development of cancer: Proposal for a new scenario. *Adv. Viral Oncol. 7*: 173–206.
19. Klein, G. (1987). In defense of the "old" Burkitt lymphoma scenario. *Adv. Viral Oncol. 7*: 207–211.
20. Manolov, G., and Manolova, Y. (1972). Marker band in one chromosome 14 from Burkitt lymphomas. *Nature 237*: 33–34.
21. Zech, L., Haglund, U., Nilsson, K., and Klein, G. (1976). Characteristic chromosomal abnormalities in biopsies and lymphoid cell lines from patients with Burkitt and non-Burkitt lymphomas. *Int. J. Cancer 17*: 47–56.
22. Kaiser-McCaw, B., Epstein, A. L., Kaplan, H. S., and Hecht, F. (1977). Chromosome 14 translocation in African and North American Burkitt's lymphoma. *Int. J. Cancer 19*: 482–486.
23. Manolova, Y., Manolov, G., Kieler, J., Levan, A., and Klein, G. (1979). Genesis of the 14q+ marker in Burkitt's lymphoma. *Hereditas 90*: 5–10.
24. Berger, R., Bernheim, A., Flandrin, H. J., Weh, G., Daniel, M. T., Brouet, J. C., and Colbert, N. (1979). A new translocation in Burkitt's tumor cells. *Hum. Genet. 53*: 111–112.
25. van den Berghe, H., Parloir, A., Gosseye, S., Englebienne, V., Cornu, G., and Sokal, G. (1979). Variant translocation in Burkitt lymphoma. *Cancer Genet. Cytogenet. 1*: 9–14.
26. Miyoshi, I., Hiraki, S., Kimura, I., Miyamoto, K., and Sato, J. (1979). 2/8 translocation in a Japanese Burkitt's lymphoma. *Experientia 35*: 742–743.
27. Bornkamm, G. W., Kaduk, B., Kachel, G., Schneider, U., Fresen, K. O., Schwanitz, G., and Hermanek, P. (1980). Epstein-Barr virus positive Burkitt's lymphoma in a German woman during pregnancy. *Blut 40*: 167–177.
28. Bernheim, A., Berger, R., and Lenoir, G. M. (1981). Cytogenetic studies on African Burkitt's lymphoma cell lines t(8;14), t(2;8) and t(8;22) translocations. *Cancer Genet. Cytogenet. 3*: 307–315.
29. Lenoir, G. M., Vuillaume, M., and Bonnardel, C. (1985). The use of lymphomatous and lymphoblastoid cell lines in the study of Burkitt's lymphoma. In *Burkitt's Lymphoma: A Human Cancer Model* (Lenoir, G. M., O'Conor, G. T., and Olweny, C. L. M. eds.) IARC Scientific Publication No. 60, Lyon, pp. 309–318.
30. Klein, G., Lindahl, T., Jondal, M., Leibold, W., Menezes, J., Nilsson, K., Sundstroem, C. (1974). Continuous lymphoid cell lines with characteristics of B cells (bone-marrow-derived), lacking the Epstein-Barr virus genome and derived from three human lymphomas. *Proc. Natl. Acad. Sci. U.S.A. 71*: 3283–3286.
31. Berger, R., Bernheim, A., Sigaux, F., Valensi, F., Daniel, M.-T., and Flandrin, G. (1985). Two Burkitt's lymphoma with chromosome 6 long arm deletions. *Cancer Genet. Cytogenet. 15*: 159–167.
32. Mitelman, F. (1981). Marker chromosome 14q+ in human cancer and leukemia. *Adv. Cancer Res. 34*: 141–170.
33. Sigaux, F., Berger, R., Bernheim, A., Valensi, F., Daniel, M. T., and Flandrin, G. (1984). Malignant lymphomas with band 8q24 chromosome

abnormality: A morphologic continuum extending from Burkitt's to immunoblastic lymphoma. *Br. J. Haematol. 57*: 393–405.

34. Shade, M., Woodward, M. A., and Steel, C. M. (1980). Chromosome aberrations acquired in vitro by human B-cell lines II: Distribution of breakpoints, *J. Natl. Cancer Inst. 65*: 101–109.
35. Steel, C. M., Morton, J. E. N., and Foster, E. (1985). The cytogenetics of human B lymphoid malignancy: Studies in Burkitt's lymphoma and Epstein-Barr virus-transformed lymphoblastoid cell lines. In *Burkitt's Lymphoma: A Human Cancer Model* (Lenoir, G. M., O'Conor, G. T., and Olweny, C. L. M. eds.) IARC Scientific Publication No. 60, Lyon, pp. 265–292.
36. Fialkow, P. J., Jacobson, R. J., and Papayannopoulou, T. (1977). Chronic myelocytic leukemia: Clonal origin in a stem cell common to the granulocyte, erythrocyte, platelet and monocyte/macrophage. *Am. J. Med. 63*: 125–130.
37. Kirsch, I. R., Ravetch, J. V., Kwan, S.-P., Max, E. E., Ney, R. L., and Leder, P. (1981). Multiple immunoglobulin switch region homologies outside the heavy chain constant region locus. *Nature 293*: 585–587.
38. Klein, G. (1981). The role of gene dosage and genetic transposition in carcinogenesis. *Nature 294*: 313–318.
39. Klein, G. (1983). Specific chromosomal translocations and the genesis of B-cell-derived tumors in mice and men. *Cell 32*: 311–315.
40. Neel, B. G., Jhanwar, S. C., Chaganti, R. S. K., and Hayward, W. S. (1982). Two human c-onc genes are located on the long arm of chromosome 8. *Proc. Natl. Acad. Sci. U.S.A. 79*: 7842–7846.
41. Taub, R., Kirsch, I., Morton, C., Lenoir, G. M., Swan, D., Tronick, S., Aaronson, S., and Leder, P. (1982). Translocation of the c-*myc* gene into the immunoglobulin heavy chain locus in human Burkitt lymphoma and mouse plasmacytoma cells. *Proc. Natl. Acad. Sci. U.S.A. 79*: 7837–7841.
42. Dalla-Favera, R., Bregni, M., Erikson, J., Patterson, D., Gallo, R. C., and Croce, C. M. (1982). Human c-*myc* onc gene is located on the region of chromosome 8 that is translocated in Burkitt lymphoma cells. *Proc. Natl. Acad. Sci. U.S.A. 79*: 7824–7827.
43. Hayward, W. S., Neel, B. G., and Astrin, S. M. (1981). Activation of a cellular onc gene by promoter insertion in ALV-induced lymphoid leukosis. *Nature 290*: 475–480.
44. Shen-Ong, G. L. C., Keath, E. J., Piccoli, S. P., and Cole, M. D. (1982). Novel *myc* oncogene RNA from abortive immunoglobulin gene recombination in mouse plasmacytomas. *Cell 31*: 443–452.
45. Bister, K., and Jansen, H. W. (1986). Oncogenes in retroviruses and cells. Biochemistry and molecular genetics. *Adv. Cancer Res. 47*: 99–188.
46. Colby, W. W., Chen, E. Y., Smith, D. H., and Levinson, A. D. (1983). Identification and nucleotide sequence of a human locus homologous to the v-*myc* oncogene of avian myelocytomatosis virus MC29. *Nature 301*: 722–725.
47. Bernard, O., Cory, S., Gerondakis, S., Webb, E., and Adams, J. M. (1983). Sequence of the murine and human cellular *myc* oncogenes and two modes of

myc transcription resulting from chromosome translocation in B lymphoid tumors. *EMBO J. 2*: 2375–2383.

48. Watson, D. K., Psallidopoulos, C., Samuel, K. P., Dalla-Favera, R., and Papas, T. S. (1983). Nucleotide sequence analysis of human c-*myc* locus, chicken homologue, and myelocytomatosis virus MC29 transforming gene reveals a highly conserved gene product. *Proc. Natl. Acad. Sci. U.S.A. 80*: 3642–3645.
49. Linial, M., and Groudine, M. (1985). Transcription of three c-*myc* exons is enhanced in chicken bursal lymphoma cell lines. *Proc. Natl. Acad. Sci. U.S.A. 82*: 53–57.
50. Leder, P., Battey, J., Lenoir, G., Moulding, C., Murphy, W., Potter, H., Stewart, T., and Taub, R. (1983). Translocations among antibody genes in human cancer. *Science 222*: 765–770.
51. Cory, S. (1986). Activation of cellular oncogenes in hemopoietic cells by chromosome translocation. *Adv. Cancer Res. 47*: 189–234.
52. Dani, C., Blanchard, J. M., Piechaczyk, M., El Sabouty, S., Marty, L., and Jeanteur, P. (1984). Extreme instability of c-*myc* mRNA in normal and transformed cells. *Proc. Natl. Acad. Sci. U.S.A. 81*: 7046–7050.
53. Shaw, G., and Kamen, R. (1986). A conserved AU sequence from the 3′ untranslated region of GM-CSF mRNA mediates selective mRNA degradation. *Cell 46*: 659–667.
54. Saito, H., Hayday, A. C., Wiman, K., Hayward, W. S., and Tonegawa, S. (1983). Activation of the c-*myc* gene by translocation: A model for translational control. *Proc. Natl. Acad. Sci. U.S.A. 80*: 7476–7480.
55. Bentley, D. L., and Groudine, M. (1986). Novel promoter upstream of the human c-*myc* gene and regulation of c-*myc* expression in B-cell lymphomas. *Mol. Cell. Biol. 6*: 3481–3489.
56. Gazin, C., Dupont de Dinechin, S., Hampe, A., Masson, J. M., Martin, P., Stehelin, D., and Galibert, F. (1984). Nucleotide sequence of the human c-*myc* locus: Provocative open reading frame within the first exon. *EMBO J. 3*: 383–387.
57. Bentley, D. L., and Groudine, M. (1986). A block to elongation is largely responsible for decreased transcription of c-*myc* in differentiated HL60 cells. *Nature 321*: 702–706.
58. Nepveu, A., and Marcu, K. B. (1986). Intragenic pausing and anti-sense transcription within the murine c-*myc* locus. *EMBO J. 5*: 2859–2865.
59. Siebenlist, U., Hennighausen, L., Battey, J., and Leder, P. (1984). Chromatin structure and protein binding in the putative regulatory region of the c-*myc* gene in Burkitt's lymphoma. *Cell 37*: 381–391.
60. Dyson, P. J., Littlewood, T. D., Forster, A., and Rabbitts, T. H. (1985). Chromatin structure of transcriptionally active and inactive human c-*myc* alleles. *EMBO J. 4*: 2885–2891.
61. Fahrlander, P. D., Piechaczyk, M., and Marcu, K. B. (1985). Chromatin structure of the murine c-*myc* locus: Implications for the regulation of normal and chromosomally translocated genes. *EMBO J. 4*: 3195–3202.

62. Corcoran, L. M., Cory, S., and Adams, J. M. (1985). Transposition of the immunoglobulin heavy chain enhancer to the *myc* oncogene in a murine plasmacytoma. *Cell 40*: 71–79.
63. Chung, J., Sinn, E., Reed, R. R., and Leder, P. (1986). Trans-acting elements modulate expression of the human c-*myc* gene in Burkitt lymphoma cells. *Proc. Natl. Acad. Sci. U.S.A. 83*: 7918–7922.
64. Remmers, E. F., Yang, J. Q., and Marcu, K. B. (1986). A negative transcriptional control element located upstream of the murine c-*myc* gene. *EMBO J. 5*: 899–904.
65. Yang, J. Q., Remmers, E. F., and Marcu, K. B. (1986). The first exon of c-*myc* proto-oncogene contains a novel positive control element. *EMBO J. 5*: 3553–3562.
66. Lipp, M., Schilling, R., Wiest, S., Laux, G., and Bornkamm, G. W. (1987). Target sequences for cis-acting regulation within the dual promoter of the human c-*myc* gene. *Mol. Cell. Biol. 7*: 1393–1400.
67. Eick, D., Berger, R., Polack, A., and Bornkamm, G. W. (1987). Transcription of c-*myc* in human mononuclear cells is regulated by an elongation block. *Oncogene 2*: 61–65.
68. Hann, S. R., and Eisenman, R. N. (1984). Proteins encoded by the human c-*myc* oncogene: Differential expression in neoplastic cells. *Mol. Cell. Biol. 4*: 2486–2497.
69. Persson, H., Hennighausen, L., Taub, R., DeGrado, W., and Leder, P. (1984). Antibodies to human c-*myc* oncogene product: Evidence of an evolutionarily conserved protein induced during cell proliferation. *Science 225*: 687–693.
70. Ramsay, G., Evan, G. I., and Bishop, J. M. (1984). The protein encoded by the human proto-oncogene c-*myc*. *Proc. Natl. Acad. Sci. U.S.A. 81*: 7742–7746.
71. Persson, H., and Leder, P. (1984). Nuclear localization and DNA binding properties of a protein expressed by human c-*myc* oncogene. *Science 225*: 718–721.
72. Evan, G. I., and Hancock, D. C. (1985). Studies on the interaction of the human c-*myc* protein with cell nuclei: p62 c-*myc* as a member of a discrete subset of nuclear proteins. *Cell 43*: 253–261.
73. Eisenman, R. N., Tachibana, C. Y., Abrams, H. D., and Hann, S. R. (1985). v-*myc*- and c-*myc*-encoded proteins are associated with the nuclear matrix. *Mol. Cell. Biol. 5*: 114–126.
74. Watt, R. A., Shatzman, A. R., and Rosenberg, M. (1985). Expression and characterization of the human c-*myc* DNA-binding protein. *Mol. Cell. Biol. 5*: 448–456.
75. Miyamoto, C., Chizzonite, R., Crowl, R., Rupprecht, K., Kramer, R., Schaber, M., Kumar, G., Poonian, M., and Ju., J. (1985). Molecular cloning and regulated expression of the human c-*myc* gene in Escherichia coli and Saccharomyces cerevisiae: Comparison of the protein products. *Proc. Natl. Acad. Sci. U.S.A. 82*: 7232–7236.

76. Rabbitts, P. H., Watson, J. V., Lamond, A., Forster, A., Stinson, M. A., Evan, G., Fischer, W., Atherton, E., Sheppard, R., and Rabbitts, T. H. (1985). Metabolism of c-*myc* gene products: c-*myc* mRNA and protein expression in the cell cycle. *EMBO J. 4*: 2009–2015.
77. Persson, H., Gray, H. E., Godeau, F., Braunhut, S., and Bellve, A. R. (1986). Multiple growth-associated nuclear proteins immunoprecipitated by antisera raised against human c-*myc* peptide antigens. *Mol. Cell. Biol. 6*: 942–949.
78. Spector, D. L., Watt, R. A., and Sullivan, N. F. (1987). The v- and c-*myc* oncogene proteins colocalize in situ with small nuclear ribonucleoprotein particles. *Oncogene 1*: 5–12.
79. Studzinski, G. P., Brelvi, Z. S., Feldman, S. C., and Watt, R. A. (1986). Participation of c-*myc* protein in DNA synthesis of human cells. *Science 234*: 467–470.
80. Iguchi-Ariga, S. M. M., Itani, T., Yamaguchi, M., and Ariga, H. (1987). c-*myc* protein can be substituted for SV40 T antigen in SV40 DNA replication. *Nucleic Acids Res. 15*: 4889–4899.
81. Iguchi-Ariga, S. M. M., Itani, T., Kiji, Y., and Ariga, H. (1987). Possible function of the c-*myc* product: Promotion of cellular DNA replication. *EMBO J. 6*: 2365–2371.
82. Gonda, T., Sheiness, D., and Bishop, J. M. (1982). Transcripts of the cellular homologs of retroviral oncogenes: Distribution among chicken tissues. *Mol. Cell. Biol. 2*: 617–624.
83. Pfeifer-Ohlsson, S., Rydnert, J., Goustin, A. S., Larsson, E., Betsholtz, C., and Ohlsson, R. (1985). Cell-type-specific pattern of *myc* protooncogene expression in developing human embryo. *Proc. Natl. Acad. Sci. U.S.A. 82*: 5050–5054.
84. Kelly, K., Cochran, B. H., Stiles, C. D., and Leder, P. (1983). Cell-specific regulation of the c-*myc* gene by lymphocyte mitogens and platelet-derived growth factor. *Cell 35*: 603–610.
85. Makino, R., Hayashi, K., and Sugimura, T. (1984). c-*myc* transcript is induced in rat liver at a very early stage of regeneration or by cycloheximide treatment. *Nature 310*: 697–698.
86. Goyette, M., Petropoulos, C. J., Shank, P. R., and Fausto, N. (1984). Regulated transcription of c-Ki-ras and c-*myc* during compensatory growth of rat liver. *Mol. Cell. Biol. 4*: 1493–1498.
87. Mueller, R., Bravo, R., Burckhardt, J., and Curran, T. (1985). Induction of c-*fos* gene and protein by growth factors precedes activation of c-*myc*. *Nature 312*: 716–720.
88. Hesketh, T. R., Moore, J. P., Morris, J. D. H., Taylor, M. V., Rogers, J., Smith, G. A., and Metcalfe, J. C. (1985). A common sequence of calcium and pH signals in the mitogenic stimulation of eukaryotic cells. *Nature 313*: 481–484.

89. Reed, J. C., Nowell, P. C., and Hoover, R. G. (1985). Regulation of c-*myc* mRNA levels in normal human lymphocytes by modulators of cell proliferation. *Proc. Natl. Acad. Sci. U.S.A. 82*: 4221–4224.
90. Smeland, E., Godal, T., Ruud, E., Beiske, K., Funderud, S., Clark, E. A., Pfeifer-Ohlsson, S., and Ohlsson, R. (1985). The specific induction of *myc* protooncogene expression in normal human B cells is not a sufficient event for acquisition of competence to proliferate. *Proc. Natl. Acad. Sci. U.S.A. 82*: 6255–6259.
91. Stiles, C. D., Capone, G. T., Scher, C. D., Antoniades, H. N., van Wyk, J. J., and Pledger, W. J. (1979). Dual control of cell growth by somatomedins and platelet-derived growth factor. *Proc. Natl. Acad. Sci. U.S.A. 76*: 1279–1283.
92. Armelin, H. A., Armelin, M. C. S., Kelly, K., Stewart, T., Leder, P., Cochran, B. H., and Stiles, C. D. (1984). Functional role for c-*myc* in mitogenic response to platelet derived growth factor. *Nature 310*: 655–660.
93. Kaczmarek, L., Hyland, J. K., Watt, R., Rosenberg, M., and Baserga, R. (1985). Microinjected c-*myc* as a competence factor. *Science 228*: 1313–1315.
94. Reed, J. C., Sabath, D. E., Hoover, R. G., and Prystowsky, M. B. (1985). Recombinant interleukin 2 regulates levels of c-*myc* mRNA in a cloned murine T lymphocyte. *Mol. Cell. Biol. 5*: 3361–3368.
95. Cleveland, J. L., Rapp, U. R., and Farrar, W. L. (1987). Role of c-*myc* and other genes in interleukin 2 regulated CT6 T lymphocytes and their malignant variants. *J. Immunol. 138*: 3495–3504.
96. Stern, D. F., Roberts, A. B., Roche, N. S., Sporn, M. B., and Weinberg, R. A. (1986). Differential responsiveness of *myc*- and *ras*-transfected cells to growth factors: Selective stimulation of *myc*-transfected cells by epidermal growth factor. *Mol. Cell. Biol. 6*: 870–877.
97. Kingston, R. E., Jr., Baldwin, A. S., and Sharp, P. A. (1984). Regulation of heat shock protein 70 gene expression by c-*myc*. *Nature 312*: 280–282.
98. Mougneau, E., Lemieux, L., Rassoulzadegan, M., and Cuzin, F. (1984). Biological activities of v-*myc* and rearranged c-*myc* oncogenes in rat fibroblast cells in culture. *Proc. Natl. Acad. Sci. U.S.A. 81*: 5758–5762.
99. Keath, E. J., Caimi, P. G., and Cole, M. D. (1984). Fibroblast lines expressing activated c-*myc* oncogenes are tumorigenic in nude mice and syngeneic animals. *Cell 39*: 339–348.
100. Balk, S. D., Riley, T. M., Gunther, H. S., and Morisi, A. (1985). Heparin-treated, v-*myc* transformed chicken heart mesenchymal cells assume a normal morphology but are hypersensitive to epidermal growth factor (EGF) and brain fibroblast growth factor (bFGF); cells transformed by the v-Ha-*ras* oncogene are refractory to EGF and bFGF but are hypersensitive to insulin-like growth factors. *Proc. Natl. Acad. Sci. U.S.A. 82*: 5781–5785.
101. Sorrentino, V., Drozdoff, V., McKinney, M. D., Zeitz, L., and Fleissner, E. (1986). Potentiation of growth factor activity by exogenous c-*myc* expression. *Proc. Natl. Acad. Sci. U.S.A. 83*: 8167–8171.

102. Cory, S., Bernard, O., Bowtell, D., Schrader, S., and Schrader, J. (1987). Murine c-*myc* retroviruses alter the growth requirements of myeloid cells. *Oncogene Res. 1*: 61–76.
103. Vennstroem, B., Kahn, P., Adkins, B., Enrietto, P., Hayman, M. J., Graf, T., and Luciw, P. (1984). Transformation of mammalian fibroblasts and macrophages in vitro by a murine retrovirus encoding an avian v-*myc* oncogene. *EMBO J. 3*: 3223–3229.
104. Graf, T., von Weizsaecker, F., Grieser, S., Coll, J., Stehelin, D., Patschinsky, T., Bister, K., Bechade, C., Calothy, G., and Leutz, A. (1986). v-mil induces autocrine growth and enhanced tumorigenicity in v-*myc*-transformed avian macrophages. *Cell 45*: 357–364.
105. Namba, Y., and Hanaoka, M. (1972). Immunocytology of cultured IgM-forming cells of mouse. I. Requirement of phagocytic cell factor for the growth of IgM-forming tumor cells in tissue culture. *J. Immunol. 109*: 1193–1200.
106. Metcalf, D. (1974). The serum factor stimulating colony formation in vitro by murine plasmacytoma cells: Response to antigens and mineral oil. *J. Immunol. 113*: 235–243.
107. Nordan, R. P., and Potter, M. (1986). A macrophage-derived factor required by plasmacytomas for survival and proliferation in vitro. *Science 233*: 566–569.
108. Rapp, U. R., Cleveland, J. L., Brightman, K., Scott, A., and Ihle, J. N. (1985). Abrogation of IL-3 and IL-2 dependence by recombinant murine retroviruses expressing v-*myc* oncogenes. *Nature 317*: 434–438.
109. Potter, M., Wax, J. S., Anderson, A. O., and Nordan, R. P. (1985). Inhibition of plasmacytoma development in BALB/c mice by indomethacin. *J. Exp. Med. 161*: 996–1012.
110. Potter, M. (1987). Plasmacytoma development in BALB/c mice. *Adv. Viral Oncol. 7*: 99–122.
111. Campisi, J., Gray, H. E., Pardee, A. B., Dean, M., and Sonenshein, G. E. (1984). Cell-cycle control of c-*myc* but not c-ras expression is lost following chemical transformation. *Cell 36*: 241–247.
112. Thompson, C. B., Challoner, P. B., Neiman, P. E., and Groudine, M. (1985). Levels of c-*myc* oncogene mRNA are invariant through the cell cycle. *Nature 314*: 363–366.
113. Hann, S. R., Thompson, C. B., and Eisenman, R. N. (1985). c-*myc* oncogene protein synthesis is independent of the cell cycle in human and avian cells. *Nature 314*: 366–369.
114. Zetterberg, A., and Larsson, O. (1985). Kinetic analysis of regulatory events in G1 leading to proliferation or quiescence of Swiss 3T3 cells. *Proc. Natl. Acad. Sci. U.S.A. 82*: 5365–5369.
115. Langdon, W. Y., Harris, A. W., Cory, S., and Adams, J. M. (1986). The c-*myc* oncogene perturbs B lymphocyte development in E-mu-*myc* transgenic mice. *Cell 47*: 11–18.

116. Westin, E. H., Wong-Staal, F., Gelman, E. P., Dalla-Favera, R., Papas, T. S., Lautenberger, J. A., Eva, A., Reddy, E. P., Tronick, S. R., Aaronson, S. A., and Gallo, R. C. (1982). Expression of cellular homologues of retroviral onc genes in human hematopoietic cells. *Proc. Natl. Acad. Sci. U.S.A. 79*: 2490–2494.

117. Reitsma, P. H., Rothberg, P. G., Astrin, S. M., Trial, J., Bar-Shavit, Z., Hall, A., Teitelbaum, S. L., and Kahn, A. J. (1983). Regulation of *myc* gene expression in HL60 leukemia cells by a vitamin D metabolite. *Nature 306*: 492–494.

118. Lachman, H. M., and Skoultchi, A. I. (1984). Expression of c-*myc* changes during differentiation of mouse erythroleukaemia cells. *Nature 310*: 592–594.

119. Coppola, J. A., and Cole, M. D. (1986). Constitutive c-*myc* oncogene expression blocks mouse erythroleukaemia cell differentiation but not commitment. *Nature 320*: 760–763.

120. Dmitrovsky, E., Kuehl, W. M., Hollis, G. F., Kirsch, I. R., Bender, T. P., and Segal, S. (1986). Expression of a transfected human c-*myc* oncogene inhibits differentiation of a mouse erythroleukaemia cell line. *Nature 322*: 748–750.

121. Prochownik, E. V., and Kukowska, J. (1986). Deregulated expression of c-*myc* by murine erythroleukaemia cells prevents differentiation. *Nature 322*: 848–850.

122. Graf, T., and Beug, H. (1978). Avian leukemia viruses interaction with their target cells in vivo and in vitro. *Biochim. Biophys. Acta Rev. Cancer 516*: 269–299.

123. Blanchard, J. M., Piechaczyk, M., Dani, C., Chambard, J. C., Franchi, A., Pouyssegur, J., and Jeanteur, P. (1985). c-*myc* is transcribed at high rate in G_0-arrested fibroblasts and is post-transcriptionally regulated in response to growth factors. *Nature 317*: 443–445.

124. Dony, C., Kessel, M., and Gruss, P. (1985). Post-transcriptional control of *myc* and p53 expression during differentiation of the embryonal carcinoma cell line F9. *Nature 317*: 636–639.

125. Mechti, N., Piechaczyk, M., Blanchard, J. M., Marty, L., Bonnieu, A., Jeanteur, P., and Lebleu, B. (1986). Transcriptional and post-transcriptional regulation of c-*myc* expression during the differentiation of murine erythroleukemia Friend cells. *Nucleic Acids Res. 14*: 9653–9666.

126. Dani, C., Mechti, N., Piechaczyk, M., Lebleu, B., Jeanteur, P., and Blanchard, J. M. (1985). Increased rate of degradation of c-*myc* mRNA in interferon-treated Daudi cells. *Proc. Natl. Acad. Sci. U.S.A. 82*: 4896–4899.

127. Knight, E., Anton, E. D., Fahey, D., Friedland, B. K., and Jonak, G. J. (1985). Interferon regulates c-*myc* gene expression in Daudi cells at the post-transcriptional level. *Proc. Natl. Acad. Sci. U.S.A. 82*: 1151–1154.

128. Grosso, L. E., and Pitot, H. C. (1985). Transcriptional regulation of c-*myc* during chemically induced differentiation of HL-60 cultures. *Cancer Res. 45*: 847–850.

Translocation of c-*myc* into the immunoglobulin heavy-chain locus in human acute B-cell leukemia. A molecular analysis. *EMBO J. 5*: 905–911.

159. Hayday, A. C., Gillies, S. D., Saito, H., Wood, C., Wiman, K., Hayward, W. S., and Tonegawa, S. (1984). Activation of a translocated human c-*myc* gene by an enhancer in the immunoglobulin heavy-chain locus. *Nature 307*: 334–340.
160. Dean, M., Kent, R. B., and Sonenshein, G. E. (1983). Transcriptional activation of immunoglobulin alpha heavy-chain genes by translocation of the c-*myc* oncogene. *Nature 305*: 443–446.
161. Calabi, F., and Neuberger, M. S. (1985). Chromosome translocation activates heterogeneously initiated, bipolar transcription of a mouse c-*myc* gene. *EMBO J. 4*: 667–674.
162. Eick, D., Piechaczyk, M., Henglein, B., Blanchard, J. M., Traub, B., Kofler, E., Wiest, S., Lenoir, G. M., and Bornkamm, G. W. (1985). Aberrant c-*myc* RNAs of Burkitt's lymphoma cells have longer half-lives. *EMBO J. 4*: 3717–3725.
163. Ar-Rushdi, A., Nishikura, K., Erikson, J., Watt, R., Rovera, G. and Croce, C. M. (1983). Differential expression of the translocated and the untranslocated c-*myc* oncogene in Burkitt lymphoma. *Science 222*: 390–393.
164. Piechaczyk, M., Yang, J.-Q., Blanchard, J.-M., Jeanteur, P., and Marcu, K. B. (1985). Posttranscriptional mechanisms are responsible for accumulation of truncated c-*myc* RNAs in murine plasma cell tumors. *Cell 42*: 589–597.
165. Rabbitts, P. H., Forster, A., Stinson, M. A., and Rabbitts, T. H. (1985). Truncation of exon 1 from the c-*myc* gene results in prolonged c-*myc* RNA stability. *EMBO J. 4*: 3727–3733.
166. Piechaczyk, M., Bonnieu, A., Eick, D., Remmers, E., Yang, J.-Q., Marcu, K., Jeanteur, P., and Blanchard, J. M. (1986). Altered c-*myc* RNA metabolism in Burkitt's lymphomas and mouse plasmacytomas. *Curr. Top. Microbiol. Immunol. 132*: 331–338.
167. Lenoir, G. M., Preud'homme, J. L., Bernheim, A., and Berger, R. (1982). Correlation between immunoglobulin light chain expression and variant translocation in Burkitt's lymphoma. *Nature 298*: 474–476.
168. Magrath, J., Erikson, J., Whang-Peng, J., Sieverts, H., Armstrong, G., Benjamin, D., Triche, T., Alabaster, O., and Croce, C. M. (1983). Synthesis of kappa light chains by cell lines containing an 8;22 chromosomal translocation derived from a male homosexual with Burkitt's lymphoma. *Science 222*: 1094–1098.
169. Hollis, G. F., Mitchell, K. F., Battey, J., Potter, H., Taub, R., Lenoir, G. M., and Leder, P. (1984). A variant translocation places the gamma immunoglobulin genes 3′ to the c-*myc* oncogene in Burkitt's lymphoma. *Nature 307*: 752–755.
170. Denny, C. T., Magrath, G. F., Hollis, I. T., and Kirsch, I. R. (1985). Burkitt lymphoma cell line carrying a variant translocation creates new DNA at the breakpoint and violates the hierachy of immunoglobulin gene rearrangement. *Mol. Cell. Biol. 5*: 3199–3207.

171. Hartl, P., and Lipp, M. (1987). Generation of a variant t(2;8) translocation of Burkitt's lymphoma by site-specific recombination via the kappa light-chain joining signals. *Mol. Cell. Biol. 7*: 2037–2045.
172. Klobeck, G., Combriato, G., and Zachau, H. G. (1987). N segment insertion and region-directed somatic hypermutation in a kappa gene of a t(2;8) chromosomal translocation. *Nucleic Acids Res. 15*: 4877–4888.
173. Sun, L. K., Showe, L. C., and Croce, C. M. (1986). Analysis of the 3′ flanking region of the human c-*myc* gene in lymphomas with the t(8;22) and t(2;8) chromosomal translocations. *Nucleic Acids Res. 14*: 4037–4050.
174. Taub, R., Kelly, K., Battey, J., Latt, S., Lenoir, G. M., Tantravahi, U., Tu, Z., and Leder, P. (1984). A novel alteration in the structure of an activated c-*myc* gene in a variant t(2;8) Burkitt lymphoma. *Cell 37*: 511–520.
175. Graham, M., and Adams, J. M. (1986). Chromosome 8 breakpoint far 3′ of the c-*myc* oncogene in a Burkitt's lymphoma 2;8 variant translocation is equilvalent to the murine *pvt*-1 locus. *EMBO J. 5*: 2845–2851.
176. Cory, S., Graham, M., Webb, E., Corcoran, L., and Adams, J. M. (1985). Variant (6;15) translocations in murine plasmacytomas involve a chromosome 15 locus at least 72 kb from the c-*myc* oncogene. *EMBO J. 4*: 675–681.
177. Graham, M., Adams, J. M., and Cory, S. (1985). Murine T lymphomas with retroviral inserts in the chromosomal 15 locus for plasmacytoma variant translocations. *Nature 314*: 740–743.
178. Villeneuve, L., Rassart, E., Jolicoeur, P., Graham, M., and Adams, J. M. (1986). Proviral integration site Mis-1 in rat thymomas correspond to the *pvt*-1 translocation breakpoint in murine plasmacytomas. *Mol. Cell. Biol. 6*: 1834–1837.
179. Mengle-Gaw, L., and Rabbitts, T. H. (1987). A human chromosome 8 region with abnormalities in B cell, HTLV-I+ T cell and c-*myc* amplified tumours. *EMBO J. 6*: 1959–1965.
180. Manolov, G., Manolova, Y., Klein, G., Lenoir, G. M., and Levan, A. (1986). Alternative involvement of two cytogenetically distinguishable breakpoints on chromosome 8 in Burkitt's lymphoma associated translocations. *Cancer Genet. Cytogenet. 20*: 95–99.
181. Lenoir, G. M., Lipp, M., Bechet, J. M., Hartl, P., Bornkamm, G. W., Philip, T., Lavoue, M. F., and Ladgag, J. (1987). Constitutional c-*myc* duplication in two cancer patients and their families (submitted for publication).
182. Rabbitts, T. H., Hamlyn, P. H., and Baer, R. (1983). Altered nucleotide sequences of a translocated c-*myc* gene in Burkitt lymphoma. *Nature 306*: 760–765.
183. Rabbitts, T. H., Forster, A., Hamlyn, P. H., and Baer, R. (1984). Effect of somatic mutation within translocated c-*myc* gene in Burkitt's lymphoma. *Nature 309*: 592–597.
184. Murphy, W., Sarid, J., Taub, R., Vasicek, T., Battey, J., Lenoir, G. M., and Leder, P. (1986). A translocated human c-*myc* oncogene is altered in a conserved coding sequence. *Proc. Natl. Acad. Sci. U.S.A. 83*: 2939–2943.

185. Battey, J., Moulding, C., Taub, R., Murphy, W., Stewart, T., Potter, H., Lenoir, G. M., and Leder, P. (1983). The human c-*myc* oncogene: Structural consequences of translocation into the IgH locus in Burkitt lymphoma. *Cell 34*: 779–787.
186. Wiman, K. G., Clarkson, B., Hayday, A. C., Saito, H., Tonegawa, S., and Hayward, W. S. (1984). Activation of a translocated c-*myc* gene: Role of structural alterations in the upstream region. *Proc. Natl. Acad. Sci. U.S.A. 81*: 6798–6802.
187. Taub, R., Moulding, C., Battey, J., Murphy, W., Vasicek, T., Lenoir, G. M., and Leder, P. (1984). Activation and somatic mutation of the translocated c-*myc* gene in Burkitt lymphoma cells. *Cell 36*: 339–348.
188. Pelicci, P. G., Knowles, D. M., Magrath, I., and Dalla-Favera, R. (1986). Chromosomal breakpoints and structural alterations of the c-*myc* locus differ in endemic and sporadic forms of Burkitt lymphoma. *Proc. Natl. Acad. Sci. U.S.A. 83*: 2984–2988.
189. Showe, L. C., Moore, R. C. A., Erikson, J., and Croce, C. M. (1987). MYC oncogene involved in a t(8;22) chromosome translocation is not altered in its putative regulatory regions. *Proc. Natl. Acad. Sci. U.S.A. 84*: 2824–2828.
190. Szajnert, M. F., Saule, S., Bornkamm, G. W., Wajcman, H., Lenoir, G. M., and Kaplan, J.-C. (1987). Clustered somatic mutations in and around first exon of non-rearranged c-*myc* in Burkitt lymphoma with t(8;22) translocation. *Nucleic Acids Res. 15*: 4553–4565.
191. Otsu, M., Katamine, S., Uno, M., Yamaki, M., Ono, Y., Klein, G., Sasaki, M. S., Yaoita, Y., and Honjo, T. (1987). Molecular characterization of novel reciprocal translocation t(6;14) in an Epstein-Barr virus-transformed B cell precursor. *Mol. Cell. Biol. 7*: 708–717.
192. Stewart, T. A., Pattengale, P. K., and Leder, P. (1984). Spontaneous mammary adenocarcinomas in transgenic mice that carry and express MTV/*myc* fusion genes. *Cell 38*: 627–637.
193. Adams, J. M., Harris, A. W., Pinkert, C. A., Corcoran, L. M., Alexander, W. S., Cory, S., Palmiter, R. D., and Brinster, R. L. (1985). The c-*myc* oncogene driven by immunoglobulin enhancers induces lymphoid malignancy in transgenic mice. *Nature 318*: 533–538.
194. Leder, A., Pattengale, P. K., Kuo, A., Stewart, T. A., and Leder, P. (1986). Consequences of widespread deregulation of the c-*myc* gene in transgenic mice: Multiple neoplasms and normal development. *Cell 45*: 485–495.
195. Potter, M., Mushinski, J. F., Mushinski, E. B., Brust, S., Wax, J. S., Wiener, F., Babonits, M., Rapp, U. R., and Morse, H. C. (1987). Avian v-*myc* replaces chromosomal translocation in murine plasmacytomagenesis. *Science 235*: 787–789.
196. Lee, W., Schwab, M., Westaway, D., and Varmus, H. E. (1985). Augmented expression of normal c-*myc* is sufficient for cotransformation of rat embryo cells with a mutant ras gene. *Mol. Cell. Biol. 5*: 3345–3356.

197. Baumbach, W. R., Keath, E. J., and Cole, M. D. (1986). A mouse c-*myc* retrovirus transforms established fibroblast lines in vitro and induces monocyte-macrophage tumors in vivo. *J. Virol. 59*: 276–283.
198. Martin, P., Henry, C., Ferre, F., Duterque-Coquillaud, M., Lagrou, C., Ghysdael, J., Debuire, B., and Stehelin, D. (1986). Transformation of quail embryo fibroblasts by a retrovirus carrying a normal human c-*myc* gene. *EMBO J. 5*: 1529–1533.
199. Erikson, J., ar-Rushdi, A., Drwinga, H. L., Nowell, P. C., and Croce, C. M. (1983). Transcriptional activation of the translocated c-*myc* oncogene in Burkitt lymphoma. *Proc. Natl. Acad. Sci. U.S.A. 80*: 820–824.
200. Maguire, R. T., Robins, T. S., Thorgeirsson, S. S., and Heilman, C. A. (1983). Expression of cellular *myc* and *mos* genes in undifferentiated B cell lymphomas of Burkitt and non-Burkitt types. *Proc. Natl. Acad. Sci. U.S.A. 80*: 1947–1950.
201. Keath, E. J., Kelekar, A., and Cole, M. D. (1984). Transcriptional activation of the translocated c-*myc* oncogene in mouse plasmacytomas: Similar RNA levels in tumor and proliferating normal cells. *Cell 37*: 521–528.
202. Alexander, W. S., Schrader, J. W., and Adams, J. M. (1987). Expression of the c-*myc* oncogene under control of an immunoglobulin enhancer in E-mu-*myc* transgenic mice. *Mol. Cell. Biol. 7*: 1436–1444.
203. Yang, J.-Q., Bauer, S., Mushinski, J. F., and Marcu, K. B. (1985). Chromosome translocations clustered 5′ of the murine c-*myc* qualitatively affect promoter usage: Implications for the site of normal c-*myc* regulation. *EMBO J. 4*: 1441–1447.
204. Dunnick, W., Shell, B. E., and Dery, C. (1983). DNA sequence near the site of reciprocal recombination between a c-*myc* oncogene and an immunoglobulin switch region. *Proc. Natl. Acad. Sci. U.S.A. 80*: 7269–7273.
205. Schwartz, R. C., Stanton, L. W., Riley, S. C., Marcu, K. B., and Witte, O. N. (1986). Synergism of v-*myc* and v-Ha-*ras* in the in vitro neoplastic progression of murine lymphoid cells. *Mol. Cell. Biol. 6*: 3221–3231.
206. Lombardi, L., Newcomb, E. W., and Dalla-Favera, R. (1987). Pathogenesis of Burkitt lymphoma: Expression of an activated c-*myc* oncogene causes the tumorigenic conversion of EBV-infected human B lymphoblasts. *Cell 49*: 161–170.
207. Kelekar, A., and Cole, M. D. (1986). Tumorigenicity of fibroblast lines expressing the adenovirus E1a, cellular p53, or normal c-*myc* genes. *Mol. Cell. Biol. 6*: 7–14.
208. Zerlin, M., Julius, M. A., Cerni, C., and Marcu, K. B. (1987). Elevated expression of an exogenous c-*myc* gene is insufficient for transformation and tumorigenic conversion of established fibroblasts. *Oncogene 1*: 19–27.
209. Lachman, H. M., Cheng, G. H., and Skoultchi, A. I. (1986). Transfection of mouse erythroleukaemia cells with *myc* sequences changes the rate of

induced commitment to differentiate. *Proc. Natl. Acad. Sci. U.S.A. 83*: 6480–6484.

210. Croce, C. M., Erikson, J., Huebner, K., and Nishikura, K. (1985). Coexpression of translocated and normal c-*myc* oncogenes in hybrids between Daudi and lymphoblastoid cells. *Science 227*: 1235–1238.

211. Nishikura, K., Erikson, J., ar-Rushdi, A., Huebner, K., and Croce, C. M. (1985). The translocated c-*myc* oncogene of Raji Burkitt lymphoma cells is not expressed in human lymphoblastoid cells. *Proc. Natl. Acad. Sci. U.S.A. 82*: 2900–2904.

212. Darveau, A., Sonenberg, J., and Pelletier, N. (1985). Differential efficiencies of in vitro translation of mouse c-*myc* transcripts differing in the 5′ untranslated region. *Proc. Natl. Acad. Sci. U.S.A. 82*: 2315–2319.

213. Butnick, N. Z., Miyamoto, C., Chizzonite, R., Cullen, B. R., Ju, G., and Skalka, A. (1985). Regulation of the human c-*myc* gene: 5′ noncoding sequences do not affect translation. *Mol. Cell. Biol. 5*: 3009–3016.

214. Feo, S., Harvey, R., Showe, L., and Croce, C. M. (1986). Regulation of translocated c-*myc* genes transfected into plasmacytoma cells. *Proc. Natl. Acad. Sci. U.S.A. 83*: 706–709.

215. Polack, A., Eick, D., Koch, E., and Bornkamm, G. W. (1987). Truncation does not abrogate transcriptional downregulation of the c-*myc* gene by sodium butyrate in Burkitt's lymphoma cells. *EMBO J. 6*: 2959–2964.

216. Anisimova, E., Saemundsen, A. K., Roubal, J., Vonka, V., and Klein, G. (1982). Effects of n-butyrate on Epstein-Barr virus-carrying lymphoma lines. *J. Gen. Virol. 58*: 163–171.

217. Croce, C. M. (1987). Role of chromosome translocations in human neoplasia. *Cell 49*: 155–156.

218. Dyson, P. J., and Rabbitts, T. H. (1985). Chromatin structure around the c-*myc* gene in Burkitt lmphomas with upstream and downstream translocation points. *Proc. Natl. Acad. Sci. U.S.A. 82*: 1984–1988.

219. Moulding, C., Rapaport, A., Goldman, P., Battey, J., Lenoir, G. M., and Leder, P. (1985). Structural analysis of both products of a reciprocal translocation between c-*myc* and immunoglobulin loci in Burkitt lymphoma. *Nucleic Acids Res. 13*: 2141–2152.

220. Gelmann, E. P., Psallidopoulos, M. C., Papas, T. S., and Dalla-Favera, R. (1983). Identification of reciprocal translocation sites within the c-*myc* oncogene and immunoglobulin mu locus in a Burkitt lymphoma. *Nature 306*: 799–803.

221. van Dongen, J. J. M., Versnel, M. A., Geurts van Kessel, A. H. M., Smit, E. M. E., Hooijkaas, H., and Hagemeijer, A. (1985). Immunoglobulin chain expression in Burkitt lymphoma derived cell lines. In: *Leukemia: Recent Advances in Biology and Treatment.* (Gale, R. and Golde D. eds.) Alan R. Liss, Inc., pp. 481–489.

EIGHT

Oncogene Activation in Human T-Cell and Non-Burkitt B-Cell Malignancies

Frank G. Haluska,
Yoshihide Tsujimoto, and
Carlo M. Croce
The Wistar Institute of Anatomy and Biology
Philadelphia, Pennsylvania

INTRODUCTION

In the past several years, diverse avenues of investigation on the molecular basis of malignancy have converged. Boundaries between once separated disciplines have dissolved, and a satisfying unification of the science of human neoplasia has emerged. Nowhere has this been more apparent than in the melding of cytogenetic and molecular perspectives to study chromosome aberrations consistently associated with various forms of human cancer. It has been understood for more than a quarter-century that nonrandom chromosomal anomalies, and particularly translocations, characterize many human tumors. This was first shown by Nowell and Hungerford (1), who discovered the Philadelphia chromosome (Ph^1) of chronic myelogenous leukemia (CML). More recently, characteristic chromosomal rearrangements were shown to be a feature of Burkitt's lymphoma by Manolov and Manolova (2), and by George Klein and his colleagues (3).

These karyotypic findings laid the foundation for the elucidation of the molecular genetics of these malignancies. Indeed, our understanding of Burkitt's lymphoma and CML now constitutes a paradigm for the molecular cytogenetic investigation of human malignancies in general.

The utility of this paradigm lies in the breadth and scope of its applicability. Approaches similar to those used in the study of Burkitt's lymphoma in particular have been adapted to other lymphoid malignancies. The strategy employed generally has taken the following form. Characteristic cytogenetic abnormalities are identified in a specific types of leukemia or lymphoma. Often the abnormality is a translocation, and in many cases one of the cytogenetic loci for the immunoglobulin (Ig) or T-cell receptor (TCR) genes is implicated. In such instances, well-described deoxyribonucleic (DNA) probes derived from these genes are applied to the molecular cloning of the translocated chromosomal regions. Surrounding sequences are then screened for expression, with the objective being the isolation of new genes activated consequent to their pathological rearrangement.

In this chapter, we will discuss the successful extension of this strategy to the molecular analysis of several translocation breakpoints from both B-cell and T-cell malignancies. For two reasons these studies bear special emphasis. First, they have enabled the identication of new genes thought to be central to the process of oncogenesis, and have shed light on the mechanisms which function to activate these genes. Second, the studies have provided insight into the circumstances whereby translocations occur. We begin by considering the translocations consistently observed in various lymphoid malignancies.

Cytogenetics of Lymphoid Malignancy

The initial discoveries of tumor-specific chromosomal abnormalities lent support to the proposition that somatic cell genetic changes were responsible for cellular transformation. Findings from the field of molecular virology later substantiated this view. Furthermore, with the cytological localization of the cellular proto-oncogenic homologies of viral oncogenes, it became clear that characteristic tumor-associated translocation breakpoints involved regions carrying such genes. Such cytogenetic analyses first demonstrated involvement of the *myc* gene in Burkitt's lymphoma (4). *myc* localizes to chromosome 8 band q24.1 (5,6). This band is uniformly rearranged in Burkitt's tumors; however, the reciprocally involved chromosome varies (4). In the majority of cases, a t(8;14)(q24;q32) translocation is involved. Variant translocations are found in less than 25% of cases. These comprise t(2;8)(p11;q24) or t(8;22)(q24;q11) translocations. Strikingly, the chromosome region rearranged with the *myc* locus is always the location of an immunoglobulin gene. The heavy chain locus (IgH) is at 14q32 (7). The light chain genes, Igκ and Igλ are at chromosomes 2p11 and 22q11, respectively (8,9). Molecular investigations have demonstrated the direct involvement of each of the Ig loci in the translocations. In each case, the *myc* gene is abnormally juxtaposed to Ig elements, which activate *myc* expression in *cis* (4). Moreover, it is apparent that translocations occur as a consequence of the propensity of Ig genes for physiological rearrangement during normal B-cell ontogeny (10). Enzymes whose function it is to facilitate VDJ rearrangement or isotype switching make mistakes. As a result, chr. 8 sequences are recognized by the recombinases and translocations ensue.

In light of these observations, it is reasonable to ask if similar mechanisms operate in other lymphoid neoplasms. Are the Ig loci involved in tumor-specific translocations in non-Burkitt tumors? In fact, the cytogenetic locations of the IgH genes are frequently involved. A translocation identical to Burkitt's lymphoma t(8;14) is observed in some cases of acute lymphoblastic leukemia (ALL) (11). In the most common B-cell neoplasm, follicular lymphoma, a t(14;18)(q32;q21) is observed in more than 85% of cases (12). This is illustrated in Fig. 1. Several B-cell malignancies carry the t(11;14)(q13;q32) translocations, including chronic lymphocytic leukemia (CLL), diffuse large cell lymphomas, diffuse small cell lymphomas, and multiple myelomas (12a,13). Murine plasmacytomas exhibit translocations similar to those of Burkitt's lymphomas (14). Involvement of chromosomal bands where the Ig loci, and in particular the heavy chain genes, reside is a recurrent feature of B-cell malignancies.

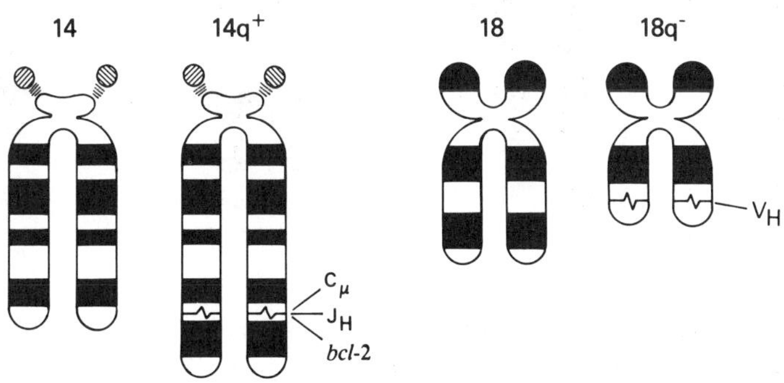

Figure 1 Schematic representation of the t(14;18)(q32;q21) chromosomal translocation observed in follicular lymphomas. Note the juxtaposition of J_H and *bcl*-2 sequences on the 14q+ chromosome.

T-cell neoplasms exhibit a similar nonrandom distribution of chromosome breakpoints. The most frequently involved region is chromosome 14q11, the cytogenetic location of the TCR α-chain genes (14a). These genes are organized in much the same manner as the IgH genes and rearrange during T-cell differentiation is a tissue-specific fashion. This suggests an analogy between translocations observed in B and T cells: A crucial role is played in both cases by rearranging receptor genes. The spectrum of translocations observed in T-cell malignancies includes t(14;14)(q11;q32) or inv(14) inversions (15,16,17), t(8;14)(q24;q11) translocations (11), t(10;14)(q24;q11) translocations (18), and t(11;14)(p13;q11) translocations (11). The translocations which involve the TCRα locus are illustrated in Fig. 2. Less frequently, the α chain of the TCR, located at chr. 7q35 (18a), is involved in translocations such as the recently described t(7;9)(q35;q34) translocation (19). In ataxia telangiectasia (20), translocations are observed between the chromosomal bands carrying all of the TCR genes (α, β, and γ); individuals with this affliction suffer a high incidence of lymphoid cancers.

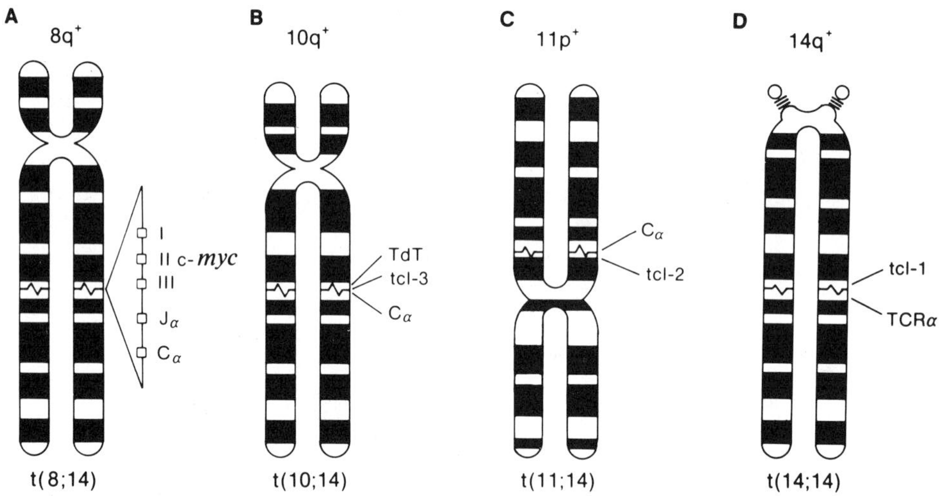

Figure 2 Translocations commonly observed in various T-cell leukemias and lymphomas. In A, the t(8;14)(q24;q11) translocation is illustrated; we have cloned the breakpoint from this tumor and demonstrated the juxtaposition of sequences 3′ of *myc* and the TCR J_α segment. In B and C, translocations which we have studies utilizing somatic cell hybrid techniques, are illustrated; the locations of putative T-cell oncogenes is illustrated.

Thus, lymphoid malignancies commonly carry translocations which appear to involve the Ig and TCR genes. These genes normally are expressed specifically and at relatively high levels in their respective lineages; moreover, they must undergo rearrangement to allow their utilization (21). These features of the normal biology of Ig and TCR genes are central to the pathogenesis of chromosome translocations, as we will discuss below.

Cloning the t(11;14) Translocation Breakpoint: *bcl*-1

The first non–Burkitt translocations to come under molecular scrutiny was the t(11;14) translocation of CLL. In studies utilizing somatic cell hybrids between CLL cells and murine partners, it was initially demonstrated that the breakpoint on chr. 14 directly involved the IgH locus (22). In fact, Southern blot experiments showed that the breakpoint involves the heavy chain joining (J_H) segments (22). This led to the suggestion that the chr. 11 region involved in the translocation constitutes a gene which we denoted *bcl*-1 (B-cell leukemia/lymphoma-1), and that this gene is activated through its rearrangement with IgH sequences (22).

Subsequently, probes for the J_H segments were employed to clone the DNA surrounding several CLL breakpoints (23). It was shown that these breakpoints cluster upstream of J_H segments on chr. 14 and within a short stretch of nucleotides on chr. 11 (24). The latter finding further suggests that some element near the breakpoint on chr. 11 confers a selective advantage on neoplastic cells by virtue of its activation through translocation. However, no transcript has yet been identified from this region. Thus, *bcl*-1 remains a putative gene.

The t(14;18) Translocation Breakpoint: *bcl*-2

The best studied gene implicated in the pathogenesis of non–Burkitt lymphoma is *bcl*-2. This gene is located on chr. 18 at band q21, and is involved in the t(14;18) translocation of follicular lymphoma, which is the most common B-cell neoplasm. As in the case of *bcl*-1, the cloning of the t(14;18) breakpoint was facilitated by utilizing J_H probes. The region of chr. 18 involved in the t(14;18) translocation was first cloned from the 380 cell line (25). This cell line was derived from a patient with acute lymphoblastic leukemia and carries t(8;14) and t(14;18) translocations (26) (Fig. 3). By screening a genomic library made from 380 genomic DNA with J_H probes, two sets of clones were obtained (25). These correspond to translocation breakpoints from both 14q+ chromosomes. Thus both J_H alleles in this neoplastic clone were involved in translocations. Deoxyribonucleic acid from the 380 t(14;18) clone was then employed to

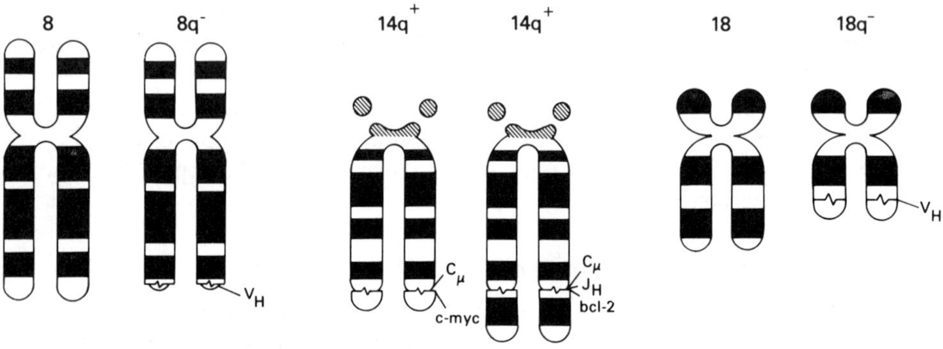

Figure 3 Involvement of both chromosomes 14 in the t(8;14) and t(14;18) translocations of the acute lymphoblastic leukemia cell line 380. The t(8;14) translocation positions *myc* upstream of the C_α gene, whereas the t(14;18) similarly positions *bcl*-2.

investigate translocations in follicular lymphomas, and we were able to demonstrate that a common segment of DNA is interrupted by translocation in many follicular lymphoma (FL) cases (27). In fact, greater than 60% of FL breakpoints are situated within an approximately 100-bp segment of chr. 18, and a second cluster lies several kilobases away (27). In addition, clustering of breakpoints on chr. 14 5′ of J_H segments was demonstrated (25,28), as had been demonstrated for the t(11;14) translocation involving *bcl*-1. Subsequently, these results were confirmed by several independent groups of investigators, both for additional cases of FL and for diffuse histocytic lymphomas (29,30).

Strikingly, probes from the region of chromosome 18 abnormally juxtaposed to the chr. 14 J_H segments recognized several transcripts on Northern blots (27,29,30). In fact, expression of these sequences in ribonucleic acid (RNA) from several B-cell, T-cell, myeloid, and erythroleukemia cell lines has been demonstrated. This gene was designated *bcl*-2 (B-cell leukemia/lymphoma-2) to underscore its importance in B-cell oncogenesis (25).

The *bcl*-2 gene was further investigated by studying its transcript. Complementary DNA (cDNA) clones were constructed from polyadenylated RNA from the 380 cell line (31). Using probes spanning the *bcl*-2 gene, it was determined that *bcl*-2 is expressed as three transcripts of 8.5, 5.5, and 3.5 kilobases (31). All three transcripts contain common sequences which constitute the first exon. However, only the two larger transcripts comprise second exon sequences as well. Sequencing cDNA clones of the

5.5- and 3.5-kb transcripts revealed the presence of one reading frame shared by two transcripts; however, the sequences diverge at their 3′ ends; that is, at the carboxyterminals of the encoded proteins. The 5.5-kb transcript codes for a 239 amino acid protein with a predicted molecular weight of 25 kd, called *bcl*-2α. (The 8.5-kb transcript also codes for *bcl*-2α, but carries a longer 3′ untranslated tract.) This protein encompasses both *bcl*-2 exons. A second protein, *bcl*-2β, is encoded by the 3.5-kb transcript. This transcript is polyadenlated at a site 3′ of the first exon. The resulting *bcl*-2β protein is 205 amino acid residues in length, with a molecular mass of approximately 22 kd (31).

In all cases of follicular lymphoma so far examined which carry translocations involving *bcl*-2, the coding capacity of the gene is undisturbed. The translocation-associated *bcl*-2 proteins are identical to their normal counterparts. This suggests that the mechanism which operates to perturb *bcl*-2 function does so at the level of transcription. This proposition also follows from the architecture of the translocation junctions. The clustering of breakpoints 5′ of J_H segments in all cases leaves the heavy chain enhancers nearby the translocated *bcl*-2 locus. This parallels many translocations involving *myc* on chr. 8 and argues that *cis* transcriptional activation is the major mode of oncogene activation in B-cell malignancies. It should be noted, however, that in some FL samples, aberrant-sized messenger RNAs (mRNAs) are observed (31,32). These may constitute *bcl*-2/Ig chimeric transcripts. Analysis of one of these transcripts demonstrated no alteration in *bcl*-2 coding regions (32). Thus if post-transcriptional processes are at work in *bcl*-2 activation, they play a minor role.

What is the function of the *bcl*-2 proteins? This is not yet clear. The *bcl*-2α protein is more highly conserved across species boundaries than *bcl*-2β, suggesting that the former protein plays the crucial role in the cell (33). *bcl*-2α lacks a transmembrane domain, but subcellular fractionation experiments demonstrated its association with the cell membrane (34). This raises the possibility of its involvement of transmembrane or intracellular signal pathways. Moreover, *bcl*-2 transcription is modulated in response to mitogenic stimulation of normal B and T lymphocytes (35). Taken together, these data allow us to speculate that *bcl*-2 proteins function in controlling B-cell proliferation. Abnormal regulation of their expression as a consequence of translocation is thus a crucial stop toward B-cell transformation.

Translocations Which Involve the T-Cell Receptor Genes

The elucidation of the structure and function of the TCR family of genes has been taken advantage of by many investigators seeking to understand translocations in T-cell malignancies. Several features of these genes have facilitated the study of their pathogenetic roles. First, they are highly tissue specific in their pattern of expression. Molecular elements within the TCR gene complexes must engender this degree of specificity and may function to activate genes placed nearby. Second, the TCR genes are exceptionally large. Their loci span hundreds or thousands of kilobases of DNA. Third, these genes recombine during abnormal T-lymphoid ontogeny, and thus are susceptible to aberrant recombination as well. Of course, all of these features are shared by the Ig genes; the analogy is quite apparent. For this reason the analysis of translocations of the T-cell receptor genes has taken the same form as that of B cells.

This is the most evident in translocations near *myc*. The t(8;14)(q24;q11) translocation, the karyotype of which is shown in Fig. 4, was first examined using somatic cell hybrid techniques (36). It was shown that a region 3′ of *myc* was rearranged as a consequence of the translocation

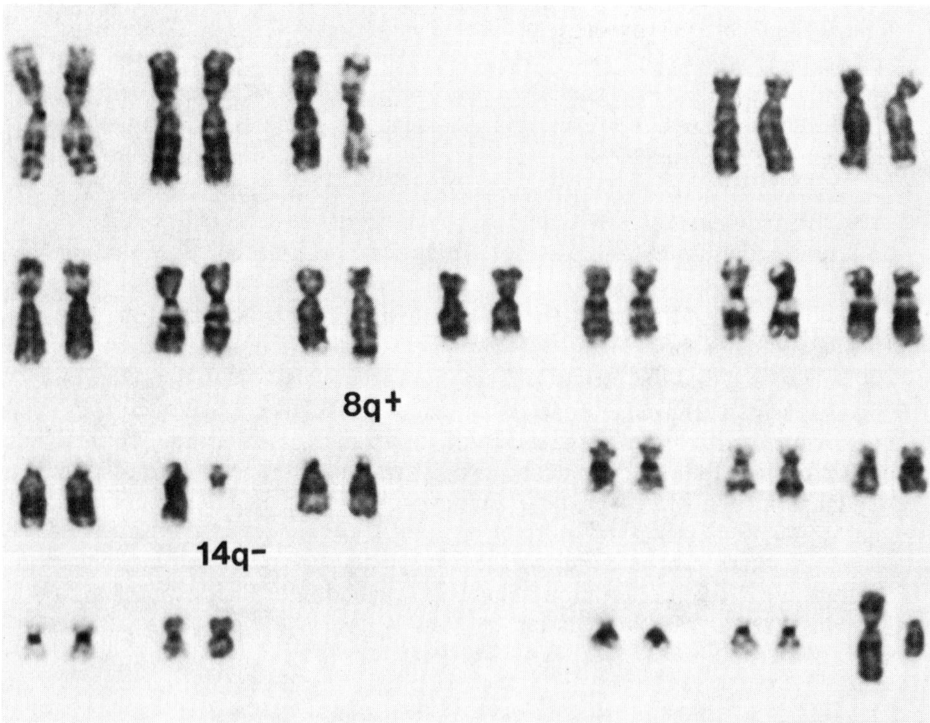

Figure 4 The karyotype of the T-cell acute lymphoblastic leukemia carrying the t(8;14)(q24;q11) translocation.

in a T-cell leukemia cell line. In a second line, no rearrangement of *myc* was detectable, but interruption of the TCRα locus, probably in the region of J_α, could be demonstrated (36). Furthermore, hybrids carrying the translocated *myc* gene expressed it inappropriately, in a manner previously shown for Burkitt's lymphoma (36). This suggested that the TCRα gene could rearrange 3′ of *myc* just as in the variant Burkitt translocations. The proposed architecture was independently confirmed using in situ hybridization (37). This translocation is illustrated in Fig 5.

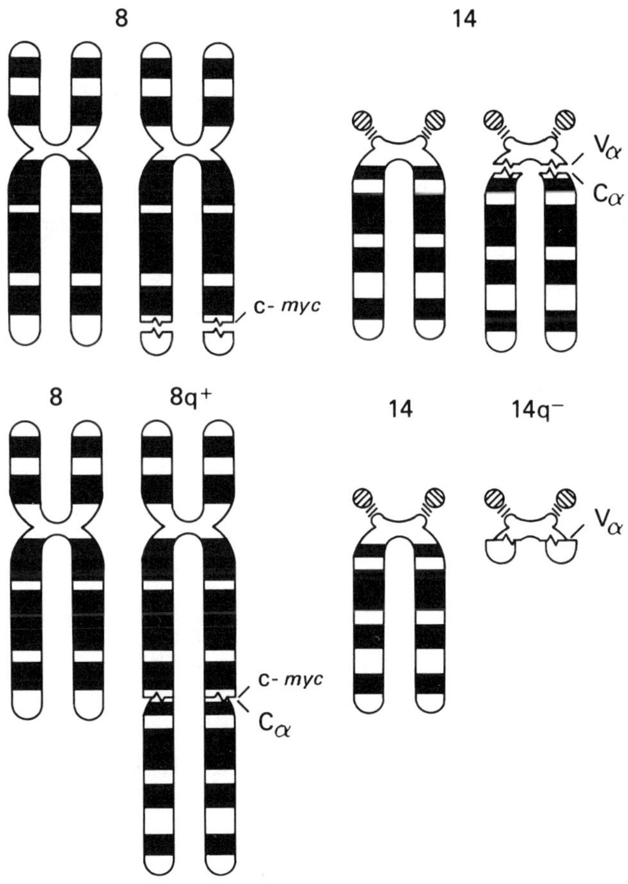

Figure 5 The molecular architecture of the T-cell t(8;14) translocation. The C_α locus is translocated 3′ of the *myc* gene in this rearrangement.

Cloning of the t(8;14) breakpoint verified the interruption of the TCR-J_α region (38–40). In two lines, the break was shown to occur directly upstream of J_α segments and 3′ of *myc* (38,40). The abnormal proximity of the *myc* and α-chain genes provides an explanation for the dysregulated expression of the translocation-associated *myc* allele observed in somatic cell hybrids carrying the $8q^+$ chromosome (36).

Our group has analyzed two other translocations using somatic cell hybrids. In both the t(10;14)(q24;q11) translocation (41) and t(11;14)(p13;q11) translocation (42), it appears that the TCRα locus is interrupted in the J segments. Therefore, it is likely that genes important to the genesis of T-cell malignancy may be found near the sites of translocation on chromosomes 10 and 11, and that they become activated in *cis* by a process similar to that which activates *myc*.

Many T-cell neoplasms carry either inv(14)(q11;q32) inversions or t(14;14)(q11;q32) translocations (15–17). Can the TCR α chain recombine with IgH? Or are other genes involved? A priori, the latter is likely to be the case. Translocations must confer a selective or proliferative advantage upon cells which carry them. This advantage has been shown in other instances to derive from activation of an oncogene or putative oncogene. Thus, one would expect new loci to be involved in the t(14;14) and inv(14;14) abnormalities as well. Initial work on the inv(14), however, suggested the activation of no new genes. The cloning by several groups of the breakpoint at 14q11 of both T-cell–(43–45) and B-cell–associated (46) inversions showed the presence of V_H-J_α fusions. These studies led to speculation that either the rearrangement led to the production of a hybrid receptor gene which could either function in a transforming capacity, or else it was simply an aberrant V-J join of no proliferative consequence (43–46). Which of these alternatives is correct is not yet clear, but further investigation of these rearrangements has now suggested that in most cases, a gene proximal of the IgH genes at 14q32 must be involved (20,47). Our laboratory previously designated this putative gene *tcl*-1 (T-cell leukemia/lymphoma-1) (14a) (Fig. 2). The study of several t(14;14) and inv (14) abnormalities has demonstrated that TCR-J_α segments join to regions proximal to (3′ of) IgH. The detailed characterization of this gene awaits more extensive cloning studies.

Finally, studies on the involvement of the TCR β-chain genes in translocations are now emerging. Cloning of the rearrangement associated with a t(7;9)(q35;q34) translocation in a T-lymphoblastic tumor line has recently enabled the identification of a new gene on chr. 9, which is far from the *abl* locus (19).

The aforementioned work serves to illustrate the power and utility of the approach which applies our knowledge of the immunoglobulin superfamily genes to identify new genes implicated in oncogenesis. We now turn to a discussion of the mechanisms which give rise to translocations of these loci.

Translocation Scenarios in Lymphoid Malignancies

It has become clear that the most likely mechanism leading to chromosome translocations in T and B cells is recombinase error (also reviewed in Ref. 10). Several lines of evidence support this proposition. First, the distribution of chromosome breakpoints correlates with sites of recombinase activity. In Burkitt's lymphomas, breakpoints of the IgH genes preferentially occur 5′ of D_H or J_H segments (48,49), or in switch regions (50); variant translocations also occur near J segments (51). The t(11;14) and t(14;18) breakpoints also cluster 5′ of J_H segments on the $14q^+$ chromosome (23,28); the 11q− and 18q− chromosomes exhibit D_H involvement (52,53). In TCR translocations, the 5′ ends of J_α segments or D_β-J_β regions are involved (19). All of these sites are those located at which VDJ recombination occurs physiologically. Clustering of breakpoints 3′ of J_H regions is illustrated in Fig. 6.

Second, nucleotide sequence analysis has revealed features near translocation breakpoints indicative of VDJ recombinase activity. This is shown for follicular lymphomas in Fig. 7. These features include the presence of N regions and heptamer-nonamer motifs near the breaks (23,28,38,48,49). N regions are short spans of nucleotides added de novo to VDJ joins, probably by the enzyme terminal deoxynucleotidyl transferase (TdT) (54). Heptamer-nonamers are signals thought to be recognized by the putative VDJ recombinase enzymes (21). These features are highly conserved among immunoglobulin and TCR genes. Their presence

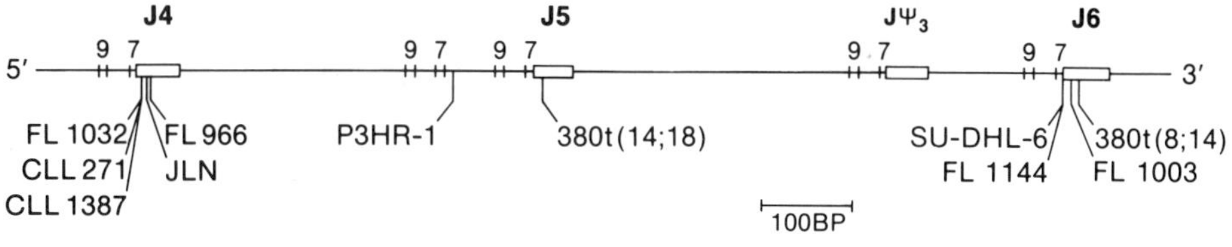

Figure 6 Clustering of chromosome breakpoints 5′ of J_H segments in various lymphoid malignancies. JLN and FL indicate follicular lymphoma; CLL, chronic lymphocytic leukemia; DHL, diffuse histiocytic leukemia carrying t(14;18); P3HR-1 is an endemic Burkitt's lymphoma; 380 is an acute lymphoblastic leukemia line.

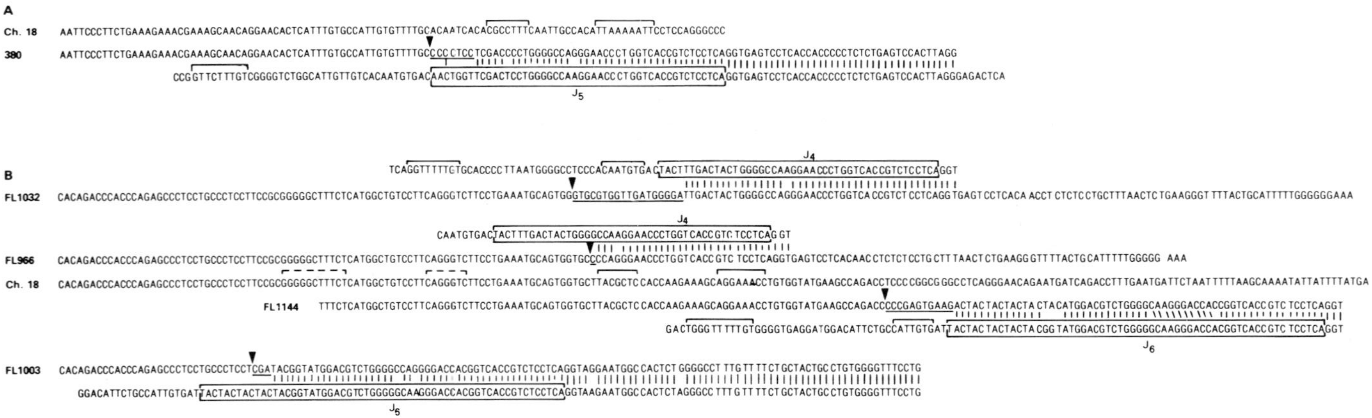

Figure 7 Sequences of breakpoints derived from samples carrying t(14;18) translocations. For each case, the position of the breakpoint is indicated by the arrow. Heavy chain J_H segments are bracketed. Heptamer-nonamer motifs are also bracketed, and N regions are indicated by underlines.

at translocation junctions, albeit in less strictly conserved forms, argues for their playing a fundamental role in the translocation process. Figure 8 demonstrates one possible version of what that role might be.

Third, it is quite clear that the recombinase system must function aberrantly from the study of the inv(14) abnormality (43–46). As already mentioned, this inversion consists of a functional Ig V_H-TCR J_α joining. Normally, such recombinations do not occur. Thus, this rearrangement allows one to ascribe wide limits to the fidelity with which the recombinase system functions.

In short, the immunoglobulinlike genes are capable of generating a response to a tremendously diverse variety of antigens. This capacity

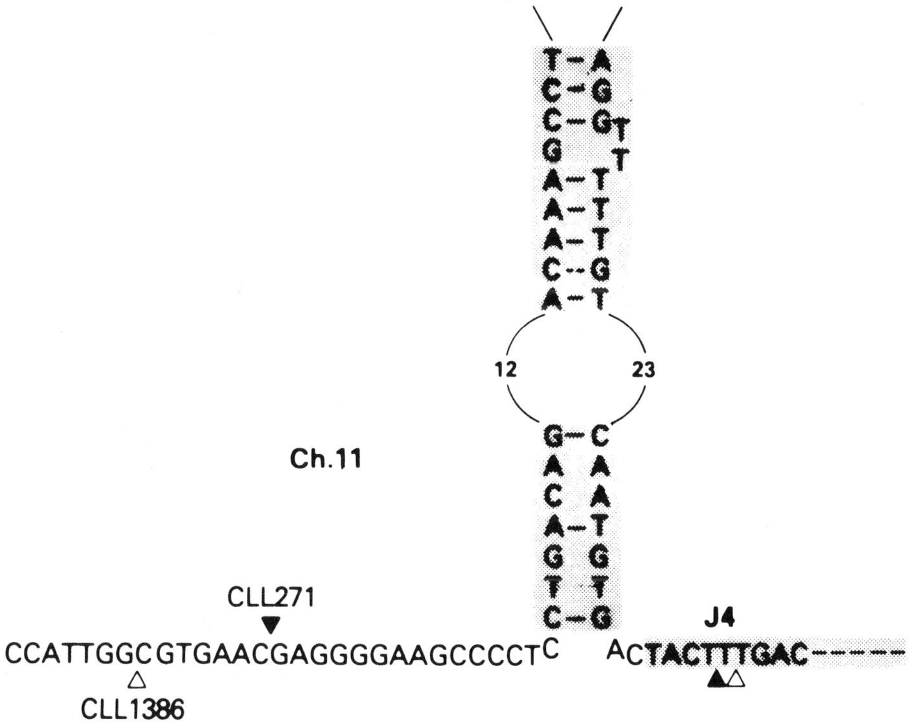

Figure 8 Possible role of heptamer-nonamer signal sequences in the genesis of the t(11;14) translocation of CLL. The breakpoints of two CLLs on chr. 11 are indicated by the triangles. It is possible that the heptamer-nonamer from chr. 11 (on the left, in gray) may pair with the heptamer-nonamer from chr. 14 (on the right) to form a stem and loop structure as shown. This is thought to take place in physiological VDJ joining; its occurrence during the course of translocation may indicate the mistaken operation of the recombinase.

requires genomic rearrangement, and it has been bought evolutionarily at the price of an increased likelihood of translocation. It is probable that translocations occur with some low frequency, and that they result simply in nonproductive Ig or TCR rearrangements. However, when they juxtapose genes important to the control of cellular proliferation and differentiation with the activating Ig or TCR elements, malignancy may ensue.

CONCLUSIONS

The link between cytogenetic abnormality and molecular derangement, first demonstrated for Burkitt's lymphoma, has now been forged for other B- and T-lymphoid cancers as well. These investigations have deepened our understanding of the malignant phenotype in general. In fact we are now witnessing the application of the cytogenetic and molecular approach to solid tumors (e.g., retinoblastoma), and to other genetic diseases (e.g., chronic granulomatoid disease) (55). The future may hold an application of this molecular understanding to cancer diagnosis and eventually to therapy.

ACKNOWLEDGMENTS

We would like to thank Ms. Charlotte Long for preparation of the manuscript. F.G.H. is a Monica Shander Fellow at the Wistar Institute, and is a trainee of the Medical Scientist Training Program of the University of Pennsylvania School of Medicine (NIH T32 GM 07170). This work was supported by grants from the National Institutes of Health Outstanding Investigator's Grant CA 39860 (CMC), CA 25875 (CMC), NIH Training Program in Basic Cancer Research CA 09171 (FGH).

REFERENCES

1. Nowell, P. C., and Hungerford, D. A. (1960). A minute chromosome in human chronic granulocytic leukemia. *Science 132*: 1497.
2. Manolov, G., and Manolova, Y. (1972). Marker band in one chromosome 14 from Burkitt lymphomas. *Nature 237*: 33–34.
3. Zech, L., Haglund, U., Nillson, K., and Klein, G. (1976). Characteristic chromosomal abnormalities in biopsies and lymphoid-cell lines from patients with Burkitt and non-Burkitt lymphomas. *Int. J. Cancer 17*: 47–56.
4. Croce, C. M., Erikson, J., Haluska, F. G., Finger, L. R., Showe, L. C., and Tsujimoto, Y. (1986). Molecular genetics of human B- and T-cell neoplasia. *Cold Spring Harbor Symp. Quant. Biol. 51*: 891–898.

5. Dalla-Favera, R., Gregni, M., Erikson, J., Patterson, D., Gallo, R. C., and Croce, C. M. (1982). Human c-*myc* oncogene is located on the region of chromosome 8 that is translocated in Burkitt lymphoma cells. *Proc. Natl. Acad. Sci. U.S.A. 79*: 7824–7827.
6. Taub, R., Kirsch, I., Morton, C., Lenoir, G., Swan, D., Tronick, S., Aaronson, S., and Leder, P. (1982). Translocation of the c-*myc* gene into the immunoglobulin heavy chain locus in human Burkitt lymphoma and murine plasmacytoma cells. *Proc. Natl. Acad. Sci. U.S.A. 79*: 7837–7841.
7. Croce, C. M., Shander, M., Martinis, J., Cicurel, L., D'Ancona, G. G., Dolby, T. W., and Koprowski, H. (1979). Chromosomal location of the genes for human immunoglobulin heavy chains. *Proc. Natl. Acad. Sci. U.S.A. 76*: 3416–3419.
8. Malcolm, S., Barton, P., Murphy, C., Ferguson-Smith, M. A., Bentley, D. L., and Rabbitts, T. H. (1982). Localization of human immunoglobulin κ light chain variable region genes to the short arm of chromosome 2 by *in situ* hybridization. *Proc. Natl. Acad. Sci. U.S.A. 74*: 4957–4961.
9. Erikson, J., Martinis, J., and Croce, C. M. (1981). Assignment of the genes for human λ immunoglobulin chains to chromosome 22. *Nature 294*: 173–175.
10. Haluska, F. G., Tsujimoto, Y., and Croce, C. M. (1987). Mechanisms of chromosome translocation in B- and T-cell neoplasia. *Trends. Genet. 3*: 11–15.
11. Williams, D. L., Look, A. T., Melvin, S. L., Roberson, P. K., Dahl, G., Flake, T., and Stass, S. (1984). New chromosomal translocations correlate with specific immunotypes of childhood acute lymphoblastic leukemia. *Cell 36*: 101–109.
12. Yunis, J. J., Frizzera, G., Oken, M. M., McKenna, J., Theologides, A., and Arnesen, M. (1987). Multiple recurrent genomic defects in follicular lymphoma. *N. Engl. J. Med. 316*: 79–84.
12a. Yunis, J. J. (1983). The chromosomal basis of human neoplasia. *Science 221*: 227–236.
13. Van Den Berghe, H., Vermaelen, K., Louwagie, A., Criel, A., Mecucci, C., and Vaerman, J. P. (1984). High incidence of chromosome abnormalities in IgG3 myeloma. *Cancer Genet. Cytogenet. 11*: 381–387.
14. Klein, G. (1983). Specific chromosomal translocations and the genesis of B-cell-derived tumors in mice and men. *Cell 32*: 311–315.
14a. Croce, C. M., Isobe, M., A., Palumbo, A., Puck, J., Ming, J., Tweardy, D., Erikson, J., and Rovera, G. (1985). Gene for α-chain of human T-cell receptor: Location on chromosome 14 region involved in T-cell neoplasms. *Science 227*: 1044–1047.
15. Hecht, F., Morgan, R., Hecht, B. K.-M., and Smith, S. D. (1984). Common region on chromosome 14 in T-cell leukemia and lymphoma. *Science 226*: 1445–1447.
16. Ueshima, Y., Rowley, J. D., Variakojis, D., Winter, J., and Gordon, L. (1984). Cytogenetic studies on patients with chronic T-cell leukemia/lymphoma. *Blood 63*: 1028–1038.

17. Zech, L., Gahrton, G., Hammarstrom, L., Juliusson, G., Mellstedt, H., Robert, K. H., and Smith, C. I. E. (1984). Inversion of chromosome 14 marks human T-cell chronic lymphocytic leukemia. *Nature 308*: 858-860.
18. Dube, I. D., Raimondi, S. C., Pi, D., and Kalousek, D. K. (1986). A new translocation, t(10;14)(q24;q11), in T-cell neoplasia. *Blood 67*: 1181–1184.
18a. Isobe, M., Erikson, J., Emanuel, B. S., Nowell, P. C., and Croce, C. M. (1985). Location of gene for β subunit of human T-cell receptor at band 7q35, a region prone to rearrangements in T-cells. *Science 228*: 580–582.
19. Reynolds, T. C., Smith, S. D., and Sklar, J. (1987). Analysis of DNA surrounding the breakpoints of chromosomal translocations involving the β T-cell receptor gene in human lymphoblastic neoplasms. *Cell 50*: 107–117.
20. Kennaugh, A. A., Butterworth, S. V., Hollis, R., Baer, R., Rabbitts, T. H., and Taylor, A. M. R. (1986). The chromosome breakpoint at 14q32 in an ataxia telangiectasia t(14;14) T cell clone is different from the 14q32 breakpoint in Burkitt's and an inv(14) T cell lymphoma. *Hum. Genet. 73*: 254–259.
21. Tonegawa, S. (1983). Somatic generation of antibody diversity. *Nature 302*: 575–581.
22. Erikson, J., Finan, J., Tsujimoto, Y. Nowell, P. C., and Croce, C. M. (1984). The chromosome 14 breakpoint in neoplastic B-cells with the t(11;14) translocation involves the immunoglobulin heavy chain locus. *Proc. Natl. Acad. Sci. U.S.A. 81*: 4144–4148.
23. Tsujimoto, Y., Jaffe, E., Cossman, J., Gorham, J., Nowell, P. C., and Croce, C. M. (1985). Clustering of breakpoints on chromosome 11 in human B-cell neoplasms with the t(11;14) chromosome translocation. *Nature 315*: 340–343.
24. Tsujimoto, Y., Yunis, J., Onorato-Showe, L., Erikson, J., Nowell, P. C., and Croce, C. M. (1984). Molecular cloning of the chromosomal breakpoint of B-cell lymphomas and leukemias with the t(11;14) chromosome translocation. *Science 224*: 1403–1406.
25. Tsujimoto, Y., Finger, L. R., Yunis, J., Nowell, P. C., and Croce, C. M. (1984). Cloning of the chromosome breakpoint of neoplastic B-cells with the t(14;18) chromosome translocation. *Science 226*: 1097–1099.
26. Pegoraro, L., Palumbo, A., Erikson, J., Fauda, M., Giovanazzo, B., Emanuel, B. S., Rovera, G., Nowell, P. C., and Croce, C. M. (1984). A 14;18 and a 8;14 chromosome translocation in a cell line derived from an acute B-cell leukemia. *Proc. Natl. Acad. Sci. U.S.A. 81*: 7166–7170.
27. Tsujimoto, Y., Cossman, J., Jaffe, E., and Croce, C. M. (1985). Involvement of the *bcl*-2 gene in human follicular lymphoma. *Science 228*: 1440–1443.
28. Tsujimoto, Y., Gorham, J., Cossman, J., Jaffe, E., and Croce, C. M. (1985). The t(14;18) chromosome translocations involved in B-cell neoplasms result from mistakes in VDJ joining. *Science 229*: 1390–1393.

29. Bakhshi, A., Jensen, J. P., Goldman, P., Wright, J. J., McBride, W., Epstein, A. L., and Korsmeyer, S. J. (1985). Cloning of the chromosomal breakpoint of t(14;18) human lymphomas: Clustering around J_H on chromosome 14 and near a transcriptional unit on 18. *Cell 41*: 899–906.
30. Cleary, M. L., and Sklar, J. (1985). Nucleotide sequence of a t(14;18) chromosomal breakpoint in follicular lymphoma and demonstration of a breakpoint-cluster region near a transcriptionally active locus on chromosome 18. *Proc. Natl. Acad. Sci. U.S.A. 82*: 7439–7444.
31. Tsujimoto, Y., and Croce, C. M. (1986). Analysis of the structure products of *bcl*-2, the gene involved in human follicular lymphoma. *Proc. Natl. Acad. Sci. U.S.A. 83*: 5214–5218.
32. Cleary, M. L., Smith, S. D., and Sklar, J. (1986). Cloning and structural analysis of cDNAs for *bcl*-2 and a hybrid *bcl*-2/immunoglobulin transcript resulting from the t(14;18) translocation. *Cell 47*: 19–28.
33. Negrini, M., Sinini, E., Kozak, C., Tsujimoto, Y., and Croce, C. M. Molecular analysis of *mbcl*-2: Structure and expression of the muring gene homologous to the human gene involved in follicular lymphoma. *Cell 49*: 455–463.
34. Tsujimoto, Y., Ikegaki, N., and Croce, C. M. (1987). Identification of the protein product of *bcl*-2, the gene involved in human follicular lymphoma. *Oncogene 2*: 1–7.
35. Reed, J. C., Tsujimoto, Y., Alpers, J. D., Croce, C. M., and Nowell, P. C. (1987). Regulation of *bcl*-2 proto-oncogene expression during normal human lymphocyte proliferation. *Science 236*: 1295–1299.
36. Erikson, J., Finger, L., Sun, L., ar-Rushdi, A., Nishikura, K., Minowada, J., Finan, J., Emanuel, B. S., Nowell, P. C., and Croce, C. M. (1986). Deregulation of c-*myc* by translocation of the T-cell receptor in T-cell leukemias. *Science 232*: 884–887.
37. Shima, E. A., LeBleu, M. M., McKeithan, T. W., Minowada, J., Showe, L. C., Mak, T. W., Minden, M. D., Rowley, J. D., and Diaz, M. O. (1986). Gene encoding the α-chain of the T-cell receptor is moved immediately downstream of c-*myc* in a chromosomal 8;14 translocation in a cell line from a human T-cell leukemia. *Proc. Natl. Acad. Sci. U.S.A. 83*: 3439–3443.
38. Finger, L. R., Harvey, R. C., Moore, R. C. A., Showe, L. C., and Croce, C. M. (1986). A common mechanism of chromosomal translocation in T- and B-cell neoplasia. *Science 234*: 982–985.
39. Mathieu-Mahul, D., Caubet, J. F., Bernheim, A., Mauchauffe, M., Palmer, E., Berger, R., and Larsen, C.-J. (1985). Molecular cloning of a DNA fragment from human chromosome 14 (14q11) involved in T-cell malignancies. *EMBO J. 4*: 3427–3433.
40. McKeithan, T. W., Shima, E. A., LeBleu, M. M., Minowada, J., Rowley, J. D., and Diaz, M. O. (1986). Molecular cloning of the breakpoint junction of a human chromosomal 8;14 translocation involving the T-cell receptor α-chain gene and sequences on the 3′ side of *myc*. *Proc. Natl. Acad. Sci. U.S.A. 83*: 6636–6640.

41. Kagan, J., Finan, J., Letofsky, J., Besa, E. C., Nowell, P. C., and Croce, C. M. (1987). α-chain locus of the T-cell antigen receptor is involved in the t(10;14) chromosome translocation of T-cell acute lymphocytic leukemia. *Proc. Natl. Acad. Sci. U.S.A. 84*: 4543–4546.
42. Erikson, J., Williams, D. L., Finan, J., Nowell, P. C., and Croce, C. M. (1985). Locus of the α-chain of the T-cell receptor is split by chromosome translocation in T-cell leukemias. *Science 229*: 784–787.
43. Baer, R., Chen, K.-C., Smith, S. D., and Rabbitts, T. H. (1985). Fusion of an immunoglobulin variable gene and a T-cell receptor constant gene in the chromosome 14 inversion associated with T-cell tumors. *Cell 43*: 705–713.
44. Denny, C. T., Yoshikai, Y., Mak, T. W., Smith, S. D., Hollis, G. F., Kirsch, I. R. (1986). A chromosome 14 inversion in a T-cell lymphoma is caused by site-specific recombination between immunoglobulin and T-cell receptor loci. *Nature 320* 549–551.
45. Baer, R., Forster, A., and Rabbitts, T. H. (1987). The mechanism of chromosome 14 inversion in a human T-cell lymphoma. *Cell 50*: 97–105.
46. Denny, C. T., Hollis, G. F., Hecht, F., Morgan, R., Link, M. P., Smith, S. D., and Kirsch, I. R. (1986). Common mechanism of chromosome inversion in B- and T-cell tumors: Relevance to lymphoid development. *Science 234*: 197–200.
47. Mengle-Gaw, L., Willard, H. F., Smith, C. I. E., Hammarstrom, L., Fischer, P., Sherrington, P., Lucas, G., Thompson, P. W., Baer, R., and Rabbitts, T. H. (1987). Human T-cell tumours containing chromosome 14 inversion or translocation with breakpoints proximal to immunoglobulin joining regions at 14q32. *EMBO J. 6*: 2273–2280.
48. Haluska, F. G., Finver, S., Tsujimoto, Y., and Croce, C. M. (1986). The t(8;14) chromosomal translocation occurring in B-cell malignancies results from mistakes in V-D-J joining. *Nature 324*: 158–160.
49. Haluska, F. G., Tsujimoto, Y., and Croce, C. M. (1987). The t(8;14) chromosome translocation of the Burkitt lymphoma cell line Daudi occurred during immunoglobulin gene rearrangement and involved the heavy chain diversity region. *Proc. Natl. Acad. Sci. U.S.A. 84*: 6835–6939.
50. Gelmann, E. P., Psallidopoulos, M. C., Papas, T., and Dalla-Favera, R. (1983). Identification of reciprocal translocation sites within the c-*myc* oncogene and immunoglobulin μ locus in a Burkitt lymphoma. *Nature 306*: 799.
51. Lipp, M., and Hartl, P. (1986). Possible role of immunoglobulin recombination sequences in the genesis of variant t(2;8) translocations of Burkitt lymphoma. *Curr. Topics Microbiol. Immunol. 132*: 162.
52. Bakhshi, A., Wright, J. J., Graninger, W., Seto, M., Owens, J., Cossman, J., Jensen, J. P., Goldman, P., and Korsmeyer, S. J. (1987). Mechanism of the t(14;18) chromosomal translocation: Structural analysis of both derivative 14 and 18 reciprocal partners. *Proc. Natl. Acad. Sci. U.S.A. 84*: 2396–2400.

53. Tsujimoto, Y., Louie, E., Bashir, M. M., and Croce, C. M. The reciprocal partners of both the t(14;18) and the t(11;14) translocations involved in B-cell neoplasms are rearranged by the same mechanism. *Oncogene* (in press).
54. Desiderio, S. V., Yancopoulos, G. D., Paskind, M., Thomas, E., Boss, M. A., Landau, N., Alt, F. W., and Baltimore, D. (1984). Insertion of N regions into heavy-chain genes is correlated with expression of terminal deoxytransferase in B cells. *Nature 311*: 752–755.
55. Orkin, S. (1986). Reverse genetics and human disease. *Cell 47*: 845–850.

NINE

The Philadelphia Chromosome and the *bcr*/c-*abl* Translocation in Chronic Myelogenous and Acute Leukemia

A. De Klein and A. Hermans
Erasmus University
Rotterdam, The Netherlands

N. Heisterkamp and J. Groffen
Childrens Hospital of Los Angeles
Los Angeles, California

G. Grosveld
Erasmus University
Rotterdam, The Netherlands

INTRODUCTION

Extensive cytogenetic studies have revealed that a considerable number of human tumors, in particular leukemias and lymphomas, are associated with consistent, specific chromosomal aberrations (Mitelman, 1985; Yunis, 1983). These observations suggested, that genes located at the specific breakpoint regions of these chromosomal abnormalities can play a role in the malignant transformation of a normal cell into a tumor cell (Klein, 1981). Attractive candidates for such genes are the cellular proto-oncogenes (Bishop, 1985; Varmus, 1984). Recent data indicate that the protein products of these proto-oncogenes are involved in the regulation of normal growth and differentiation. Alterations of these gene products, e.g., mutations and/or rearrangements caused by chromosomal aberrations, could modify the gene product and interfere with the normal cellular function, ultimately leading to transformation (Bishop, 1987; Weinberg, 1985). The chromosomal location of many proto-oncogenes has been determined by cytogenetic methods and a striking concordance has been shown for the positions of proto-oncogenes and consistent chromosomal breakpoint regions (Rowley, 1983; Yunis, 1983). Ample evidence has been provided for the involvement of the c-*myc* oncogene in the specific chromosomal translocations observed in Burkitt's lymphoma and mouse plasmacytoma (see Chap. 5). Similarly, the c-*abl* oncogene proved to be directly involved in the Philadelphia translocation observed in chronic myelogenous leukemia and acute leukemias.

THE PHILADELPHIA CHROMOSOME IN CHRONIC MYELOGENOUS LEUKEMIA

Cytogenetic Characterization

Chronic myelogenous leukemia (CML) is a clonal disorder of pluripotent hematopoietic stem cells. It was the first human neoplasm in which a consistent chromosomal aberration was discovered: the Philadelphia chromosome (Ph^1) (Nowell and Hungerford, 1960). This chromosome (or 22q −) is found in 96% of all CML patients and is the result of either a standard (9;22) translocation (90% of the cases) (Rowley, 1973) or a variant translocation (3–8% of the cases), involving other chromosomes as well (Heim et al., 1985). In a minority (3–7%) of the CML cases, Ph^1 is not present. (Ph^1-negative CML) (Rowley and Testa, 1982).

The c-*abl* oncogene is normally located at chromosome 9q34 (Heisterkamp et al., 1982), but as a result of the Ph^1 translocation (Fig. 1), it is translocated to the 22q − chromosome (De Klein et al., 1982). Molecular cloning of the breakpoint region of chromosome 22 resulted in the identification of a breakpoint cluster region (*bcr*) (Groffen et al., 1984). This *bcr* is disrupted and the distal (3 ′) *bcr* sequences are translocated to the 9q + derivative chromosome (Groffen et al., 1983), together with the c-*sis* oncogene, located at chromosome 22q13 (Bartram et al., 1984). In cytogenetic variant Ph^1 translocations, a similar consistent translocation of the c-*abl* oncogene to the proximal (5 ′) *bcr* sequences has been demonstrated (Bartram et al., 1983; De Klein and Hagemeijer, 1984; Hagemeijer et al., 1985). This juxtaposition of c-*abl* and *bcr* sequences was not only found in Ph^1-positive leukemic CML cells, but also in the leukemic cells of some Ph^1-negative CML patients (Bartram et al., 1985; Ganesan et al., 1986; Morris et al., 1986). Clinical and hematological features of the latter Ph^1-negative CML patients are indistinguishable from Ph^1-positive CML patients. This is in contrast to other Ph^1-negative CML patients, who lack the *bcr*/c-*abl* juxtaposition and probably represent myelodysplasia and reactive myeloproliferative conditions other than CML, with an overall poorer prognosis (Pugh et

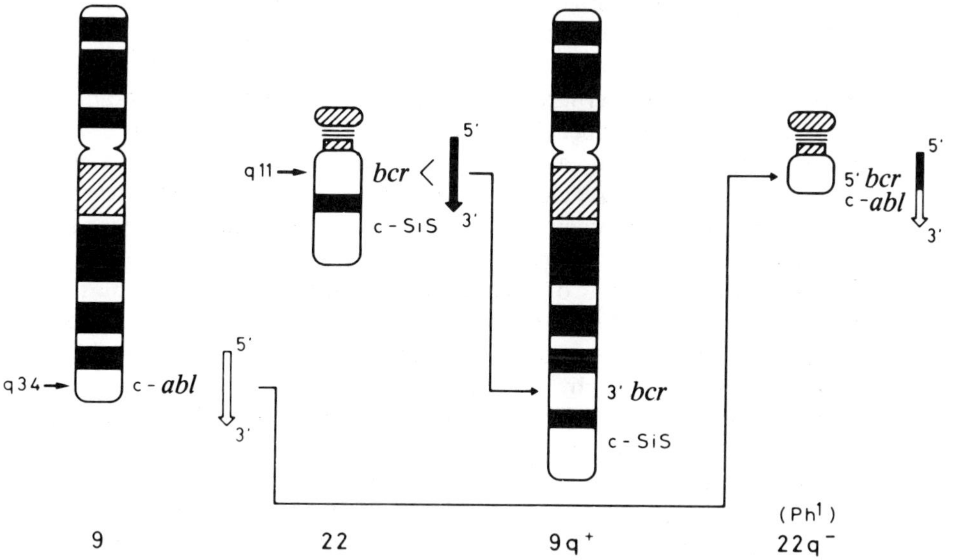

Figure 1 Schematic representation of the standard Ph[1] translocation t(9;22)(q34;q11). Part of the long (q) arm of chr. 22, 22q11–22qter, is translocated to the q arm of chr. 9, and a part of the terminal chr. 9 band (9q34-qter) is translocated to the shortened chromosome 22q−, or Ph[1]. The localization and orientation of the marker genes are indicated.

al., 1985; Travis et al., 1986). These results indicate that the translocation of the c-*abl* oncogene to the *bcr* sequences is a critical event, and both the c-*abl* and *bcr* sequences may play a pivotal role in the pathogenesis of CML.

Molecular Characterization

The Human c-*abl* Gene

Before discussing the molecular events affecting the configuration of the *bcr* and c-*abl* genes in CML, the normal structure of these genes will be described.

The proto-oncogene c-*abl* was initially identified as the cellular homologue of the viral-transforming gene (v-*abl*) of Abelson murine leukemia virus (A-MuLV) (Goff et al., 1980). The c-*abl* gene was found to be evolutionary conserved; the deoxyribonucleic acid (DNA) of Drosophila (Hoffmann-Falk et al., 1983; Shilo and Weinberg, 1981), Nematoda (Goddard et al., 1986), mouse (Ben Neriah et al., 1986a; Goff and Baltimore,

1982; Wang et al., 1984), cat (Schalken et al., 1985), and man (Heisterkamp et al., 1983) all contain c-*abl* homologous sequences. The giant c-*abl* locus in man covers 225 kb of DNA and has a rather unique structure (Fig. 2) (A. Bernards, personal communication; Heisterkamp et al., 1983). It is transcribed into two major messenger ribonucleic acids (mRNAs) of 6 and 7 kb, of which the structure was elucidated by complementary DNA (cDNA) cloning (Shtivelman et al., 1986). This revealed the existence of two alternative 5′ exons (1A and 1B), that are spliced to a common set of 10 exons (exon$_2$ to exon$_{11}$), representing the body of the *abl* gene (Fig. 2). The region of homology with v-*abl* starts within the third exon and extends to the 5′ part of exon$_{11}$. The most 3′ 2 kb of exon$_{11}$ contains untranslated sequences. The body exons cover some 50 kb of genomic DNA, preceded by the two alternative first exons$_{1A}$ and exon$_{1B}$ at a distance of 19 and 194 kb, respectively. Transcription from these two first exons is directed by their individual promoter sequences. These putative promoters lack TATA and CAAT boxes, but do contain multiple GGGCGG repeats within a GC-rich surrounding, characteristic for the SP1 transcription factor binding site (Dynan et al., 1986). Furthermore, no differential expression of the 6- and 7-kb transcripts has been observed; both are expressed at a constant low level in all tissues examined (Westin, 1982). These findings are consistent with a role of c-*abl* as a "housekeeping" gene in all cells, like hypoxanthine phosphoribosyltransferase (HPRT) and

The human c-*abl* gene

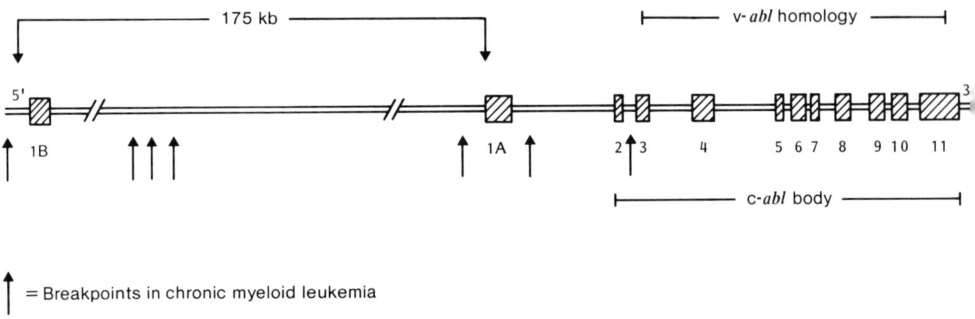

Figure 2 The human c-*abl* gene. The two alternative first exons, 1B and 1A, and the c-*abl* body exons$_{2-11}$ are indicated as hatched boxes. Distances between exons$_{1A}$ and exon$_{1B}$ and the position of the v-*abl* homologous part of the gene are shown above the map. The cloned and analyzed breakpoints are indicated by arrows below the map. =//= represents a gap of DNA that has not been cloned.

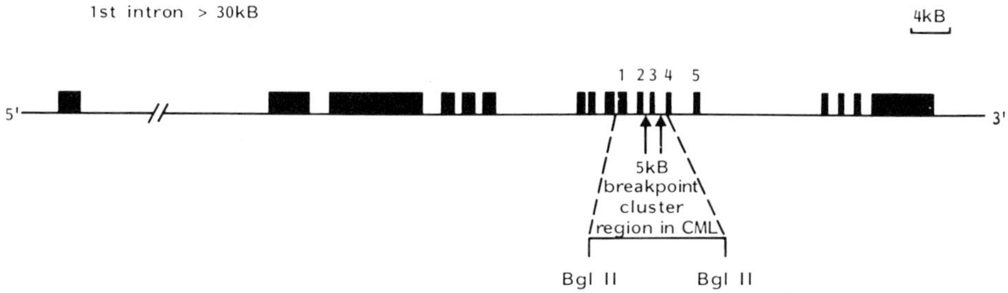

Figure 3 The human *bcr* gene. The black boxes indicate approximate positions of exons. —//— indicates a gap of unknown size in cloned sequences. Exons$_{1-4}$ are part of the breakpoint cluster region (*bcr*). Arrows point to documented breakpoints in CML.

adenosine deaminase (ADA), which have a similar type of promoter structure (Melton et al., 1986; Valerio et al., 1985).

Additional c-*abl* transcripts have been described (of 2.5 and 10 kb) in human leukemias (de Kretser et al., 1986). Furthermore, a 12-kb mRNA is transcribed from an Abelson-related gene (Arg). This gene is located on chr. 1q24-q25 and part of it has recently been isolated (Kruh et al., 1986). In mouse testis, a 4.5-kb c-*abl* mRNA is specifically expressed at a high level in haploid spermatids (Ponzetto and Wolgemuth, 1985). cDNA cloning experiments reveal that the germ cell–specific c-*abl* mRNA is generated by curtailment at the 3′ end through the use of an uncommon polyadenylation site situated 1 kb upstream from the normal polyA signal. The open reading frame in the 4.5-kb mRNA remains unaltered (D. Meijer, submitted).

The human c-*abl* gene encodes a 145-kd protein (p145$^{c\text{-}abl}$), which can be immunoprecipitated by c-*abl* antibodies directed against internal and carboxyterminal domains of the protein. Immunoprecipitated p145$^{c\text{-}abl}$ can carry out in vitro tyrosine-specific kinase reactions by both trans- and autophosphorylation mechanisms (Konopka and Witte, 1985). In cell fractionation experiments, both a membrane-bound and a cytoplasmic pool of c-*abl* proteins is observed. Those two pools probably represent the translational products of the 7-kb (type 1B) and 6-kb (type 1A) mRNAs, respectively. Type 1A mRNA contains an open reading frame of 1130 aa, whereas type 1B has a 1148-aa open reading frame, starting with Met-Gly at its NH_2-terminal. The Met-Gly sequence is a potential myristilation site and NH_2-terminal myristic acid addition to the protein is thought to anchor it to the inner side of the cell membrane (Cross et al., 1984). The 1A-type *abl* protein on the other hand lack such a myristilation site (Shtivelman et al., 1986). Therefore, the

1A-type *abl* protein is probably part of the soluble cytoplasmatic fraction.

A second open reading frame (p18) was found in the 3′ untranslated region of the mouse v-*abl* gene, which is virtually identical in sequence to the mouse c-*abl* gene (Wang et al., 1984). However, antibodies raised against bacterially expressed p18 open reading frame sequences do not detect a protein product in mouse cells (Konopka and Witte, 1985). Furthermore, direct sequence comparison between mouse and human c-*abl* cDNAs shows no conservation of the p18 open reading frame in man (A. Hermans, unpublished data).

In conclusion, the c-*abl* gene encodes two polypeptides displaying a tyrosine kinase enzymatic activity in vitro. The c-*abl* proteins lack several characteristics of receptor polypeptides; there are no signal peptides, no extracellular or transmembrane domains, and they have a cytoplasmic subcellular localization (Shtivelman et al., 1986).

The Human *bcr* Gene

The human *bcr* gene on chr. 22 was discovered by cloning of a chimeric breakpoint fragment from a CML patient (Heisterkamp et al., 1983). From this fragment, a chr. 22–specific probe was prepared, and subsequent Southern blot analysis of the DNA of a number of CML patients showed that chr. 22 breakpoints mapped in a stretch of 5.8 kb of DNA (Groffen et al., 1984). This area on chr. 22 has been designated the breakpoint cluster region (*bcr*). The isolation of cDNAs hybridizing to *bcr* probes established this region as part of a protein-encoding locus. The *bcr* gene is oriented with its 5′ end pointing toward the centromere of chr. 22. A minimum of 18 exons have been identified to date, which are dispersed over ± 90 kb of the human genome (Groffen et al., 1986; and unpublished data). The *bcr* contains four small exons, designated b1 to b4. Almost all chr. 22 breaks in CML occur in the introns between $exon_{b2}$ and $exon_{b3}$ or $exon_{b3}$ and $exon_{b4}$ (Fig. 3). Recently, a small number of CMLs have been investigated that lack breakpoints in the *bcr*. Further analysis showed these breaks to map further upstream in the *bcr* gene (C. Bartram and L. Selleri, personal communication).

Transcription of the *bcr* gene occurs at a low level in all tissues examined, which clearly indicates that *bcr* is not specifically expressed in myeloid cells (M. von Lindern, in preparation). From the *bcr* gene, a 4.5-and a 7-kb mRNA are transcribed (Stam et al., 1985). The cDNA of the 4.5-kb mRNA has been cloned and sequence analysis identifies an open reading frame of 1271 amino acids, which fails to show homology with any known protein sequence (Hariharan and Adams, 1987; Heisterkamp et al., 1985; Mess Masson et al., 1986). Probes covering the entire 4.5-kb *bcr* cDNA all hybridize to the 7-kb *bcr* transcript. The most plausible explanation is that the 7-kb mRNA represents an alternative splicing product from the *bcr* locus, containing one or more extra exons comprising 1.5 kb of transcribed sequences.

Several investigators employed *bcr*-specific antibodies to detect *bcr* proteins by immunoprecipitation (Ben Neriah et al., 1986b; Stam et al., 1987). *bcr* phosphoproteins are reported with molecular weights of 160 and 190 kd, exhibiting an associated protein kinase activity. It has not been demonstrated, however, whether this kinase activity is intrinsic to the *bcr* gene product, or that it derives from a protein coprecipitated in a complex with p160/190 *bcr*.

The *bcr-abl* Juxtaposition

The Philadelphia translocation results in a head-to-tail joining of *bcr* and c-*abl* sequences on Ph^1 (see Fig. 1). Thus, the 5 ′ part of the *bcr* gene (centromeric) is linked to the translocated c-*abl* sequences (telomeric) in the same transcriptional orientation (see Fig. 5). This new genomic configuration consists of a relatively constant amount of *ber* gene sequences; the absence of $exon_{b3}$ (75 bp) represents the only variation, depending on the exact breakpoint in the *bcr*. (see arrows Fig. 3) (Grosveld et al., 1986; Heisterkamp et al., 1985; Shtivelman et al., 1986). The amount of c-*abl* sequences that are translocated can vary from the whole c-*abl* locus (most 5 ′ breakpoint as indicated by an arrow in Fig. 2), to only the *abl* body $exons_{3-11}$ (Fig. 2) (most 3 ′ breakpoint described: L. Hoefsloot, in preparation). This indicates, however, that in all cases of CML the tyrosine kinase domain of the c-*abl* homologous part of c-*abl* is translocated to Ph^1.

An important consideration is whether the *bcr-abl* juxtaposition on the Ph^1 influences the transcription of these genes. Northern blot analysis showed the existence of a novel 8.5-kb mRNA (Canaani et al., 1984), hybridizing both to 5 ′ *bcr* and c-*abl* probes (Grosveld et al., 1986; Stam et al., 1985). This novel 8.5-kb mRNA seems to be specific for Ph^1-positive CML cells, as it is not detected in either normal cells, different tissues, or other types of leukemia (Gale and Canaani, 1984; Grosveld et al., 1986; Romero et al., 1986). These results strongly suggested that the 8.5-kb mRNA is a chimeric molecule that contains the 5 ′ part of the *bcr* coding sequences coupled to c-*abl* body exons.

Direct proof for this hypothesis was provided by cloning of chimeric *bcr*/c-*abl* cDNAs (Grosveld et al., 1986; Mes-Masson, 1986; Shtivelman et al., 1985). These cDNAs indeed contain 5 ′ coding regions of the *bcr* gene fused to c-*abl* coding sequences (see Fig. 4) in a splice-dependent manner, following the GT-AG rule (Breathnach and Chambon, 1981). Transcription of the fusion gene is initiated from the *bcr* promoter and terminates at

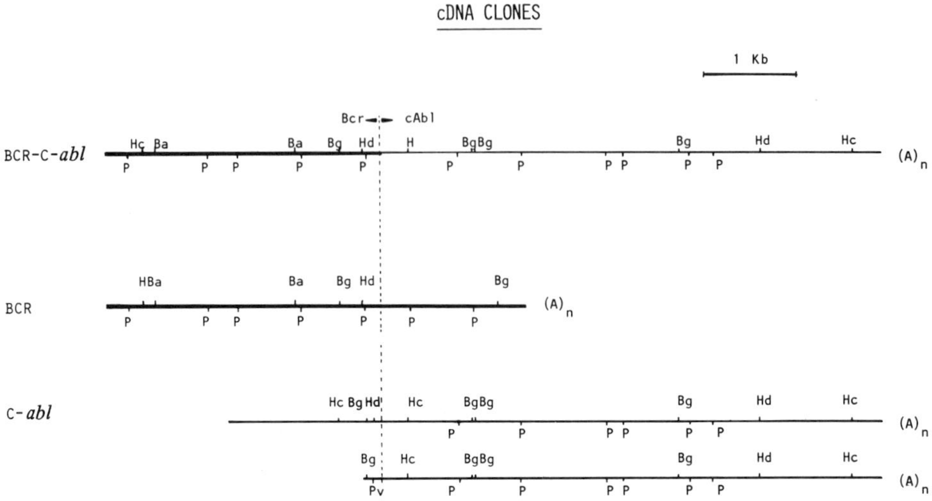

Figure 4 Restriction maps of full-length human *bcr/abl*, *bcr*, and *abl* cDNAs. The four bars from top to bottom represent the full-length cDNAs of: *bcr/abl*, 4.5-kb *bcr*, type B *abl*, and type A *abl*. The stippled line across the figure indicates the position of the breakpoint in the *bcr/abl* cDNA, the *bcr* cDNA, and the two *abl* cDNAs. The c-*abl* sequences to the right of the stippled line represent the body exons of the gene. Ba = BamHI, Bg = BglII, Hc = HindII, Hd = HindIII, P = PstI.

the 3′ end of the c-*abl* gene (Fig. 4). The mature 8.5-kb mRNA is produced by splicing of the precursor RNA, in which the versatility of the splicing system accomodates for the large variation in intron size that is present between the *bcr* and c-*abl* exons in different patients. The breakpoint on chr. 22 defines whether *bcr* $exon_{b2}$ or $exon_{b3}$ will be spliced to the first available c-*abl* exon with a splice-acceptor site, which is almost always *abl* $exon_2$. One exception appeared to be a patient in which the chr. 9 breakpoint occurred between *abl* $exon_2$ and $exon_3$, resulting in a *ber* $exon_{b2}$-*abl* $exon_3$ joining (L. Hoefsloot, in preparation). This indicates that the 8.5-kb mRNA can differ in the presence or absence of one *bcr* or one *abl* exon ($exon_{b3}$: 75 nucleotides; *abl* $exon_2$: 174 nucleotides in size). Deoxyribonucleic acid sequence data, however, revealed that all these different splice combinations yield RNA with one long *bcr-abl* open reading frame because the *bcr* gene open reading frame is in phase with the c-*abl* open reading frame (a schematic representation is depicted in Fig. 5).

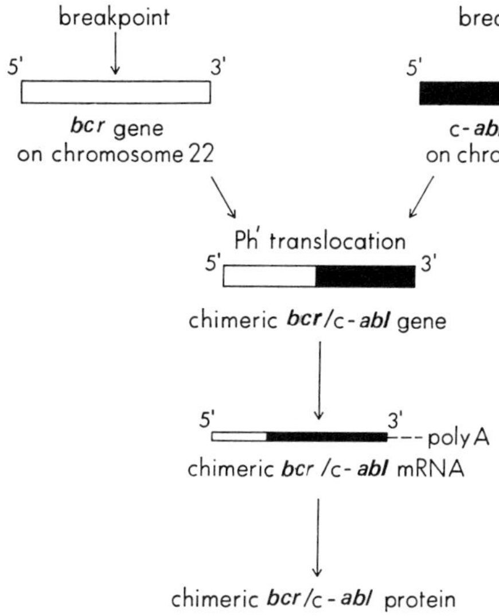

Figure 5 Schematic representation of the consequences of the Philadelphia translocation.

Translation of the 8.5-kb mRNA results in a *bcr-abl* fusion protein of 210 kd (p210$^{bcr\text{-}abl}$), which was shown to be present in several CML-derived cell lines and Ph^1-positive CML patients (Ben Neriah et al., 1986b; Stam et al., 1987). This p210$^{bcr\text{-}abl}$ contains 902/927 aa from *bcr*, and 1104/930 aa derived from c-*abl*, and is distinct in size from the normal p145$^{c\text{-}abl}$ and p160^{bcr}.

p210$^{bcr\text{-}abl}$ is like its viral counterpart p160$^{gag\text{-}abl}$, a fusion protein in which the NH_2-terminal part of *abl* has been replaced by NH_2-terminal *bcr* or *gag* residues, respectively. p160$^{gag\text{-}abl}$ has a tyrosine kinase activity which is directly associated with its transforming capacity (Prywes, 1985a,b). Interestingly, p210$^{bcr\text{-}abl}$ closely resembles the in vitro kinase properties of p160$^{gag\text{-}abl}$ (Konopka et al., 1984), and the c-*abl* tyrosine kinase domain is always present in p210$^{bcr\text{-}abl}$. However, important differences between the human and the viral c-*abl* fusion proteins need to be considered. In the viral protein, the NH_2-terminal *gag* sequences provide a myristilation site, which is indispensible for the transforming capacity of p160$^{gag\text{-}abl}$ (Rein et al., 1986). The NH_2-terminal of the *bcr* gene does not provide a potential myristilation site, and lacks any sequence homology with gag sequences. Furthermore, full-length *bcr-abl* cDNAs under control of various promoters (*bcr* promoter, Moloney murine leukemia virus long terminal repeat (LTR) simian vacuolating virus 40) fail to transform NIH3T3 fibroblasts in vitro (A. Hermans, unpublished observations). Thus, the possibility that p210$^{bcr\text{-}abl}$ exclusively transforms hematopoietic/myeloid cells needs to be investigated.

These observations clearly establish that on Ph^1 in the leukemic cells of CML patients, the *bcr-abl* juxtaposition results in the consistent formation of a *bcr-abl* hybrid mRNA, which is translated into a p210$^{bcr\text{-}abl}$ fusion protein (Fig. 5). This strongly suggests a crucial role for this protein product in the pathogenesis of CML.

Ph^1 IN ACUTE LEUKEMIA

Although Ph^1 is strongly associated with CML, its presence has also been reported in other hematological malignancies, including different subtypes of acute leukemia, in which no preceding chronic phase has been observed (Beard et al., 1976; Bloomfield et al., 1978; Sandberg, 1980). These de novo acute leukemias closely resemble the acute phase (blast crisis) of CML, and the clinical distinction between blast crisis of CML and acute leukemia is not always clear (Beard et al., 1976; Catovsky, 1979). However, the blast crisis of CML is usually accompanied by additional nonrandom chromosomal aberrations such as trisomy 8 or 19, or a second Philadelphia chromosome or isochromosome 17q (Champlin and Golde, 1985), Furthermore, the persistence of Ph^1-negative cells in the bone marrow during the acute phase and the disappearance of Ph^1 during remission are typical characteristics of cases presenting as Ph^1-positive acute leukemia (Sandberg, 1980).

In adult acute lymphoblastic leukemia (ALL), Ph^1 is the most frequently observed chromosomal abnormality, with an incidence of 17–25% (LeBeau and Rowley, 1984). A lower incidence has been reported for childhood ALL (2–6%) (Chessels et al., 1979; Priest et al., 1980) and acute myeloblastic leukemia (AML) (•1%) (Abe and Sandberg, 1979; Yunis et al., 1984). Cytogenetically, Ph^1 of ALL and AML is indistinguishable from Ph^1 of CML and is usually the result of a t(9;22)(q34;q11). As in CML, a consistent translocation was observed of the c-*abl* oncogene to Ph^1 in the Ph^1-positive leukemic ALL cells (De Klein et al., 1986; Erikson et al., 1986). However, molecular studies showed a heterogeneous picture using *bcr* probes and Southern blot analysis; some of the Ph^1-positive ALL patients showed *bcr* rearrangements, whereas other Ph^1-positive ALL patients lack such rearrangements (De Klein et al., 1986; Erikson et al., 1986; Rodenhuis et al., 1985). In the leukemic cells of those ALL patients with *bcr* rearrangements, the additional 8.5-kb chimeric *bcr*/c-*abl* mRNAs as well the p210$^{bcr\text{-}abl}$ fusion were present. In the ALL patients without *bcr* rearrangement, only the normal *bcr* and c-*abl* mRNA species were found (Chan et al., 1987; De Klein et al., 1986; Erikson et al., 1986), or as in two cases, additional c-*abl* mRNA transcripts of 6.5 and 7.4 kb were present (Clark et al., 1987; Kurzrock et al., 1987). Although lacking *bcr* rearrangements, these ALL patients express a novel p180- to p190-kd c-*abl* protein ($p190^{c\text{-}abl}$) with enhanced tyrosine kinase activity (Chan et al., 1987; Clark et al., 1987; Kurzrock et al., 1987). Since in one Ph¹-positive ALL patient, who expresses the $p190^{c\text{-}abl}$, the breakpoint in the c-*abl* oncogene is located 3′ of the c-*abl* first $exon_{1A}$ Chan et al., 1987), it is conceivable that the $p190^{c\text{-}abl}$ ALL-specific protein is a fusion product between the protein encoded by the c-*abl* body exons and other chr. 22 sequences. In situ hybridization experiments and Southern blot analysis of somatic cell hybrids suggested that these chr. 22 sequences are located proximal (5′) of the breakpoint cluster region of the *bcr* gene (Erikson et al., 1986). It is not known whether these sequences are located within or to the 5′ side of the *bcr* gene.

Initially it was suggested that only the pediatric Ph¹-positive ALL patients would have chr. 22 breakpoints outside the *bcr* (Erikson et al., 1986; Rodenhuis et al., 1985). However, also adult Ph¹-positive ALL patients lack *bcr* rearrangements (De Klein et al., 1986) and express the novel $p190^{c\text{-}abl}$ (Chan et al., 1987; Clark et al., 1987). Clark et al. (1987) demonstrated that the $p190^{c\text{-}abl}$ has a similar autophosphorylation pattern as the normal $p145^{c\text{-}abl}$, and it is expressed at elevated levels in the leukemic Ph¹-positive ALL cells. Enhanced tyrosine kinase activity or elevated protein levels of $p145^{c\text{-}abl}$ has been reported in one Ph¹-negative ALL patient (Chan et al., 1987). This could indicate that elevated tyrosine kinase activity rather than altered substrate specificity (as suggested for the $p210^{bcr\text{-}abl}$ and the viral $p160^{gag\text{-}abl}$) is important for the pathogenesis in ALL. This suggests that in some Ph¹-positive ALL patients, the change in the c-*abl* associated tyrosine kinase is caused by a different mechanism than the one found in CML patients. Thus, it is thought that Ph¹-positive ALL patients, who have molecular characteristics indistinguishable from CML patients, in fact are patients with a lymphoid blast crisis of CML, evolving from a clinically silent or short chronic phase (Chan et al., 1987; Kurzrock et al., 1987). However, these assumptions are based on the partial analysis of a limited number of Ph¹-positive ALL patients. Investigation of more Ph¹-positive hematopoietic malignancies and follow-up for a longer period will be necessary to corroborate the clinical and/or biological importance of these molecular differences among the Ph¹-positive leukemia patients.

CONCLUSIONS

Although the presence of the p210$^{bcr\text{-}abl}$ fusion protein is highly characteristic for Ph^1-positive CML, reports by Lisker et al. (1980) and Fialkow et al. (1981) suggest that acquisition of Ph^1 is not the initial abnormality in CML. Thus, other genes might be involved in the pathogenesis of CML. Several of these genes have been identified. By DNA-mediated transfection of NIH3T3 cells it was shown that some CML patients and CML-derived cell lines contain an activated N or K-*ras* gene (Eva et al., 1983; Hirai et al., 1985). Amplification and rearrangement of c-*myc* has been found in the acute phase of a CML patient (McCarthy et al., 1984), and may play a role in the progression of the disease. A similar role has been suggested for the expression of c-*sis* during accelerated/blast phase, but not in the chronic phase of CML (Romero et al., 1986). Moreover, several other as yet unidentified genes are specifically expressed in CML (Mars et al., 1985; Calabretta et al., 1986). In Ph^1-positive ALL, lacking breakpoints in the *bcr*, a novel *abl* protein, p190$^{c\text{-}abl}$, has been described. This finding suggests that alternative mechanisms of c-*abl* activation exist and may be important in the development of human acute lymphoid rather than chronic myeloid malignancies. Therefore, analysis of the biological effects of p210$^{bcr\text{-}abl}$ versus p190$^{c\text{-}abl}$ on normal hematopoietic cell proliferation is strongly indicated. Expression of full-length cDNAs in in vitro hematopoietic culture systems and in transgenic mice will be necessary to define the precise role of these proteins and hence of the Ph translocation in the pathogenesis of CML and ALL.

ACKNOWLEDGMENTS

The authors gratefully acknowledge Prof. D. Bootsma for continuous support, Rita Boucke for help in preparation of the manuscript, and Tar van Os for printing the illustrations. Part of this work was supported by the Netherlands Cancer Society (Koningin Wilhelmina Fonds).

REFERENCES

Abe, S., and Sandberg, A. (1979). Chromosomes and causation of human cancer and leukemia XXXII. *Cancer 43*: 2352–2364.

Bartram, C. R., de Klein, A., Hagemeijer, A., van Agthoven, T., Geurts, van Kessel, A., Bootsma, D., Grosveld, G., Ferguson-Smit, M. A., Davies, T., Stone, M., Heisterkamp, N, Stephenson, J. R., and Groffen, J. (1983).

Translocation of c-*abl* oncogene correlates with the presence of a Philadelphia chromosome in chronic myelocytic leukemia. *Nature 306*: 277–280.

Bartram, C. R., de Klein, A., Hagemeijer, A., Grosveld, G., Heisterkamp, N., and Groffen, J. (1984). Localization of the human c-*sis* oncogene in Ph[1]-positive and Ph[1]-negative chronic myelocytic leukemia by using in situ hybridization. *Blood 63*: 223–225.

Bartram, C. R., Kleihauer, E., De Klein, A., Grosveld, G. C., Teyssier, J. R., Heisterkamp, N., and Groffen, J. (1985). c-*abl* and *bcr* are rearranged in a Ph[1]-negative CML patient. *EMBO J. 4*: 683–686.

Beard, M., Durrant, J., Catovsky, D., Wiltshaw, E., Amess, J., Brearley, R., Krik, B., Wrigley, P., Janossy, G., Greaves, M., and Galton, D. A. G. (1976). Blast crisis of chronic myeloid leukaemia (CML) I. Presentation simulating acute lymphoid leukaemia (ALL). *Br. J. Haematol. 34*: 167–178.

Ben-Neriah, Y., Bernards, A., Paskin, M., Daley, G. Q., and Baltimore, D. (1986a). Alternative 5′ exons in c-*abl* mRNA. *Cell 44*: 577–586.

Ben-Neriah, Y., Daley, G. Q., Mes-Masson, A.-M., Witte, O. N., and Baltimore, D. (1986b). The chronic myelogenous leukemia-specific p210 protein is the product of the *bcr/abl* hybrid gene. *Science 233*: 212–214.

Bishop, J. M. (1985). Viral oncogenes. *Cell 42*: 23–38.

Bishop, J. M. (1987). The molecular genetics of cancer. *Science 253*: 305–311.

Bloomfield, C., Lindquist, L., Brunning, R., Yunis, J., and Coccia, P. (1978). The Philadelphia chromosome in acute leukemia. *Virchows Arch.* (*Cell Pathol.*) *29*: 81–91.

Breathnach, R., and Chambon, P. (1981). Organization and structure of eucaryotic split genes coding for proteins. *Ann. Rev. Biochem. 50*: 349–383.

Callabretta, B., Venturelli, D., Kaczmarek, L., Narni, F., Talpaz, M., Anderson, B., Beran, M., and Baserga, R. (1986). Altered expression of Gl-specific genes in human malignant myeloid cells. *Proc. Natl. Acad. Sci. U.S.A. 83*: 1495–1498.

Canaani, E., Gale, R. P., Steiner-Saltz, D., Berrebi, A., Aghai, E., and Januszewicz, E. (1984). Altered transcription of an oncogene in chronic myeloid leukemia. *Lancet* 593–595.

Catovsky, D. (1979). Ph[1]-positive acute leukemia and chronic granulocytic leukaemia: One or two diseases. *Br. J. Haematol. 42*: 493–498.

Champlin, R. E., and Golde, D. W. (1985). Chronic myelogenous leukemia: Recent advances. *Blood 65*: 1039–1047.

Chan, L. C., Karhi, K. K., Rayter, S. I., Heisterkamp, N., Eridani, S., Powles, R., Lawler, S. D., Groffen, J., Foulkes, J. G., Greaves, M. F., and Wiedemann, L. M. (1987). A novel *abl* protein expressed in Philadelphia chromosome positive acute lymphoblastic leukemia. *Nature 325*: 635–637.

Chessels, J. M., Janossy, G., Lawler, S. D., and Secker Walker, L. M. (1979). The Ph[1] chromosome in childhood leukaemia. *Br. J. Haematol. 41*: 25–41.

Clark, S. S., Mc Laughlin, J., Crist, W. M., Champlin, R., and Witte, O. N. (1987). Unique forms of the *abl* tyrosine kinase distinguish Ph[1]-positive CML from Ph[1]-positive ALL. *Science 235*: 85–88.

Cross, F. R., Garber, E. A., Pellman, D., and Hanafusa, H. (1984). A short sequence in the p60[src] N-terminus is required for p60[src] myristilation and membrane association and for cell transformation. *Mol. Cell. Biol. 4*: 1834–184.

De Klein, A., and Hagemeijer, A. (1984). Cytogenetic and molecular analysis of the Ph[1] translocation in chronic myeloid leukemia. *Cancer Surveys 3*: 515–529.

De Klein, A., Geurts van Kessel, A., Grosveld, G., Bartram, C. R., Hagemeijer, A., Bootsma, D., Spurr, N. K., Heisterkamp, N., Groffen, J., and Stephenson, J. R. (1982). A cellular oncogene is translocated to the Philadelphia chromosome in chronic myelocytic leukaemia. *Nature 300*: 765–767.

De Klein, A., Hagemeijer, A., Bartram, C. R., Houwen, R., Hoefsloot, L., Carbonell, F., Chan, L., Barnett, M., Greaves, M., Kleihauer, E., Heisterkamp, N., Groffen, J., and Grosveld, G. (1986). *bcr* rearrangement and translocations of the c-*abl* oncogene in Philadelphia positive acute lymphoblastic leukemia. *Blood 68*: 1369–1375.

de Kretser, T., Adams, F., Devereux, L., Garson, M., Michael, P., and Keith, S. (1986). Elevation of c-*abl* mRNA in human leukemic B lymphoblasts. *Leuk. Res. 12*: 1391–1399.

Dynan, W. S., Sazer, S., Tjian, R., and Schimke, R. (1986). Transcription factor Spl recognizes a DNA sequence in the mouse dihydrofolate reductase promoter. *Nature 319*: 246–248.

Erikson, J., Griffen, C. A., Ar-Rushid, A., Valtieri, M., Hoxie, J., Finan, J., Emanuel, B. S., Rovera, G., Nowell, P. C., and Croce, C. M. (1986). Heterogeneity of chromosome 22 breakpoints in Philadelphia positive (Ph^+) acute lymphocytic leukemia. *Proc. Natl. Acad. Sci. U.S.A. 83*: 1807–1811.

Eva, A., Tronick, S. R., Gol, R. A., Pierce, J. H., and Aaronson, S. A. (1983). Transforming genes of human hematopoietic tumors: Frequent detection of ras-related oncogenes whose activation appears to be independent of tumor phenotype. *Proc. Natl. Acad. Sci. U.S.A. 80*: 4926–4930.

Fialkow, P. J., Martin, P. J., Najfeld, V., Penfold, G. K., Jacobson, R. J., and Hansen, J. A. (1981). Evidence for a multistep pathogenesis of chronic myelogenous leukemia. *Blood 58*: 158–163.

Gale, R. P., and Canaani, E. (1984). An 8-kilobase *abl* RNA transcript in chronic myelogenous leukemia. *Proc. Natl. Acad. Sci. U.S.A. 81*: 5648–5652.

Ganesan, T. S., Rassool, F., Guo, A. P., Th'ng, K. H., Dowding, C., Hibbin, J. A., Young, B. D., White, H., Kumaran, T. O., Galton, D. A. G., and Goldman, J. M. (1986). Rearrangement of the *bcr* gene in Philadelphia chromosome-negative chronic myeloid leukemia. *Blood 68*: 957–960.

Goddard, J. M., Weiland, J. J., and Capecchi, M. R. (1986). Isolation and characterization of caenorhabditis elegans DNA sequences homologous to the v-*abl* gene. *Proc. Natl. Acad. Sci. U.S.A. 83*: 2172–2176.

Goff, S. P., and Baltimore, D. (1982). The cellular oncogene of the Abelson murine leukemia virus genome. *Adv. Viral Oncol. 1*: 127–139.

Goff, S. P., Gilboa, E., Witte, O. N., and Baltimore, D. (1980). Structure of the Abelson murine leukemia virus genome and the homologous cellular gene: Studies with cloned viral DNA. *Cell 22*: 777–785.

Groffen, J., Heisterkamp, N., Stephenson, J. R., Geurts van Kessel, A. G., De Klein, A., Grosveld, G., and Bootsma, D. (1983). c-*sis* is translocated from chromosome 22 to chromosome 9 in chronic myelocytic leukemia. *J. Exp. Med. 158*: 9–15.

Groffen, J., Stephenson, J. R., Heisterkamp, N., De Klein, A., Bartram, C. R., and Grosveld, G. (1984). Philadelphia chromosomal breakpoints are clustered within a limited region, *bcr*, on chromosome 22. *Cell 36*: 93–99.

Groffen, J. Heisterkamp, N., Stam, K., de Klein, A., and Grosveld, G. (1986). Activation of c-*abl* as a result of the Ph^1 translocation in chronic myelocytic leukemia. *Adv. Viral Oncol.*

Grosveld, G., Verwoerd, T., van Agthoven, T., de Klein, A., Ramachandran, K. L., Heisterkamp, N., Stam, K., and Groffen, J. (1986). The chronic myelocytic cell line K562 contains a breakpoint in bcr and produces a chimeric *bcr*/c-*abl* transcript. *Mol. Cell. Biol. 6*: 607–616.

Hagemeijer, A., De Klein, A., G8odde-Salz, Turc-Carel, C., Smit, E. M. E., van Agthoven, T., and Grosveld, G. (1985). Translocation of c-*abl* to masked Ph in chronic myeloid leukemia. *Cancer Genet. Cytogenet. 18*: 95–104.

Hariharan, I. K., and Adams, J. M. (1987). cDNA sequence for human *bcr*, the gene that translocates to the *abl* oncogene in chronic myeloid leukaemia. *EMBO J. 6*: 115–119.

Heim, S., Billstr8om, R., Kristoffersson, U., Mandahl, Str8ombeck, B., and Mitelman, F. (1985). Variant Ph translocations in chronic myeloid leukemia. *Cancer Genet. Cytogenet. 18*: 215–227.

Heisterkamp, N., Groffen, J., Stephenson, J. R., Spurr, N. K., Goodfellow, P. N., Solomon, E., Carritt, B., and Bodmer, W. F. (1982). Chromosomal localization of human cellular homologues of two viral oncogenes. *Nature 299*: 747–749.

Heisterkamp, N., Stephenson, J. R., Groffen, J., Hansen, P. F., de Klein, A., Bartram, C. R., and Grosveld, G. (1983). Localization of the c-*abl* oncogene adjacent to the translocation breakpoint in chronic myelocytic leukemia. *Nature 306*: 239–242.

Heisterkamp, N., Stam, K., Groffen, J., de Klein, A., and Groffen, G. (1985). Structural organization of the *bcr* gene and its role in the Ph^1 translocation. *Nature 315*: 758–761.

Hira, H., Tanaka, S., Azuma, M., Anruka, Y., Kobayashi, Y., Fujisawa, M., Okabe, T., Urabe, A., and Takaku, F. (1985). Transforming genes in human leukemia cells. *Blood 66*: 1371–1378.

Hoffmann-Falk, H., Einat, D., Shilo, B. Z., and Hoffman, F. M. (1983). Drosophila melanogaster DNA clones, homologous to vertebrate oncogenes: Evidence for a common ancester to the *src* and *abl* cellular genes. *Cell 32*: 589–598.

Klein, G. (1981). The role of gene dosage and genetic transpositions in carcinogenesis. *Nature 294*: 313–318.

Kanopka, J. B., and Witte, O. N. (1985). Activation of the *abl* oncogene in murine and human leukemias. *Bioch.et Biophys. Acta 823*: 1–17.

Konopka, J. B., Watanbe, S. M., and Witte, O. M. (1984). An alteration of the human c-*abl* protein in K562 leukemia cells unmasks associated tyrosine kinase activity. *Cell 37*: 1035–1042.

Kruh, G. D., King, C. R., Kraus, M. H., Popescu, N. C., Amsbaugh, S. C., McBride, W. O., and Aaronson, S. A. (1986). A novel human gene closely related to the *abl* proto-oncogene. *Science 234*: 1545–1548.

Kurzrock, R., Shtalrid, M., Romero, P., Kloetzer, W. S., Talpas, M., Trujillo, J. M., Blick, M., Beran, M., and Gutterman, J. U. (1987). A novel c-*abl* protein product in Philadelphia-positive acute lymphoblastic leukaemia. *Nature 325*: 631–635.

LeBeau, M. M., and Rowley, J. R. (1984). Recurring chromosomal abnormalities in leukemia and lymphoma. *Cancer Surveys 3*: 371–394.

Lisker, R., Casas, L., Mutchinick, O., Perez-Chavez, F., and Labardini, J. (1980). Late-appearing Philadelphia chromosome in two patients with chronic myelogenous leukemia. *Blood 56*: 812–814.

Mars, W., Florine, D., Talpaz, M., and Sauders, G. (1985). Preferentially expressed genes in chronic myelogenous leukemia. *Blood 65*: 1218–1225.

Melton, D. W., McEwan, C., McKie, A. B., and Reid, A. M. (1986). Expression of the mouse HPRT gene: Deletional analysis of the promoter region of an X-chromosome linked housekeeping gene. *Cell 44*: 319–328.

Mes-Masson, A.-M., McLaughlin, J., Daley, G. Q., Paskind, M., and Witte, O. N. (1986). Overlapping cDNA clones define the complete coding region for the $p210^{c\text{-}abl}$ gene product associated with chronic myelogenous leukemia cells containing the Philadelphia chromosome. *Proc. Natl. Acad. Sci. U.S.A. 83*: 9768–9772.

McCarthy, D., Rassool, F., Goldman, J., Graham, S., and Birnie, G. (1984). Genomic alterations involving the c-*myc* proto-oncogene locus during the evolution of a case of chronic granulocytic leukaemia. *Lancet 2*: 1362–1365.

Mitelman, F. (1985). Catalog of chromosome aberrations in cancer. In *Progress and Topic in Cytogenetics,* vol. 5 (Sandberg, A. A., ed.)

Morris, C. M., Reeve, A. E., Fritzgerald, P. H., Hollings, P. E., Beard, M. E. J., and Heaton, D. C. (1986). Genomic diversity correlates with clinical variation in Ph^1-negative chronic myeloid leukemia. *Nature 330*: 281–283.

Nowell, P. C., and Hungerford, D. A. (1960). A minute chromosome in human chronic granulocytic leukemia. *Science 132*: 1497.

Ponzetto, C., and Wolgemuth, D. J. (1985). Haploid expression of a unique c-*abl* transcript in the mouse male germ line. *Mol. Cell. Biol. 5*: 1791–1794.

Priest, J. R., Robinson, L. L., McKenna, R. W., Lindquist, L. L., Warkentin, P. I., LeBien, T. W., Woods, W. G., Kersey, J. H., Coccia, P. F., and Nesbit, M. E. (1980). Philadelphia chromosome positive childhood acute lymphoblastic leukemia. *Blood 56*: 15–22.

Prywes, R., Hoag, J., Rosenberg, N., and Baltimore, D. (1985a). Protein stabilization explains the *gag* requirement for transformation of lymphoid cells by Abelson murine leukemia virus. *J. Virol. 54*: 123–132.

Prywes, R., Foulkes, J. G., and Baltimore, D. (1985b). The minimum transforming region of v-*abl* is the segment encoding protein-tyrosine kinase. *J. Virol. 54*: 114–122.

Pugh, W. C., Pearson, M., Vardiman, J. W., and Rowley, J. D. (1985). Philadelphia chromosome-negative chronic myelogenous leukemia: A morphological reassesement. *Br. J. Haematol. 60*: 457–467.

Rein, A., McClure, M., and Schultz, A. (1986). The myristilation site is required for transformation by the *gag-abl* product of Abelson murine leukemia virus. 14th Int. Cancer Congress, Augest, Budapest, Hungary.

Rodenhuis, S., Smets, L. A., Slater, R. M., Bchrendt, H., and Veerman, A. J. P. (1985). Distinguishing the Philadelphia chromosome of acute lymphoblastic leukemia from its counterpart in chronic myelogenous leukemia. *N. Engl. J. Med. 313*: 51–52.

Romero, P., Blick, M., Talpaz, M., Murphy, E., Hester, J., and Gutterman, J. (1986). c-*sis* and c-*abl* expression in chronic myelogenous leukemia and other hematologic malignancies. *Blood 67*: 839–841.

Rowley, J. D. (1973). A new consistent chromosomal abnormality in chronic myelogenous leukaemia identified by quinacrine fluorescence and Giemsa staining. *Nature 243*: 290–293.

Rowley, J. D. (1983). Human oncogene locations and chromosome aberrations. *Nature 301*: 290–291.

Rowley, J. D., and Testa, J. R. (1982). Chromosome abnormalities in malignant hematologic disease. *Adv. Canc. Res. 36*: 103–148.

Sandberg, A. A. (1980). *The Chromosomes in Human Cancer and Leukemia.* Elsevier/North Holland, New York.

Schalken, J. A., van den Ouweland, A. W. M., Bloemers, H. P. J., and van de Ven, J. W. M. (1985). Characterization of the feline c-*abl* proto-oncogene. *Biochem. Biophys. Acta 824*: 104–112.

Shilo, B. Z., and Weinberg, R. A. (1981). DNA sequences homologous to vertebrate oncogenes are conserved in *Drosophila melanogaster. Proc. Natl. Acad. Sci. U.S.A. 78*: 6789–6792.

Shtivelman, E., Lifshitz, B., Gale, R. P., and Canaani, E. (1985). Fused transcript of *abl* and *bcr* genes in chronic myelogenous leukaemia. *Nature 315*: 550–554.

Shtivelman, E., Lifshitz, B., Gale, R. P., Roe, B. A., and Canaani, E. (1986). Alternative splicing of RNAs transcribed from the human *abl* gene and from the *bcr-abl* fused gene (1986). *Cell 47*: 277–284.

Stam, K., Heisterkamp, N., Grosveld, G., de Klein, A., Verma, R. S., Coleman, M., Dosik, H., and Groffen, J. (1985). Evidence of a new chimeric *bcr*/c-*abl* mRNA in patients with chronic myelocytic leukemia and the Philadelphia chromosome. *N. Engl. J. Med. 313*: 1429–1433.

Stam, K., Heisterkamp, N., Reynolds, Jr., F. H., and Groffen, J. (1987). Evidence that the ph1 gene encodes a 160.000 dalton phosphoprotein with associated kinase activity. *Mol. Cell. Biol.* 1955–1960.

Travis, L. B., Pierre, R. V., and DeWald, G. W. (1986). Ph^1-negative chronic granulocytic leukemia: A nonentity. *Am. J. Clin. Pathol. 85*: 186–193.

Valerio, D., Duyvesteyn, M. G. C., Dekker, B. M. M., Weeda, G., Berkvens, T. M., van der Voorn, L., van Ormondt, H., and van der Eb, A. J. (1985). Adenosine deaminase: Characterization and expression of a gene with a remarkable promoter. *EMBO J. 4*: 437–443.

Varmus, H. E. (1984). The molecular genetics of cellular oncogenes. *Ann. Rev. Genet. 18*: 553–612.

Wang, J. Y. J., Ledley, F., Goff, S., Lee, R., Groner, Y., and Baltimore, D. (1984). The mouse c-*abl* locus: Molecular cloning and characterization. *Cell 36*: 349–356.

Weinberg, R. A. (1985). The action of oncogenes in the cytoplasm and nucleus. *Science 230*: 770–776.

Westin, E. H., Wong-Staal, F., Gelamnn, E. P., Dalla Favera, R., Papas, T. S., Lautenberg, J. A., Eva, M., Reddy, E. P., Tronick, S. R., Aaronson, S. A., and Gallo, R. C. (1982). Expression of cellular cells. *Proc. Natl. Acad. Sci. U.S.A. 79*: 2490–2494.

Yunis, J. J. (1983). The chromosomal basis of human neoplasia. *Science 221*: 227–236.

Yunis, J. J., Brunning, R. D., Howe, R. B., and Lobell, A. (1984). High-resolution chromosomes as an independent prognostic indicator in adult acute nonlymphocytic leukemia. *N. Engl. J. Med. 311*: 812–818.

TEN

Oncogene Amplification and Tumor Progression

Steven J. Collins and Mark Groudine
Fred Hutchinson Cancer Research Center and University of Washington School of Medicine Seattle, Washington

INTRODUCTION

There is considerable evidence that cancer results from a genetic mutation or series of mutations. Studies with the X-linked glucose-6-phosphate dehydrogenase (G-6-PD) marker indicate that most human malignancies are clonal (1), suggesting the occurrence of a rare event(s) such as a somatic mutation in their development. Individuals with inherited defects in deoxyribonucleic acid (DNA) repair, such as Bloom's syndrome and xeroderma pigmentosa, are more susceptible to certain malignancies than normals (2). Most carcinogens are thought to act by binding to and altering DNA. Moreover, specific chromosome abnormalities are frequently demonstrated in certain malignancies, indicating the presence of specific genetic changes in these particular cancers. Until recently, the specific genes effected by mutations producing cancer were completely unknown. This situation has changed markedly in the past 5 years with the isolation and characterization of specific human genes (cellular oncogenes or proto-oncogenes) that appear to be intimately related to malignant transformation. Genomic amplification, point mutations and chromosome rearrangements involving these particular (onco)genes have been described in various human cancers and appear to be specific for malignant versus normal cells. This chapter will focus on the relationship between the presence of genomic amplification of particular cellular oncogenes and the development of human malignancies. The frequency of occurrence of oncogene amplification in different types of human cancers, the possible selective advantage that the presence of such oncogene amplification confers on the tumor cells, and the relationship between the presence of such oncogene amplification to the progression and prognosis of different human cancers will be discussed.

GENE AMPLIFICATION IN METHOTREXATE-RESISTANT CELLS

The prototype model system for the study of gene amplification in mammalian cells is the dihydrofolate reductase (DHFR) gene amplification that occurs in vitro when cells are grown under selective pressure in the presence of methotrexate. When certain rodent cells are cultured in progressively increasing concentrations of methotrexate, resistant cells are obtained which exhibit genomic amplification of the DHFR gene (3). With progressive increases in methotrexate concentration the copy number of the DHFR gene in highly resistant cells can be as high as 1000, and this amplified DNA can represent several percent of the total genome. This gene amplification is frequently associated with aberrant chromosome markers, including localized expansions of a single chromosome region, termed homogenous staining regions (HSRs) and small, paired chromosomal elements, termed double minutes (DMs). The amplified DHFR genes have been localized to both types of these chromosome markers in methotrexate-resistant cells (4,5). In general, stable methotrexate resistance is found in cells exhibiting HSRs, whereas cells exhibiting DMs display unstable resistance, since the unequal distribution of DMs at mitosis results in random loss of the amplified DHFR genes in progeny cells.

The mechanism by which such genomic amplification occurs in methotrexate-resistant cells remains unclear. Treatment of cultured cells with a number of different agents has been shown to increase the frequency of methotrexate-resistant cells exhibiting DHFR gene amplification. These agents include hydroxyurea (6), UV irradiation (7), the carcinogen *N*-acetoxy-*N*-acetylaminofluorene (7), the tumor promoter TPA (8), and transient hypoxia (9). It has been noted that one effect these agents have in common is the transient inhibition of DNA synthesis (9), and it has been postulated that if DNA synthesis is inhibited in the presence of active RNA and protein synthesis, removal of this block to DNA synthesis results in overreplication of DNA in a single cell cycle (10). Such overreplication of DNA in actively proliferating cells exposed to DNA-damaging agents could lead to random amplification of different genes. In the presence of selective pressure such random gene amplification could lead to selective growth advantage for some cells with specific genes being amplified (10).

Gene amplification also appears to occur more readily in genomically unstable, tumorigenic cells than in normal diploid cells. This has been demonstrated by comparing the response to methotrexate of the diploid nontumorigenic Chinese hamster embryo fibroblastic cell line CHEF/18 with the closely related but tumorigenic CHEF/16 cell line. When these cell lines were cultured in increasing concentrations of methotrexate, the tumorigenic CHEF/16 cells developed many more copies of the DHFR gene and displayed more chromosome abnormalities than the nontumorigenic CHEF/18 cells (11). This observation suggests that gene amplification may be more tightly regulated in normal versus transformed cells, and that one measure of genomic instability in transformed cells is the increased propensity to develop gene amplification under selective pressure.

These observations involving DHFR gene amplification in cultured methotrexate-resistant rodent cells offer considerable insight into the mechanisms, genetic structure, and pathogenetic significance of the oncogene amplification that has been observed in different types of human tumors. There are several significant parallels between experimental findings in the methotrexate-resistant cells and various observations regarding human tumors. These include the following:

1. Aberrant chromosome structures, including HSRs and DMs, are frequently noted on karyotypic examination of human tumor cells. These aberrant chromosome structures are virtually identical to similar structures noted in the methotrexate-resistant cells harboring amplified DHFR genes. In certain tumors, as noted below, there is direct evidence that these HSRs and DMs harbor amplified oncogene sequences.

2. The observation that the frequency of DHFR gene amplification in methotrexate-resistant cells is markedly augmented by treatment with carcinogens and tumor-promoting agents suggests that tumor initiation and progression by such agents may be related to their ability to promote (onco)gene amplification in specific target cells. Similarly, the enhanced frequency of DHFR amplification noted in hypoxic methotrexate-resistant cells suggests that the hypoxic state, which is frequently noted in portions of solid tumors with a compromised blood supply, may predispose such

tumors to the development of progressive (onco)gene amplification and further tumor evolution (9).

3. The observation that DHFR gene amplification occurs much more frequently in tumorigenic than in nontumorigenic cells suggests that tumor cells with their inherent genomic instability are predisposed to the development of gene amplification. This is consistent with the fact that while amplification of genomic sequences has been frequently observed in mammalian tumor cells, it has rarely, if ever, been noted in normal mammalian tissue.

4. Cultured cells harboring DHFR gene amplification have a distinct selective advantage in methotrexate-containing media. Although the physiological function of many oncogene products is presently unknown, by analogy to the methotrexate-resistant cells it is possible that the presence of specific oncogene amplification in tumor cells also provides such cells with a selective growth advantage over cells that do not harbor such oncogene amplification.

Thus, many of the observations in methotrexate-resistant cells harboring amplified DHFR genes are relevant to observations on human tumors. Specific oncogene amplification has been noted in a variety of different human cancers, including the leukemias, childhood neuroblastomas, lung cancer, various squamous cell cancers, and breast cancer. Each of these malignancies will be discussed separately below with particular emphasis on the frequency of occurrence of oncogene amplification in these various types of cancers and the relationship of the presence of such gene amplification to the pathogenesis and progression of the disease.

Oncogene Amplification in Leukemia

The first example of amplification of a particular cellular oncogene in a human malignancy was the observation that the c-*myc* oncogene was amplified some 20- to 30-fold in the HL-60 human promyelocytic leukemia cell line (12,13). This cell line was derived from a patient with acute promyelocytic leukemia (14), and can be induced to differentiate both to mature granulocytes upon exposure to agents such as dimethysulfoxide (DMSO) or retinoic acid (15,16) and to macrophagelike cells upon exposure to TPA (17). The c-*myc* oncogene is localized to the distal portion of the q arm of chromosome 8, and an aberrant staining region localized to 8q+ which by in situ hybridization hybridizes to a c-*myc* probe has been noted in cultured HL-60 cells (18). In association with this genomic amplification of c-*myc* HL-60 cells also display relatively high levels of c-*myc* ribonucleic acid (RNA) and protein product.

What is the significance of this genomic amplification of c-*myc* in HL-60 cells? Amplification of this cellular oncogene has also been noted in the fresh primary leukemic cells of the patient from whom the HL-60 cell culture was derived (13), indicating that the HL-60 c-*myc* amplification is not an in vitro artifact that arose with continuous cell culture. The normal physiological function of c-*myc* remains to be defined, but there is considerable circumstantial evidence that c-*myc* is somehow involved in controlling cell proliferation. The c-*myc* oncogene is defined by virtue of its homology to the transforming sequences of the avian MC-29 retrovirus, which primarily causes myeloid tumors in chickens. The c-*myc* product is localized to the nucleus (19), and normal resting cells when stimulated to divide express enhanced levels of c-*myc* prior to the initiation of S phase (20). In addition this oncogene acts in synergy with members of the *ras* family of oncogenes to malignantly transform primary rat fibroblast cultures in cotransfection studies (21). It has been suggested that c-*myc* may function in controlling the expression of certain genes that are essential for rendering cells competent to divide, or may be directly involved in DNA replication or RNA processing, but its exact physiological role remains to be defined. It is noteworthy that the steady-state level of c-*myc* RNA rapidly drops when HL-60 cells are induced to terminally differentiate with granulocytic or macrophage inducers.

It is also important to note that mutations involving other oncogenes have also been observed in HL-60 cells. For example, HL-60 DNA is capable of malignantly transforming NIH 3T3 cells in transfection assays, and this activity has been traced to a point mutation in the HL-60 N-*ras* oncogene (22,23). In addition, a significant deletion of the p53 oncogene has been observed in HL-60 (24). These latter findings further complicate the assessment of how c-*myc* amplification is related to the initiation and/or progression of the HL-60 leukemia. It is possible that the genomic amplification and overexpression of c-*myc* in HL-60 may have been an initiating event in the development of this malignancy and resulted in maintaining immature myeloid cells in a continuous state of proliferation. This subsequently could have increased the possibility of mutations in other genes such as p53 and N-*ras* which eventually could have resulted in full-blown malignancy. This is purely speculative, and the role each of these mutations may have played in the initiation and progression of the HL-60 leukemia remains to be defined. Nevertheless, these observations in HL-60 of mutations involving multiple different oncogenes serve to emphasize that the pathogenesis of malignancy is a multistage phenomenon: Leukemia probably results not from a single mutation but from a series of mutations.

Our initial observation of c-*myc* amplification in HL-60 cells prompted us to screen other fresh and cultured leukemic cells by Southern blot hybridization for the presence of an amplified *myc* oncogene. Of some 30 such leukemic samples screened none demonstrated any *myc* amplification. Using a similar approach involving over 100 fresh leukemia and lymphoma samples Rothberg et al. demonstrated *myc* amplification in only one other sample, a Burkitt's lymphoma (25). Other examples of c-*myc* amplification in human leukemia include the observation of amplified *myc* sequences in the blast phase of chronic myelogenous leukemia (26) and the presence of c-*myc* amplification in the leukemic cells of an elderly patient with acute myelogenous leukemia associated with the presence of DMs (27). These reports are anecdotal, and it appears that c-*myc* amplification in human leukemia is a relatively rare event. Nevertheless, it is clear from Rothberg's study as well as the work of others that enhanced expression of c-*myc* can occur in certain leukemia or lymphoma cells in the absence of c-*myc* genomic amplification (25), and in such malignancies this overexpression of c-*myc* could have contributed to the initiation or progression of the malignancy.

Amplification of the c-*abl* cellular oncogene has been noted in certain chronic myelogenous leukemia (CML) cells. Over 90% of cases of CML exhibit the Philadelphia chromosome (Ph^1), which results from a reciprocal translocation involving the distal portions of the q arms of chromosomes 9 and 22, and which is the most specific chromosome abnormality associated with any human malignancy. The c-*abl* oncogene is defined by virtue of its homology to v-*abl*, the transforming sequences of the Abelson murine leukemia virus. In CML, this cellular oncogene is translocated from its usual position on the distal end of chr. 9 to a relatively restricted region on the Ph^1, termed the breakpoint cluster region, or *bcr* (28). As a result of this translocation, a hybrid *bcr-abl* transcript (8 kb) is generated which codes for a *bcr-abl* fusion protein (p210) with enhanced tyrosine kinase activity (29–31). Although the physiological function of the c-*abl* oncogene is unknown, these findings indicate that abnormalities in the structure and expression of this oncogene may be critical to the pathogenesis of CML. We previously noted a four- to eightfold amplification of the *bcr-abl* fusion gene in the K-562 cell line, which was derived from a patient in CML blast crisis (32,33). This genomic amplification is associated with enhanced expression of the 8-kb *bcr-abl* fusion transcript. Interestingly the lambda immunoglobulin constant region locus is also amplified some four- to eightfold in this cell line, and in situ hybridization suggests that both the c-*abl* and C lambda immunoglobulin genes are tandemly amplified on an aberrant marker chromosome in K-562 (34). These observations suggest that both the *bcr-abl* fusion gene and the lambda immunoglobulin constant region locus reside on the same amplified unit in K-562. However, while K-562 cells exhibit enhanced expression of the *bcr-abl* fusion transcript, this cell line does not display any transcripts related to the lambda immunoglobulin constant region genes. These observations indicate that genomic amplification of a particular gene can occur in the absence of expression of the gene.

How frequent is amplification of the aberrant Philadelphia chromosome associated *bcr-abl* fusion gene in CML? Is the inevitable progression of CML from chronic phase to blast crisis associated with amplification and/or enhanced expression of the *bcr-abl* gene? In addition to K-562, we have noted enhanced expression of the *bcr-abl* hybrid transcript in the CML blast crisis cell lines EM-2 and KCL-22 (35). However, our Southern blot analysis indicated that these particular cell lines do not harbor amplified *bcr-abl* genes (35). This suggests that genetic mechanisms other than genomic amplification can also lead to enhanced expression of the *bcr-abl* fusion gene in CML. We have also analyzed the DNA from leukemic cells of several patients in blast crisis exhibiting multiple Ph^1 chromosomes per metaphase. The acquisition of multiple Ph^1 chromosomes is the most common karyotypic abnormality that arises during the evolution of CML from chronic phase to blast crisis. A restriction endonuclease analysis of leukemic cell DNA from these patients indicated that the extra Ph^1 chromosomes arose from duplication of the preexisting Ph^1's rather than from new 9:22 translocation events (36). Moreover, this analysis indicated that the level of *bcr-abl* gene amplification was directly related to the number of Ph^1's per metaphase, and suggested that a single copy of the *bcr-abl* fusion gene rather that multiple copies was present on each of the multiple Ph^1 chromosomes. In one of these patients, who presented in lymphoid blast crisis and displayed three Ph^1's per metaphase, we were able to isolate both chronic phase granulocytes and blast crisis cells. Although the level of the *bcr-abl* fusion transcript was some eight- to 16-fold higher in the lymphoid blast crisis cells versus the chronic phase granulocytes, nevertheless a restriction endocuclease analysis indicated that the *bcr-abl* fusion gene was amplified to a similar degree in both (37). This observation indicates that both the lymphoid blast crisis cells and the terminally differentiated granulocytes from this patient harbor multiple Ph^1 chromosomes, and suggests that the development of multiple Ph^1 chromosomes per se cannot be the sole genetic event that leads to the blast crisis phenotype. One would therefore predict that there are other genetic factors besides multiple Ph^1 chromosomes that distinguish the blast crisis from the chronic phase CML cells.

We have also quantitated the level of the aberrant *bcr-abl* fusion transcript in fresh patient CML cells at various stages of the disease to determine whether the progression of CML from chronic phase to blast crisis is associated with enhanced expression of this hybrid transcript. Chronic phase cells invariably displayed relatively low levels of the *bcr-abl* transcript. However, we have noted considerable heterogeneity in the level of this transcript in blast crisis cells with some blast crisis patients exhibiting relatively high levels of the fusion transcript comparable to levels expressed by K-562, whereas other blast crisis cells display relatively low levels comparable to that usually noted in chronic phase cells (38). Thus, enhanced expression of the *bcr-abl* fusion transcript is not necessarily associated with the progression of CML from chronic phase to blast crisis.

These observations on *bcr-abl* gene amplification and expression in CML can be summarized as follows. Amplification of the *bcr-abl* fusion gene occurs in CML, but usually results from the development of multiple Ph[1] chromosomes harboring a single copy of this hybrid gene rather than from tandem amplification of the gene on a single chromosome. The progression of CML from chronic phase to blast crisis is not necessarily accompanied by amplification or enhanced expression of the *bcr-abl* gene, and other genetic events or mutations perhaps involving other oncogenes in addition to the Ph[1] translocation might explain the evolution of CML to blast crisis.

N-*myc* AMPLIFICATION IN CHILDHOOD NEUROBLASTOMA

Neuroblastoma is the third most common malignancy in childhood, arising in approximately 1 in 10,000 live births and is the most common cause of cancer mortality in the first 5 years of life. The disease appears to arise in embryonic neural tissue. Numerous neuroblastoma cell lines have been derived from the more aggressive of these tumors, and it had been previously noted that such cell lines frequently harbor DMs and HSRs (39). A gene with limited homology to c-*myc* was noted to be amplified up to 700-fold in certain of these neuroblastoma cell lines, and this gene has been termed N-*myc* (40,41). Chromosome fractionation and in situ hybridization studies have provided direct evidence that the DMs and HSRs in these cell lines harbor amplified N-*myc* sequences (41,42). High levels of N-*myc*-related RNA are noted in the cell lines harboring N-*myc* genomic amplification. The N-*myc* gene has been mapped to chr. 2p23-24, but the HSRs harboring the amplified N-*myc* sequences have been frequently noted to be present on multiple different chromosomes in neuroblastoma cell lines (42). Thus, both translocation and amplification of N-*myc* sequences occurs in such cell lines. Although the N-*myc* gene is approximately 8 kb in size, the amplified unit in neuroblastoma has been estimated to be from 290–430 kb (43). Therefore, as is the case with the amplified DHFR gene in methotrexate-resistant cells, there are considerable number of flanking sequences that are coamplified with the N-*myc* gene in these neuroblastoma cell lines.

What is the significance of the N-*myc* gene amplification in neuroblastoma tumors? As with c-*myc*, the normal physiological role of N-*myc* is presently unclear. The N-*myc* gene was originally identified by virtue of its homology to c-*myc*, and there are considerable functional and structural similarities between these two distinct genes. The gene products of both N-*myc* and c-*myc* are localized to the nucleus. Both genes have similar transforming potential when cotransfected with *ras* genes in rat embryo fibroblast cotransformation assays (21,44). When certain neuroblastoma cell lines are induced to differentiate to mature neurons with retinoic acid, the steady-state level of N-*myc* RNA is decreased (45). This phenomenon is similar to the decrease in c-*myc* expression noted in HL-60 cells induced to differentiate to granulocytes with retinoic acid.

c-*myc* and N-*myc* share a similar exon/intron structure with their protein products exhibiting regions of significant homology. Both genes have a large untranslated first exon which may play a presently undefined regulatory role. Although there is significant homology in the translated portions of both genes, there is virtually no homology in this untranslated first exon between N-*myc* and c-*myc*, suggesting a divergence in the regulatory patterns of the two genes (46). Indeed the two genes exhibit significant differences in expression in normal tissue. Murine N-*myc* expression is present in virtually all mouse newborn tissues, but is particularly prominent (at least 20-fold greater) in newborn forebrain, hindbrain, kidney, and intestine (47). N-*myc* expression diminishes significantly in these tissues by 2 weeks of age. N-*myc* expression is also relatively high in pre–B cells. In contrast, c-*myc* expression in these same tissues does not vary by more than threefold. Activated expression of N-*myc* in neural origin tumors such as neuroblastoma may parallel these normal patterns of expression, since both brain and newborn intestines have a large population of immature, developing neurons (47). These observations suggest the N-*myc* and c-*myc* may perform a similar physiological function, perhaps related to the control of cell proliferation, but there is distinct tissue specificity regarding the regulation of expression of these genes which might be reflected in the types of tumors where enhanced expression or genomic amplification of N-*myc* and c-*myc* occurs.

Although the physiological role of the N-*myc* gene product in normal and malignant cells remains to be defined, there is now considerable evidence that the presence of N-*myc* amplification in fresh neuroblastoma tumors correlates with more aggressive disease. Childhood neuroblastoma is clinically staged by anatomical criteria, with stage I disease confined to the organ or structure of origin; stage II tumors extending beyond this organ, but not crossing the midline; stage III tumors extending beyond the midline; and stage IV tumors exhibiting distant metastases. Patients with stage I or II disease generally have a good prognosis with 75–90% 2-year disease-free survival with conventional radiotherapy/chemotherapy, whereas stage III or IV disease carries a significantly worse prognosis, with only a 10–30% 2-year disease-free survival. Patients with stage IV-S disease have a good prognosis despite anatomically extensive disease, as these tumors are frequently associated with spontaneous regression. In a survey of primary neuroblastoma tumors Brodeur and Seeger et al. demonstrated a significant correlation between the presence of N-*myc* genomic amplification and the biological aggressiveness of neuroblastomas (48,49). In a series of 89 patient tumor samples N-*myc* amplification was demonstrated in 0 of eight stage I tumors, two of 16 stage II, and 32 of 60 stages III and IV tumors. Zero of five of the good prognosis stage IVS tumors exhibited N-*myc* amplification. There was a close correlation between patient survival and the N-*myc* copy number in tumors. The probability of progression-free survival after conventional therapy at 18 months after diagnosis was 70%, 30%, and 5% in patients whose tumors exhibited no N-*myc* amplification, three- to 10-fold amplification, or greater than 10-fold amplification, respectively. Thus, there appears to be a significant correlation between genomic amplification of N-*myc*, anatomical progression, and disease aggressiveness of primary neuroblastomas. Presently, at many cancer centers in the United States the copy number of N-*myc* in newly diagnosed neuroblastoma primary tumors is routinely determined and those patients, regardless of anatomical stage, whose tumors exhibit an increased N-*myc* copy number are treated with more aggressive therapy including bone marrow transplantation.

The above data suggest that N-*myc* amplification is associated with neuroblastoma tumor progression rather than tumor initiation since early stage tumors are histologically malignant, but infrequently exhibit N-*myc* genomic amplification. Nevertheless, it is presently unclear whether these early stage neuroblastomas harboring a single copy N-*myc* gene express elevated levels of N-*myc*, or whether there are subtle changes such as point mutations in the regulatory or coding region portions of N-*myc* which may be involved in neuroblastoma initiation. It is also important to emphasize that the above data indicates that there are a significant number (approximately 50%) of biologically aggressive, advanced stage neuroblastomas that do not exhibit N-*myc* genomic amplification. Presumably these tumors harbor mutations or possibly amplification of other (onco)genes that lead to a decided growth advantage. For example, DNA from some neuroblastoma cells is able to malignantly transform NIH 3T3 cells in transfection assays, and the transforming gene has been demonstrated to be N-*ras* rather that N-*myc* in these cases (50). There is a clear analogy here between such neuroblastoma cells and HL-60 cells, since both exhibit genomic amplification of a member of the *myc* family of oncogenes and both harbor point mutations within the N-*ras* locus, accounting for their ability to transform NIH 3T3 cells.

Oncogene Amplification in Lung Cancer

In general, there are four histologically distinct types of human lung cancer: squamous or epidermoid cell carcinoma, which makes up some 40% of all lung cancers; small cell carcinoma comprising some 20–25% of these cancers; and both adenocarcinomas and large cell carcinomas which make up the remaining 35–40% of these tumors. Both squamous cell carcinomas and small cell carcinomas are clearly associated with smoking. The most aggressive of these types of lung cancers, displaying the highest growth fraction, the shortest doubling time, and the greatest propensity for early metastases are those of the small cell histology. Dr. John Minna's laboratory has developed over 30 different independent cell lines from primary or metastatic tumors from patients with small cell carcinoma of the lung, and the majority of these cell lines display genomic amplification of certain members of the *myc* family of oncogenes, including c-*myc*, N-*myc*, and L-*myc* (51–53).

The c-*myc* oncogene was noted to be amplified in nine of 31 of the small cell carcinoma cell lines, and the level of genomic amplification of c-*myc* varied from 20–75-fold in these cell lines (51). The cell lines which displayed such genomic amplification also exhibited relatively high levels of c-*myc*-related mRNA, and many of these cell lines harbor double minutes and homogeneous staining regions. Most of the cell lines which harbor the amplified c-*myc* gene are members of the SCLC-V subclass of small cell carcinomas which have slightly different histological characteristics from pure small cell lung carcinoma, and which display a more malignant phenotype, including a faster doubling time, higher cloning efficiency, greater x-ray resistance, and increased tumorigenicity in nude mice (51). Thus, it appears that c-*myc* amplification in these small cell carcinoma cell lines is generally associated with more aggressive disease.

Amplification of the N-*myc* oncogene was noted in seven of 31 of Minna's small cell carcinoma cell lines (52). The level of this genomic amplification ranged from 35-fold to as high as 150-fold. Normal non-malignant tissue from some of the patients from whom these cell lines were derived did not exhibit such genomic N-*myc* amplification, indicating that such amplification was specific for tumor tissue. Enhanced expression of N-*myc* mRNA was noted in those cell lines exhibiting genomic amplification of N-*myc*. In contrast to the cell lines harboring c-*myc* amplification, the small cell carcinoma cell lines displaying N-*myc* amplification did not necessarily exhibit a more malignant phenotype (52). None of these cell lines exhibit simultaneous amplification or messenger RNA (mRNA) expression of both c-*myc* and N-*myc*.

During the screening of these cell lines, a third member of the *myc* family of oncogenes, L-*myc*, was identified and molecularly cloned (53). As with N-*myc*, there are several regions of extensive (>80%) homology between L-*myc* and the second exon of c-*myc*. The L-*myc* gene has been localized to the p arm of chr. 1, and thus its location is distinct from c-*myc* (chr. 8) and N-*myc* (chr. 2). L-*myc* genomic amplification of some 10- to 20-fold was noted in five of 31 of the small cell carcinoma cell lines and this amplification is associated with enhanced expression of L-*myc*–related mRNA. None of the cell lines displaying L-*myc* amplification also harbors c-*myc* or N-*myc* amplification, and it appears that only one of these three *myc* genes is expressed in any given small cell carcinoma cell line (53).

The above studies demonstrating amplification of members of the *myc* gene family in 21 of 31 small cell lung cancers were performed on permanently established cultured cell lines. It is possible that such gene amplification is strictly an in vitro occurrence or that the presence of such gene amplification in primary tumors facilitates the in vitro establishment of such cell lines. Is a similar degree and frequency of *myc* gene amplification exhibited by primary small cell lung cancers in vivo? Minna's group has described several patients whose primary tumors exhibited a similar degree of c-*myc*, L-*myc*, or N-*myc* amplification as the cell lines that were established from these same tumors (51–53). A more extensive survey was undertaken by Dr. Bert Vogelstein's laboratory and involved studying primary and metastatic lesions from 45 individual patients with small cell lung cancer with N-*myc* and c-*myc* probes (54). These studies were facilitated by a novel DNA extraction technique that enabled small but adequate amounts of genomic DNA for blot analysis to be obtained from paraffin-embedded samples that had been previously stored in pathology archives (55). Of the 45 primary tumors, five displayed relatively high copy numbers (seven- to 35-fold) of either N-*myc* or c-*myc*, 14 exhibited two- to three-fold amplification, whereas 26 patient samples did not exhibit amplification of either of these oncogenes (54). In many of these patients, samples from both primary and metastatic lesions were available to determine whether there was any heterogeneity in the level of oncogene amplification in different tumor samples from the same patient. When primary tumors exhibited high copy numbers of either N-*myc* or c-*myc*, the metastatic tumors from the same patient also exhibited a similar degree of amplification. Conversely, metastatic lesions from patients whose primary tumors did not harbor N-*myc* or c-*myc* amplification never exhibited amplification of these oncogenes. These studies indicate that genomic amplification of N-*myc* and c-*myc* is less frequent in fresh small cell lung cancer tissue than in established small cell carcinoma cell lines, and that such gene amplification when present occurs relatively early in tumor development and does not appear to evolve during the development of metastatic lesions (54).

Oncogene Amplification in Human Breast Cancer

Breast cancer is one of the most common female malignancies and will effect approximately one in 12 women. In the United States, there are approximately 120,000 new cases and 40,000 deaths per year from this disease. Therapeutic decisions, particularly regarding the utilization of adjuvant radiotherapy or chemotherapy, depend on the major prognostic factors for this illness, which presently include the menopausal status of the patient, the size of the primary tumor, the number of axillary lymph nodes involved with tumor, and the presence or absence of hormonal receptors. Recent reports indicate that the c-*myc* and *neu* oncogenes are frequently amplified in primary breast cancer and that the presence of the *neu* oncogene amplification may carry particular prognostic significance.

In a survey of 121 human primary breast cancers, Escot et al. noted a two- to 15-fold amplification of the c-*myc* oncogene in 38 (32%) of these tumors (56). Most of those tumors exhibiting this genomic c-*myc* amplification were of the invasive ductal histological type. Tumors exhibiting this c-*myc* amplification also expressed relatively high levels of c-*myc* mRNA. In this survey there was no correlation noted between the presence of c-*myc* amplification and the estrogen or progesterone hormonal status, the axillary node status, or the histological grade of the tumor. There was a positive correlation with patient age, with c-*myc* genomic amplification being more frequent in patients over the age of 50 (56).

Genomic amplification of the *neu* oncogene has also been frequently noted in primary breast cancers. The *neu* oncogene was initially identified and isolated in Dr. Robert Weinberg's laboratory as the NIH 3T3-transforming gene of ethylnitrosourea-induced rat neuroglioblastomas (57,58). This oncogene was also cloned in other laboratories by virtue of its homology to the v-*erb*B oncogene, and its other names include HER-2 and c-*erb*B-2 (59–61). This oncogene codes for a 185,000-dalton protein with tyrosine-kinase activity and with the structure of a cell membrane growth factor receptor. The specific ligand for this receptor is not known. Point mutations involving a codon in the transmembrane domain of this protein have been identified in the ethylnitrosourea-induced rat neuroglioblastomas (62). In a survey of 189 primary human breast cancers, Slamon et al. noted genomic amplification of the *neu* oncogene from twofold to greater than 20-fold in 30% of the tumors (63). There was no correlation between gene amplification and hormone receptor status, tumor size, or patient age. However, *neu* amplification was more frequent in those patients with >3 axillary lymph nodes involved with tumor, a parameter which is the best prognostic factor for predicting patient survival. A statistical analysis indicated a positive correlation between the presence of *neu* amplification and the time to relapse and overall patient survival (63). Thus, the presence of *neu* amplification has considerable prognostic significance that is independent of axillary lymph node status. Determining the presence of *neu* amplification could therefore be of considerable clinical relevance in deciding whether to initiate adjuvant chemotherapy or radiotherapy to woman with breast cancer who present with negative axillary nodes.

There are several interesting questions raised by these studies of oncogene amplification in human breast cancer that are presently unanswered. Do some primary breast cancers exhibit simultaneous genomic amplification of both c-*myc* and *neu*, and would this signify a particularly bad prognosis? Are metastatic breast cancer lesions more likely to harbor oncogene amplification than primary tumors? (The samples from the above studies were all primary rather than metastatic breast tumors.) Do breast cancers also harbor other alterations in the *neu* oncogene such as the point mutations described in this gene in certain rat tumors (62), and how might such mutations relate to the pathogenesis of the disease?

SUMMARY AND CONCLUSIONS

It is clear from the above discussion that oncogene amplification in human cancers is not an infrequent phenomenon, and in some tumors, such as neuroblastomas and breast cancers, such amplification appears to be relatively common. It is important to emphasize that the incidence of such oncogene amplification in human cancers may be significantly underestimated simply because molecular probes representative of amplified (onco)genes are presently unavailable. In this regard, it is interesting to note that at least three different oncogenes (N-*myc*, L-*myc*, and c-*erb*B-2) were identified and isolated by virtue of their being amplified in certain human tumors. Undoubtedly there are other new oncogenes that will be identified in the future using similar approaches.

In general, there appears to be a higher incidence of oncogene amplification in established human tumor cell lines than in primary human tumors of similar histology. This appears to be particularly true for the leukemias, neuroblastomas, and small cell lung cancers. One possible explanation for this is that oncogene amplification is primarily an *in vitro* phenomenon and that such amplification progressively occurs the longer cells are grown in culture. However, there is in fact little evidence for this. In the few cases where the degree of oncogene amplification in cultured cell lines could be directly compared with the amount of amplification in the primary tumor from which the culture was derived, the levels of gene amplification were very similar in both. Moreover, there are no documented cases of a progressive quantitative increase in oncogene amplification in cultured human tumor cells. A more likely explanation to account for the higher incidence of gene amplification in human cancer cell lines is that those primary human tumors harboring specific oncogene amplification may be more readily established in continuous culture.

Why is there preferential genomic amplification of one oncogene versus another in tumors of a specific histological type? Most likely this reflects the usual pattern of expression of a particular oncogene in the normal tissue from which the tumor evolved. For example, the N-*myc* gene appears to be preferentially expressed in embryonic tissue which is enriched in developing neurons (47), and neuroblastomas, which are tumors of primitive neural origin, preferentially amplify N-*myc*. In contrast c-*myc* is expressed in multiple types of embryonic and adult normal tissue, and amplification of c-*myc* has been described in an equally wide variety of human tumors, including those of endodermal, mesenchymal, and epithelial origin (12,13,51,56,64). Certain squamous cell malignancies exhibit amplification of the EGF receptor (*erb*B oncogene)(65) and this most likely reflects the normal physiological role this receptor plays in epidermoid cell growth and differentiation. Conversely, the *neu* oncogene has the molecular structure of a specific growth factor receptor (ligand unknown), and the relatively high incidence of *neu* amplification in human breast cancer suggests that this receptor may play an important physiological role in growth and/or differentiation of normal breast epithelium.

What role does oncogene amplification play in the initiation and/or progression of human cancers? It is known that DHFR gene amplification in methorexate-resistant mouse cells is relatively unstable, and that this gene amplification is rapidly lost when selective pressure (i.e., methotrexate) is removed from the culture medium. The observation that oncogene amplification in cultured human tumor cells is quite stable is strong circumstantial evidence that such amplification is providing the tumor cells with a selective growth advantage. It is more difficult to determine whether such oncogene amplification is the actual initiating event in tumorigenesis. The observations outlined above in human neuroblastomas and breast cancer suggest that oncogene amplification is more closely associated with tumor progression rather than tumor initiation. Moreover, there is well-documented evidence of specific mutations involving several different oncogenes within an individual malignancy. For example, point mutations in the N-*ras* oncogene have been described in HL-60 cells and in certain neuroblastomas. These tumors also exhibit amplification of c-*myc* and N-*myc*, respectively. It is difficult to sort out which of these mutations is associated with tumor initiation and which with tumor progression. These observations emphasize what has been previously predicted from epidemiological data: Cancer arises not from a single mutation, but from a series of mutations; and the pathogenesis of malignancy is a multistage phenomenon. Oncogene amplification appears to be one of perhaps many important genetic events involving specific cellular genes that occurs during the progressive evolution of human tumors.

REFERENCES

1. Fialkow, P. J. (1976). Clonal origin of human tumors. *Biochem. Biophys. Acta 458*: 283–296.
2. Knudson, A. G. (1977). Genetic factors in human malignancy. In *Advances in Human Genetics.* (Harris, H., ed.). 1–25.
3. Alt, F. W., Kellems, R. E., Bertino, J. R., and Schimke, R. T. (1978). Selective multiplication of dihydrofolate reductase genes in methotrexate-resistant variants of cultured murine cells. *J. Biol. Chem. 253*: 1357–1370.
4. Nunberg, J. N., Kaufman, R. J., Schimke, R. T., Urlaub, G., and Chasin, L. (1976). Amplified dihydrofolate reductase genes are localized to a homogenously staining region of a single chromosome in a methotrexate resistant Chinese hamster ovary cell line. *Proc. Natl. Acad. Sci. U.S.A. 75*: 5553–5556.
5. Schimke, R. T., Brown, P. C., Kaufman, R. J., McGrogan, M., and Slate, D. (1981). Chromosomal and extrachromosomal localization of amplified dihydrofolate reductase genes in cultured mammalian cells. *Cold Spring Harbor Symp. Quant. Biol. 55*: 785–797.

6. Brown, P. C., Tisty, T. D., and Schimke, R. T. (1983). Enhancement of methotrexate resistance and dihydrofolate reductase gene amplification by treatment of mouse 3T3 cells with hydroxyurea. *Mol. Cell. Biol. 3*: 1097–1107.
7. Tisty, T. D., Brown, P. C., and Schimke, R. T. (1984). UV irradiation facilitates methotrexate resistance and amplification of the dihydrofolate reductase gene in cultured 3T6 mouse cells. *Mol. Cell. Biol. 4*: 1050–1056.
8. Varshavsky, A. (1981). Phorbol ester dramatically increases incidence of methotrexate-resistant colony-forming mouse cells: Possible mechanisms and relevance to tumor promotion. *Cell 25*: 561–572.
9. Rice, G. C., Hoy, C., Schimke, R. T. (1986). Transient hypoxia enhances the frequency of dihydrofolate reductase gene amplification in Chinese hamster ovary cells. *Proc. Natl. Acad. Sci. U.S.A. 83*: 5978–5982.
10. Schimke, R. T., Sherwood, S. W., Hill, A. B., and Johnston, R. N. (1986). Overreplication and recombination of DNA in higher eukaryotes: Potential consequences and biological implications. *Proc. Natl. Acad. Sci. U.S.A. 83*: 2157–2161.
11. Sager, R., Gadi, I. K., Stephens, L., and Grabowy, C. (1985). Gene amplification: An example of accelerated evolution in tumorigenic cells. *Proc. Natl. Acad. Sci. U.S.A. 82*: 7015–7019.
12. Collins, S. J., and Groudine, M. (1982). Amplification of endogenous *myc*-related DNA sequences in a human myeloid leukemia cell line. *Nature 298*: 679–681.
13. Dalla-Favera, R., Wong-Staal, F., and Gallo, R. C. (1982). Onc gene amplification in promyelocytic leukemia cell line HL-60 and primary leukemia cells of the same patient. *Nature 299*: 61–63.
14. Collins, S., Gallo, R., and Gallagher, R. (1977). Continuous growth and differentiation of human myeloid leukemic cells in suspension culture. *Nature 270*: 347–349.
15. Collins, S., Ruscetti, F., Gallagher, R., and Gallo, R. (1978). Terminal differentiation of human promyelocytic leukemia cells induced by dimethylsulfoxide and other polar compounds. *Proc. Natl. Acad. Sci. U.S.A. 75*: 2458–2462.
16. Breitman, T., Selonick, S., and Collins, S. (1980). Induction of differentiation of the human promyelocytic leukemia cell line (HL-60) by retinoic acid. *Proc. Natl. Acad. Sci. U.S.A. 77*: 2936–2940.
17. Rovera, G., Santoli, D., and Damsky, C. (1979). Human promyelocytic leukemia cells in culture differentiate into macrophage-like cells when treated with phorbol diester. *Proc. Natl. Acad. Sci. U.S.A. 76*: 2779–2783.
18. Nowell, P., Finan, J., Dalla-Favera, R., Gallo, R., ar-Rushdi, A., Romanczuk, H., Selden, J., Emanuel, B., Rovera, G., and Croce, C. (1983). Association of amplified oncogene c-*myc* with an abnormally banded chromosome 8 in a human leukemia cell line. *Nature 306*: 494–497.
19. Hann, S., Abrahms, H., Rohrschneider, L., and Eisenman, R. (1983). Proteins encoded by v-*myc* and c-*myc* oncogenes: Identification and localization in acute leukemia virus transformants and bursal lymphoma cell lines. *Cell 34*: 789–798.

20. Kelly, K., Cochran, B., Stiles, C., and Leder, P. (1983). Cell-specific regulation of the c-*myc* gene by lymphocyte mitogens and platelet-derived growth factor. *Cell 35*: 603–610.
21. Land, H., Parada, L., and Weinberg, R. (1983). Tumorigenic conversion of primary embryo fibroblasts requires at least two cooperating oncogenes. *Nature 304*: 596–600.
22. Murray, M., Cunningham, J., Parada, L., Dautry, F., Lebowitz, P., and Weinberg, R. (1983). The HL-60 transforming sequence: A ras oncogene cooexisting with altered *myc* genes in hematopoietic tumors. *Cell 33*: 749–758.
23. Bos, J., Verlaan-deVries, M., Jansen, A., Veeneman, G., and van Boom, J., van der Eb, A. (1984). Three different mutations in codon 61 of the human N-ras gene detected by synthetic oligonucleotide hybridization. *Nucleic Acids Res. 12*: 9155–9162.
24. Wolf, D., and Rotter, V. (1985). Major deletions in the gene encoding the p53 tumor antigen cause lack of p53 expression in HL-60 cells. *Proc. Natl. Acad. Sci. U.S.A. 82*: 790–794.
25. Rothberg, P., Erisman, M., Diehl, R., Rovigatti, U., and Astrin, S. (1984). Structure and expression of the oncogene c-*myc* in fresh tumor material from patients with hematopoietic malignancies. *Mol. Cell. Biol. 4*: 1096–1104.
26. McCarthy, D., Rassool, F., Goldman, J., Graham, S., and Birnie, G. (1984). Genomic alterations involving the c-*myc* proto-oncogene locus during the evolution of a case of chronic myelogenous leukemia. *Lancet 1*: 1362–1365.
27. Alitalo, K., Winqvist, R., Keski-Oja, J., Ilvonen, M., Saksela, K., Alitalo, R., Laiho, M., Knuutila, S., and de la Chapelle, A. (1985). Acute myelogenous leukemia with c-*myc* amplification and double minute chromosomes. *Lancet 2*: 1035–1038.
28. Groffen, J., Stephenson, J., Heisterkamp, N., de Klein, A., Bartram, C., and Grosveld, G. (1984). Philadelphia chromosome breakpoints are clustered within a limited region, *bcr*, on chromosome 22. *Cell 36*: 93–99.
29. Shtivelman, E., Lifshitz, B., Gale, R., and Canaani, E. (1985). Fused transcripts of abl and bcr genes in chronic myelogenous leukemia. *Nature 315*: 550–554.
30. Konopka, J., Watanabe, S., Singer, J., Collins, S., and Witte, O. (1985). Cell lines and clinical isolates derived from Ph-positive chronic myelogenous leukemia patients express c-abl proteins with a common structural alteration. *Proc. Natl. Acad. Sci. U.S.A. 82*: 1810–1814.
31. Ben-Neriah, Y., Daley, G., Mes-Masson, A., Witte, O., and Baltimore, D. (1986). The chronic myelogenous leukemia-specific p210 protein is the product of the bcr/abl hybrid gene. *Science 233*: 212–214.
32. Lozzio, C., and Lozzio, B. (1975). Human chronic myelogenous leukemia cell line with positive Philadelphia chromosome. *Blood 45*: 321–334.
33. Collins, S., and Groudine, M. (1983). Rearrangement and amplification of c-abl sequences in the human chronic myelogenous leukemia cell line K-562. *Proc. Natl. Acad. Sci. U.S.A. 80*: 4813–4817.

34. Selden, J., Emmanuel, B., Wang, E., Cannizzaro, A., Erikson, J., Nowell, P., Rovera, G., and Croce, C. (1983). Amplified C lambda and c-abl genes are on the same marker chromosome in K-562 leukemia cells. *Proc. Natl. Acad. Sci. U.S.A. 80*: 7289–7292.
35. Collins, S., Kubonishi, I., Miyoshi, I., and Groudine, M. (1984). Altered transcription of the c-abl oncogene in K-562 and other chronic myelogenous leukemia cells. *Science 225*: 72–74.
36. Collins, S. (1986). Breakpoints on chromosomes 9 and 22 in Philadelphia chromosome positive chronic myelogenous leukemia (CML). Amplification of rearranged c-abl oncogenes in CML blast crisis. *J. Clin. Invest. 78*: 1392–1396.
37. Collins, S., and Groudine, M. (1987). Chronic myelogenous leukemia: Amplification of a rearranged c-abl oncogene in both chronic phase and blast crisis. *Blood 69*: 893–898.
38. Andrews, D., and Collins, S. (1987). *Leukemia* (in press).
39. Biedler, J., Helson, L., and Spengler, B. (1973). Morphology and growth, tumorigenicity, and cytogenetics of human neuroblastoma cells in continuous culture. *Cancer Res. 33*: 2643–2652.
40. Schwab, M., Alitalo, K., Klempnauer, K., Varmus, H., Bishop, J., Gilbert, F., Brodeur, G., Goldstein, M., and Trent, J. (1983). Amplified DNA with limited homology to *myc* cellular oncogene is shared by human neuroblastoma cell lines and a neuroblastoma tumor. *Nature 305*: 245–248.
41. Kohl, N., Kanda, N., Schreck, R., Bruns, G., Latt, S., Gilbert, F., and Alt, T. (1983). Transposition and amplification of oncogene related sequences in human neuroblastomas. *Cell 35*: 359–367.
42. Schwab, M., Varmus, H., Bishop, J., Grzeschik, K., Naylor, S., Sakaguchi, A., Brodeur, G., and Trent, J. (1984). Chromosome localization in normal human cells and neuroblastomas of a gene related to c-*myc*. *Nature 308*: 288–291.
43. Kinzler, K., Zehnbauer, B., Brodeur, G, Seeger, R., Trent, J., Meltzer, and Vogelstein, B. (1986). Amplification units containing human N-*myc* and c-*myc* genes. *Proc. Natl. Acad. Sci. U.S.A. 83*: 1031–1035.
44. Schwab, M., Varmus, H., and Bishop, J. (1985). Human N-*myc* gene contributes to neoplastic transformation of mammalian cells in culture. *Nature 316*: 160–162.
45. Thiele, C., Reynolds, C., and Israel, M. (1985). Decreased expression of N-*myc* precedes retinoic acid-induced morphological differentiation of human neuroblastoma. *Nature 313*: 404–406.
46. De Pinho, R., Legouy, E., Feldman, L., Kohl, N., Yancopoulos, G., and Alt, F. (1986). Structure and expression of the murine N-*myc* gene. *Proc. Natl. Acad. Sci. U.S.A. 83*: 1827–1831.
47. Zimmerman, K., Yancopoulos, G., Collum, R., Smith, R., Kohl, N., Denis, K., Nau, M., Witte, O., Toran-Allerand, D., Gee, C., Minna, J., and Alt. F. (1986). Differential expression of *myc* family genes during murine development. *Nature 319*: 780–783.

48. Brodeur, G., Seeger, R., Schwab, M., Varmus, H., and Bishop, J. M. (1984). Amplification of N-*myc* in untreated human neuroblastomas correlates with advanced disease stage. *Science 224*: 1121–1124.
49. Seeger, R., Brodeur, G., Sather, H., Dalton, A., Siegel, S., Wong, K., and Hammond, D. (1985). Association of multiple copies of the N-*myc* oncogene with rapid progression of neuroblastomas. *N. Engl. J. Med. 313*: 1111–1116.
50. Taparowsky, E., Shimizu, K., Goldfarb, M., and Wigler, M. (1983). Structure and activation of the human N-ras gene. *Cell 34*: 581–586.
51. Little, C., Nau, M., Carney, D., Gazdar, A., and Minna, J. (1983). Amplification and expression of the c-*myc* oncogene in human lung cancer cell lines. *Nature 306*: 194–196.
52. Nau, M., Brooks, B., Carney, D., Gazdar, A., Battey, J., Sausville, E., and Minna, J. (1986). Human small-cell lung cancers show amplification and expression of the N-*myc* gene. *Proc. Natl. Acad. Sci. U.S.A. 83*: 1092–1096.
53. Nau, M., Brooks, B., Battey, J., Sausville, E., Gazdar, A., Kirsch, I., McBride, O., Bertness, V., Hollis, G., and Minna, J. (1985). L-*myc*, a new *myc*-related gene amplified and expressed in human small cell lung cancer. *Nature 318*: 69–73.
54. Wong, A., Ruppert, J., Eggleston, J., Hamilton, S., Baylin, S., and Vogelstein, B. (1986). Gene amplification of c-*myc* and N-*myc* in small cell carcinoma of the lung. *Science 233*: 461–464.
55. Goelz, S., Hamilton, S., and Vogelstein, B. (1985). Purification of DNA from formaldehyde fixed and paraffin embedded human tissues. *Biochem. Biophys. Res. Commun. 130*: 118–122.
56. Escot, C., Theillet, C., Lidereau, R., Spyratos, F., Champeme, M.-H., Gest, J., and Callahan, R. (1986). Genetic alteration of the c-*myc* protooncogene (MYC) in human primary breast carcinomas. *Proc. Natl. Acad. Sci. U.S.A. 83*: 4834–4838.
57. Schechter, A., Stern, D., Vaidyanathan, L., Decker, S., Drebin, J., and Greene, M., and Weinberg, R. (1984). The neu oncogene: An erb-B-related gene encoding a 185,000-M tumor antigen. *Nature 312*: 513–516.
58. Schechter, A., Hung, M.-C., Vaidyanathan, L., Weinberg, R., Yang-Feng, T., Franke, U., Ullrich, A., and Coussens, L. (1985). The neu gene: An erbB-homologous gene distinct from and unlinked to the gene encoding the EGF receptor. *Science 229*: 976–978.
59. Coussens, L., Yang-Feng, T., Liao, Y., Chen, E., Gray, A., McGrath, J., Seeburg, P., Libermann, T., Schlessinger, J., Franke, U., Levinson, A., and Ullrich, A. (1985). Tyrosine kinase receptor with extensive homology to EGF receptor shares chromosomal location with neu oncogene. *Science 230*: 1132–1139.
60. Yamamoto, T., Ikawa, S., Akiyama, T., Semba, K., Nomura, N., Miyajima, N., Saito, T., and Toyoshima, K. (1986). Similarity of protein encoded by the human c-erb-B-2 gene to epidermal growth factor receptor. *Nature 319*: 230–234.

61. King, C., Kraus, M., and Aaronson, S. (1985). Amplification of a novel v-erbB-related gene in a human mammary carcinoma. *Science 229*: 974–976.
62. Bargmann, C., Hung, M.-C., and Weinberg, R. (1986). Multiple independent activations of the neu oncogene by a point mutation altering the transmembrane domain of p185. *Cell 45*: 649–657.
63. Slamon, D., Clark, G., Wong, S., Levin, W., Ullrich, A., and McGuire, W. (1987). Human breast cancer: Correlation of relapse and survival with amplification of the HER-2/neu oncogene. *Science 235*: 177–182.
64. Yokata, J., Tsunetsugu-Yokata, Y., Battifora, H., LeFevre, and C., Cline, M. (1986). Alterations of myc, myb, and ras protooncogenes in cancers are frequent and show clinical correlation. *Science 231*: 261–264.
65. Yamamoto, T., Kamata, N., Kawano, H., Shimizu, S., Kuroki, T., Toyoshima, K., Rikimaru, K., Nomura, N., Ishizaki, R., Pastan, I., Gamou, S., and Shimizu, N. (1986). High incidence of amplification of the epidermal growth factor receptor gene in human squamous carcinoma cell lines. *Cancer Res. 46*: 414–416.

ELEVEN

Tumorigenic Activity of Artificially Activated Oncogenes

Herbert C. Morse, III
National Institute of Allergy and Infectious Diseases
National Institutes of Health
Bethesda, Maryland

Ulf R. Rapp
National Cancer Institute
Frederick Cancer Research Facility
Frederick, Maryland

INTRODUCTION

Over the last 10 years, it has become apparent that alterations in the structure and/or expression of a variety of cellular genes, termed c-*onc* genes, contribute to the development of neoplasia. The mechanisms by which these alterations relate to neoplasia is the subject of this volume and the multitude of approaches taken to define these relations are reviewed in the component chapters. Our efforts and those of others in this field have focused on the use of "artificially activated" c-*onc* genes to determine how they participate in normal cellular processes of growth and differentiation, and how variations in their expression result in malignant transformation. Two major systems, each with its own advantages, have been developed to study these "activated" genes—their incorporation in retroviral vectors (this chapter) and their insertion in the germ line of transgenic mice (Chap 12).

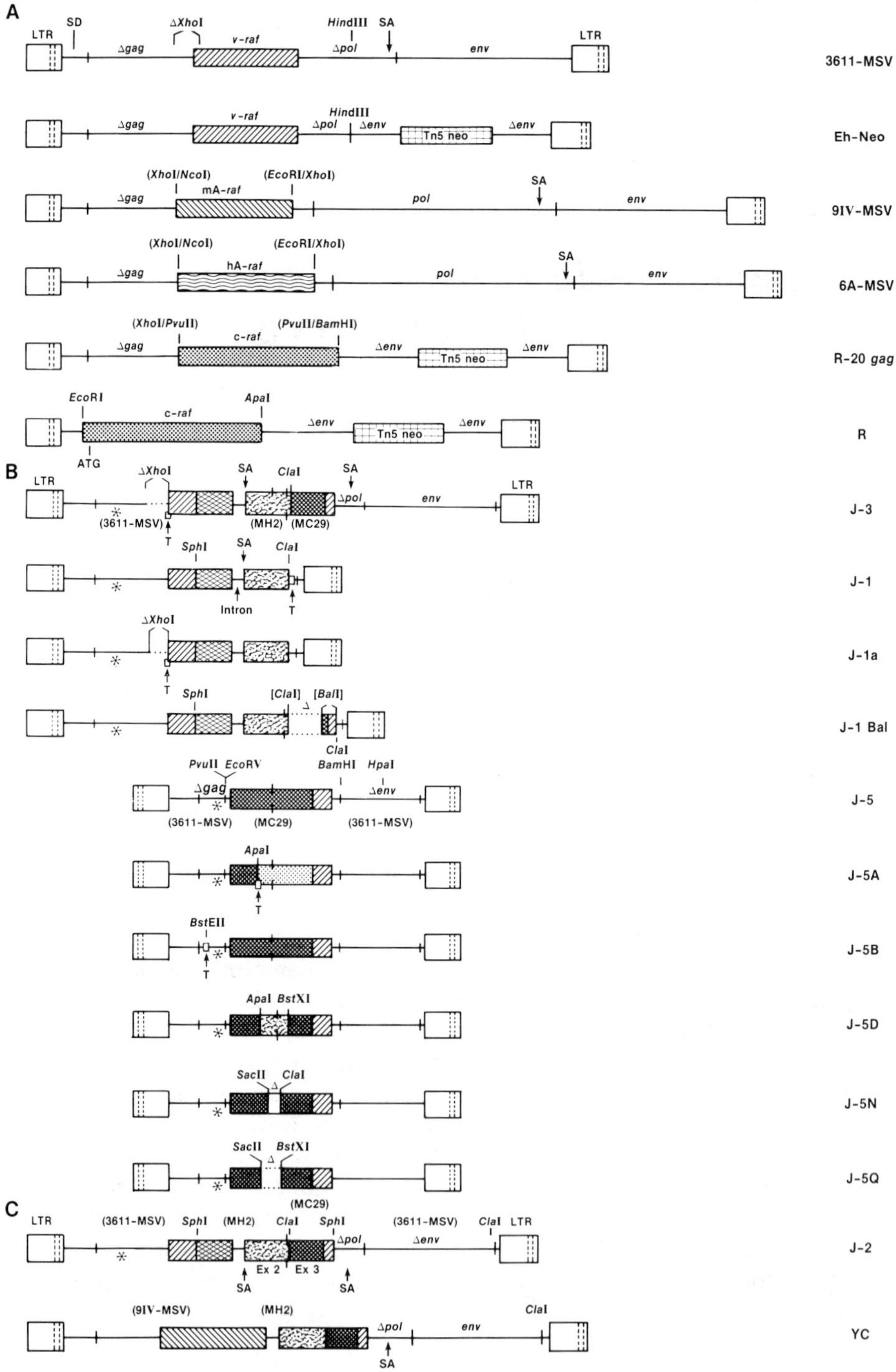
A
LTR
SD
ΔXhoI
HindIII
SA
Δgag
v-raf
Δpol
env
3611-MSV
Δenv
Tn5 neo
Eh-Neo
(XhoI/NcoI)
(EcoRI/XhoI)
mA-raf
pol
9IV-MSV
hA-raf
6A-MSV
(XhoI/PvuII)
(PvuII/BamHI)
c-raf
R-20 gag
EcoRI
ApaI
ATG
R
B
ClaI
(3611-MSV)
(MH2)
(MC29)
T
J-3
SphI
Intron
J-1
J-1a
[ClaI]
[BalI]
J-1 Bal
PvuII
EcoRV
BamHI
HpaI
J-5
J-5A
BstEII
J-5B
BstXI
J-5D
SacII
J-5N
J-5Q
C
Ex 2
Ex 3
J-2
(9IV-MSV)
YC

Our emphasis will be on the use of murine retrovirus vectors containing *raf* family genes and avian or murine *myc* genes alone or in combination. Several aspects of this system make it a remarkably strong approach to problems in neoplasia. First, the regulatory sequences in the long terminal repeats (LTRs) of the viruses that control expression of the *onc* genes are active in a wide variety of tissues, permitting an evaluation of *onc* gene effects in a spectrum of differentiated cell types. Second, by using the same LTR sequences to drive *onc* gene expression, the effects of different *onc* genes on specific types of cells can be evaluated. Third, v-*onc* sequences provide easily assayed markers for clonality in all cell types affected by their introduction, an extremely important aspect of tumor induction and evolution. Finally, the use of retroviral constructs facilitates rapid evaluation of mutations introduced to the *onc* genes that can be readily compared with mice exposed to the "parental" sequences.

VIRAL CONSTRUCTS

The specific viruses we have used in developing the studies described below and for use in future studies are presented in Fig. 1.

For the assembly of the recombinant viruses, the cloned provirus of 3611 MSV was used to provide a common vector base. Derivative viruses include: viruses carrying *raf* family oncogenes in wild type and mutant form; viruses carrying normal and mutated avian v-*myc* or mouse c-*myc* genes (Fig. 1c); the viruses containing both transforming segments of *raf* family genes and complete avian v-*myc* (Fig. 1b). The *raf* family genes that were built into viruses include v-*raf* (Rapp et al., 1983a,b), c-*raf* (Bonner et al., 1985, 1986), and A-*raf* (Beck et al., 1987; Huebner et al., 1986; Huleihel et al., 1986). v-*raf* corresponds to the C-terminal half of mouse c-*raf* from which it differs in four amino acid positions, none of which are essential for oncogenic activation (Bonner et al., 1985; Heidecker and Rapp, unpublished data). Viruses 9IV and 6A contain segments of mouse

---

Figure 1 Genomic organization of the 3611 MSV transforming virus and of the recombinant construct viruses, J-1, J-2, J-3, J-5, and J-5Q. v-*myc*–carrying retroviruses are aligned according to their content of v-*myc* sequence, and salient restriction enzyme sites are indicated. The deletion mutant, J-5Q, was derived from J-5 DNA by removing a 327 bp *Sac*II/*Bst*XI restriction fragment followed by an in-frame ligation. Introduction of termination codons is indicated by T. Specific shading delineates origin of coding and noncoding regions of v-*raf*/*mil* and v-*myc*: , 3611 MSV v-*raf*; , MH2 v-*mil*; , MH2 v-*myc*; , MC29 v-*myc* coding sequence; , MC v-*myc* noncoding sequence. Borders of retroviral genes and $exon_2$ and $exon_3$ of *myc* are indicated by vertical bars. SA indicates splice acceptor sequence, and SD, splice donor sequence.

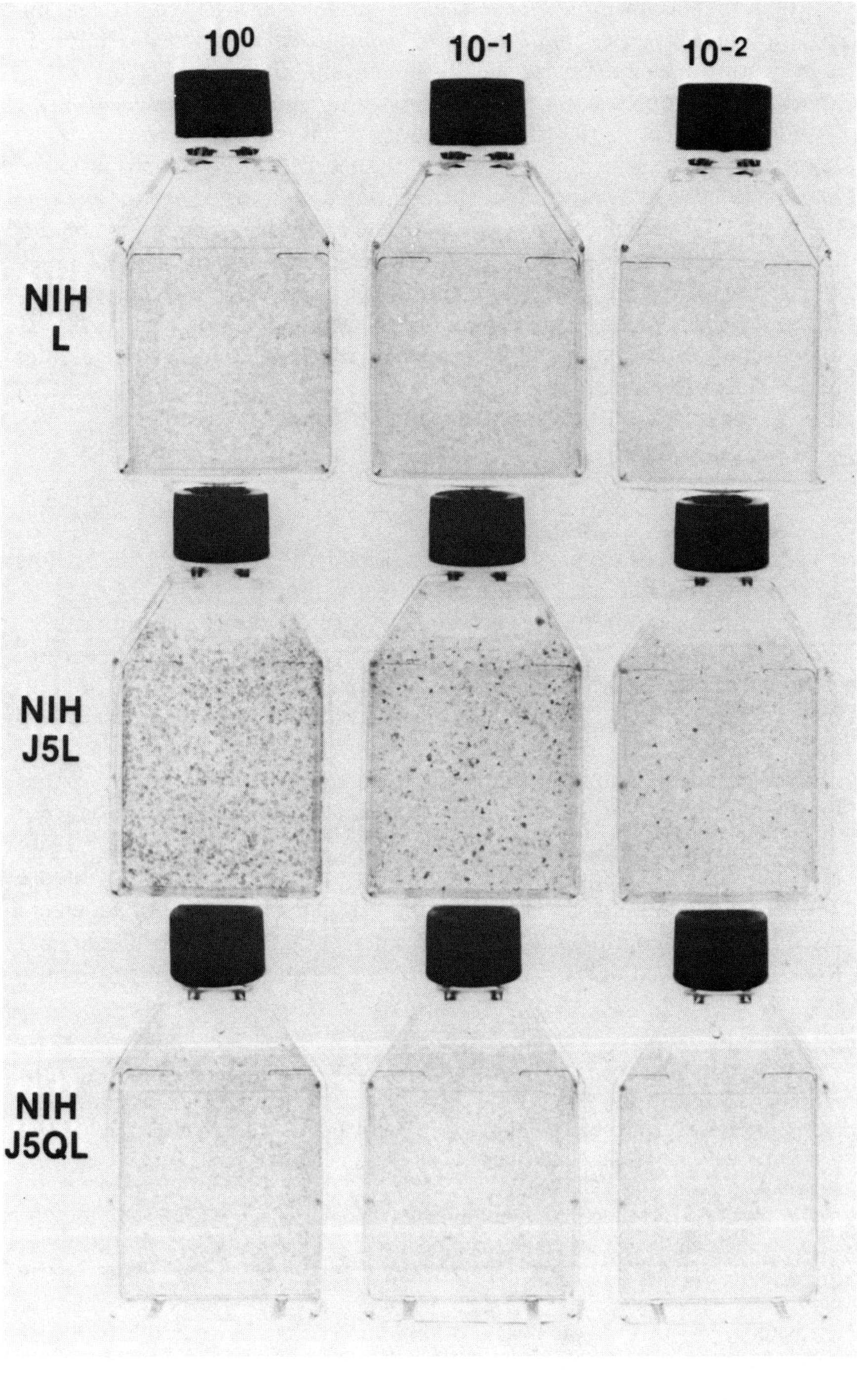
10^0
10^{-1}
10^{-2}
NIH
L
NIH
J5L
NIH
J5QL

(Huleihel et al., 1986) and human (Beck et al., 1987) A-*raf*-1, respectively, which comprise the kinase domain of A-*raf*. Several viruses were made with near full-length or full-length c-*raf*-1 complementary deoxyribonucleic acid (cDNA) (TC and EC, Fig. 1) such that c-*raf* protein was initiated either from the ATG of 3611 MSV *gag* (TC), or from the c-*raf*-1 ATG (EC) (Huleihel and Rapp, in preparation). c-*raf*-1 c-DNA was inserted in its original form and after linker insertion or site-directed mutagenesis (not shown).

Viruses carrying only *myc* genes include J-3, which expresses a hybrid MH2 (5′) MC29 (3′) avian v-*myc* from a subgenomic message, and J-5 which expresses the MC29-derived avian v-*myc* as part of a *gag-myc* fusion protein (Rapp, 1984; Rapp et al., 1985a–c). Additionally, the MC29 v-*myc* in J-5 is expressed in the absence of *gag* from a subgenomic message that uses a cryptic splice donor 5′ of the *gag* ATG, and a splice acceptor 3′ of the ATG in MC29 v-*myc*. A large series of sequence-exchange, frameshift, and deletion mutants was derived from J-5 (M. Huleihel et al., in preparation), and some of these are included in Fig. 1b. Briefly, J-5D differs from J-5 in that a segment of v-*myc* was incorporated which contains most of the MH2 v-*myc*–specific sequences present in J-3. The mutant was made as part of an effort to identify sequences specifying target cell preferences for transformation (see below). v-*myc* deletion mutants were generated with both J-3 and J-5 v-*myc* and additionally frameshift mutants were derived from J-5 (J-5A, B, Fig. 1). These mutants are being used to define regions within the v-*myc* protein important for transformation, growth factor abrogation, and c-*myc* down-regulation (Cleveland et al., 1986, 1987; Rapp et al., 1985a–c, 1987).

The third category of construct viruses include J-2 and YC (Fig. 1c) which carry two oncogenes, either v-*raf* and v-*myc* (J-2), or A-*raf* and v-*myc* (YC). The segment of mouse A-*raf* cDNA that was incorporated in place of v-*raf* of J-2 corresponds to the v-*raf* homologous portion of A-*raf* (Huleihel et al., unpublished data).

For generation of high-titered virus stocks, construct DNAs were transfected onto NIH 3T3 cells in the presence (*myc* only constructs) or absence (*raf* constructs) of PSV2 neoplasmid DNA. G418-resistant, or focus-derived, nonproducer transformed cell clones were rescued with eco- and amphotropic helper murine leukemia virus (MuLV), and the rescued virus stocks were titered on NIH 3T3 cells. Conventional focus assays were used in case of viruses carrying transforming *raf* genes and focal

---

Figure 2 Focal overgrowth induced by the v-*myc* recombinant retrovirus J-5. NIH 3T3 cells (10^5) were infected with serial dilutions of equal titers of helper virus alone (NIH Leuk) or J-5 or J-5Q viruses pseudotyped with Leuk MuLV. After 10 days the cells were fixed with methanol and stained with Geimsa.

overgrowth assays in case of *myc* viruses. The latter assay was developed, since constitutive *myc* expression does not detectably alter the morphology of infected NIH 3T3 cells, but allows such cells to continue growth in confluent monolayers which are otherwise sensitive to postconfluency inhibition of division (U. R. Rapp and M. Huleihel, in preparation). Overgrowth foci become detectable 8–10 days postinfection, and are easily scored on stained monolayers after 12–15 days (Fig. 2). v-*myc* mutant viruses which are unable to induce overgrowth foci, such as J-5Q in Fig. 2, but also J-1A, J-1 Bal, and J-5N (data not shown) were titered by determination of defective viral ribonucleic acid (RNA) in purified virus pellet harvested from rescued nonproducer cultures, or by determining the titre of neoresistance-inducing virus in case of constructs which express this selectable marker gene (Fig. 1).

IN VIVO AND IN VITRO EFFECTS OF RETROVIRAL CONSTRUCTS

Pathogenicity of v-*raf* Retroviruses

raf-family genes encode serine/threonine–specific protein kinases with distant homology to protein kinase C (Beck et al., 1987; Mark and Rapp 1984; Moelling et al., 1984; Rapp et al., 1986). Regions of greatest homology include both the kinase domain of the protein and, perhaps more significantly, the N-terminal half of the molecule. The latter homology region encompasses a cysteine-rich domain which is implicated in ligand binding in the case of protein kinase C (Knopf, personal communication). Oncogenic activation of *raf* family genes c-*raf* and A-*raf* can be achieved by N-terminal truncation which removes or destroys a presumed regulatory portion of the molecule, thereby releasing the kinase domain from negative control (Beck et al., 1987; Bonner et al., 1985, 1986; Huleihel et al., 1986; Molders et al., 1985). The truncation mode of *raf* activation is reminiscent of the proteolytic activation of protein kinase C which removes the N-terminal half of the molecule and generates a constitutively active kinase fragment (Parker et al., 1986). A second mode of oncogenic *raf* activation involves mutational alterations in the second (CR 2) of three regions (CR 1, 2, 3) in the molecule in which conservation between *raf* family genes is most pronounced (Beck et al., 1987; M. Huleihel et al., in preparation). The activating mutation may affect a proteolytic cleavage site or alter accessibility of activity-modulating phosphorylation sites, possibilities that are currently under investigation. Proteolytic activation of *raf* kinase has not yet been examined. However, the presence of a cluster of basic amino acid residues immediately upstream of the presumed adenosine triphosphate (ATP)–binding site in c-*raf* and A-*raf* indicates that proteolysis may be involved in *raf* kinase activation/down-regulation, analogous to its role in the regulation of protein kinase C activity (Kuroki, 1986). While the normal function of *raf* proteins is unknown, circumstantial evidence suggests that they function in the transduction of growth factor–induced signals from the cell surface to the nucleus (Rapp et al., 1987) where they ultimately lead to transcriptional activation of growth associated genes.

As described above, several transforming versions of c-*raf* and A-*raf* from mouse and man have been incorporated into retroviruses for somatic gene transfer experiments (Fig. 1). All of these viruses share their transcription regulatory elements with the viruses carrying avian v-*myc* genes, alone or in combination with *raf*. The most extensive data on tumor induction have been obtained with 3611 MSV, the virus in which v-*raf* was originally discovered. 3611 MSV was obtained in the course of experiments aimed at the systematic isolation of new oncogenes in culture with the help of murine leukemia virus (MuLV) Rapp, 1980; Rapp and Keski-Oja, 1982; Rapp and Todaro, 1978a,b; Rapp et al., 1975, 1983a,b, 1984, 1985). 3611 MSV was recovered from a mouse that had developed histiocytic lymphoma together with lung adenocarcinomas after infection with in vitro selected transforming virus at birth and treatment with the carcinogen butylnitrosourea (BNU) at 6 weeks of age. One tumor was transplanted serially several times before cocultivation with indicator cells in culture. The resulting virus stock contained high titers of replication-competent and replication-defective components, and was used for isolation of nonproducer transformed mouse and rat cells from which the virus was molecularly cloned (Rapp et al., 1983a,b).

Although 3611 MSV is the original virus in which the v-*raf* oncogene was recognized (Keski-Oja et al., 1982; Rapp et al., 1983a,b), it is not the only virus carrying these sequences. The avian retrovirus Mill Hill 2 (MH2) contains the avian homolog of v-*raf*, called variously v-*mil* (Coll et al., 1983; Jansen et al., 1983, 1984; Sutrave et al., 1984) or v-*mht* (Kan et al., 1983), in addition to the oncogene v-*myc*. MH2 was isolated about 50 years ago from a spontaneous ovarian tumor of a chicken (Beard, 1980), and is distinguished by the predominant induction of liver and kidney carcinomas in fowl (Alexander et al., 1979; Carr, 1960). The identification of cell-derived sequences in addition to v-*myc*, which had previously been identified in this virus, was an unexpected result that sprang from examination if molecularly cloned MH2 proviral DNA (Jansen et al., 1983, 1984). Comparison of the unidentified cell-derived sequences with v-*raf* DNA was prompted by our considerations of the similarities in disease association between 3611 MSV and MH2. The study soon revealed, first by cross-hybridization (Jansen et al., 1984) followed by direct sequence comparison

(Kan et al., 1984; Sutrave et al., 1984), that v-*mil* was indeed the avian homologue of v-*raf*.

Intraperitoneal inoculation of newborn NFS/N mice with the original tumor-derived complex induced histiocytic lymphoma, granuloma, fibrosarcoma, and erythroleukemia after a latency period of 4–8 weeks. Pseudotype virus stocks obtained by superinfection of nonproducer-transformed epithelial and fibroblastic rat as well as fibroblastic mouse cell lines with various helper MuLV, including Moloney, and several amphotropic virus strains (4070A, 1504M, Cas-Br-M) (Keski-Oja et al., 1982; Rapp et al., 1983a, 1985c), induced predominantly fibrosarcoma, erythroblastosis, and occasionally full-blown erythroleukemia with a 4- to 8-week latency and 100% incidence (Rapp et al., 1983a, 1985c). Additionally, pancreatic acinar dysplasia was observed upon systematic histological examination of 3611 MSV–inoculated mice (Fredrickson et al., in press).

The earliest lesions detected in mice injected with nonproducer-derived stocks consist of small islands of fibroblastic tumor cells on the diaphragm followed by the rapid metastasis of such cells throughout the peritoneal cavity, leading primarily to invasion of the spleen, which expands to an enormous size. Histochemical staining identified the fibroblasts in the tumors as collagen fiber producers (J. Ward and U. R. Rapp, unpublished data), which presumably accounts for the extremely hard consistency of the affected spleens. Curiously, epithelial MMCE cells transformed by 3611 MSV show a pronounced decrease in procollagen secretion relative to control cells (Keski-Oja et al., 1982), suggesting that the virus may affect fiber production in a cell type–dependent fashion.

A preliminary screen of inbred mouse strains for resistance to tumor induction by 3611 MSV showed high susceptibility in several sublines of C3H/He as well as in NFS/nude, AKR/N, DBA2, and BALB/c, and in C57BL/6, albeit at a reduced incidence (U. R. Rapp, unpublished data). Susceptibility was highest in newborn mice and rapidly decreased as they reached weaning age. Attempts to identify resistence genes to tumor induction by 3611 MSV have identified a multigenic, X-linked resistance in crosses between C57BL/6 and BALB/c (P. Klinken, unpublished data).

The avian homologue of v-*raf*, v-*mil* (*mht*), has so far not been extensively tested in the absence of MH2 v-*myc* for pathogenicity in its species of origin. The first direct evidence for the biological activity of v-*mil* came from experiments with a 3611 MSV derivative carrying a *raf*/*mil* hybrid gene (Rapp et al., 1985d). The recombinant virus, termed J-1 (Fig. 1), has the C-terminal two-thirds of v-*raf* replaced by corresponding v-*mil* sequence and tests the effects of 17 out of a total of 19 single amino acids differences with v-*mil* relative to v-*raf*. The J-1 virus-induced foci of morphological transformation in cultures of NIH 3T3 cells are less pronounced than those induced by 3611 MSV. Similarly, the average latency of tumors induced in NFS/N mice after their inoculation as newborns was increased from 6.0–8.5 weeks; their incidence and pathology, however, were indistinguishable from those tumors induced by 3611 MSV (Rapp et al., 1983a, 1985c). The continued passage of J-1 virus in culture resulted in stocks with improved focus-inducing ability, suggesting that mutations, which may affect the structure or expression of v-*raf/mil*, can increase its transforming activity (U. R. Rapp, unpublished data).

In the avian system, MH2 v-*mil* by itself appears to be incapable of transforming chicken embryo neuroretina (NR) cells (Bechade et al., 1985). However, NR cells, but not fibroblasts, are induced by v-*mil* to proliferate in liquid medium (Bechade et al., 1985). The neutrality of MH2 v-*mil* with respect to the growth behavior of chicken fibroblasts was also inferred by the use of natural or in vitro–constructed (Graf et al., 1986; Zhou et al., 1985) MH2 mutants with lesions affecting either v-*mil* or v-*myc*. In contrast, activity of v-*mil* was observed in v-*myc* virus–infected myeloid cells where it appeared to abrogate their growth factor dependence by induction of an autocrine loop (Adkins et al., 1984). However, since the entire MH2 virus was used in these abrogation experiments, it is possible that the observed induction of growth factor release by MH2 was due to differences in MH2 V-*myc* relative to other v-*myc* genes (Kan et al., 1984) which do not induce growth factors. More recently, these studies were extended by the used of deletion mutants of MH2 which inactivated either v-*mil* or v-*myc* (Graf et al., 1986). The data suggest that v-*mil* was responsible for induction of growth factor release. However, since the effect of v-*mil* deletions on the level of expression of v-*myc* was not determined, this point has not been rigorously established. Changes in the geometry of retroviral vectors can have striking effects on the ratio of spliced versus unspliced transcripts.

The basis for the difference in activity between v-*mil* and v-*raf* is not clear; one possibility is that the aminoterminal portion of v-*mil*, which extends 54 amino acids beyond v-*raf*, suppresses transforming activity. However, a LTR-activated truncated version of mouse c-*raf* (Molders et al., 1985), which directs the synthesis of a 48-kd polypeptide (A. M. Schultz, S. Oroszlan, and U. R. Rapp, submitted for publication) encompassing the entire v-*mil* coding sequence and extending its amino terminus approximately 110 amino acids, has transforming activity (Molders et al., 1985). While it is possible that this extension alleviates the aforementioned suppression, a simpler interpretation is that the extra 54 amino acids of v-*mil* do not affect transforming ability. A second possibility, the lack of activating mutations subsequent to acquisition of v-*mil* by MH2 from the cell, also seems unlikely, since the incorporation of c-*raf* cDNA into 3611 MSV DNA, such that it replaces the C-terminal two-thirds of v-*raf* (Bonner et al., 1985), is compatible with high-efficiency transformation. Moreover, construction of a recombinant virus which contains all of the v-*raf* homologous sequences derived from normal human c-*raf*-1 cDNA yields a strongly transforming virus similar to 3611 MSV (M. Huleihel and U. R. Rapp, unpublished results). Thus, it appears that v-*mil* may have been tamed by point mutations before or after transduction in MH2 or, in the course of transduction, by fusion to viral structural proteins and expression as a Δ*gag-mil* polyprotein. Wild-type MH2 virus is known to be somewhat toxic to cells in culture (Linial, 1982). It is, therefore, conceivable that either v-*mil* or v-*myc* or both had to be attenuated for the virus to survive in vitro culture. Alternatively, it has to be considered that early attempts to identify v-*mil* activity were affected by in vitro growth as well as by assay condition, since Palmieri has recently succeeded in demonstrating v-*mil*-mediated focus induction with chicken cells (Palmieri and Vogel, 1987).

In culture 3611 MSV efficiently transforms established fibroblastic and epithelial rodent cell lines (Keski-Oja et al., 1982; Rapp et al., 1983a,b) as well as primary mouse embryo fibroblasts (Rapp et al., 1986). Moreover, amphotropic pseudotypes of 3611 MSV induce foci of altered growth in human foreskin fibroblast cultures (U. R. Rapp, unpublished data). Primary bone marrow–derived (Blasi et al., 1985, 1986) or fetal liver–derived (Cleveland et al., 1986a,b; Ihle et al., 1985; Rapp, 1985; Rapp et al., 1985a,c) mouse cells grown in regular medium (DMEM supplemented with 10% FCS) are resistant to transformation by 3611 MSV. However, the infection of primary fetal liver cells with 3611 MSV in the presence of interleukin-3 (IL-3) does facilitate establishment of IL-3–dependent mast cell lines demonstrated that v-*raf*, like v-*ras* and v-*mos* (Cleveland et al., 1986; Huebner et al., 1986; Rapp et al., 1985), has an immortalizing function in myeloid lineage cells under these culture conditions. A simple explanation for these findings is that c-*myc* expression, or that of an equivalent nuclear oncogene, in addition to v-*raf* or a *raf*-equivalent function, is required for a complete growth cycle. However, induction of c-*myc* in hematopoietic cells requires mitogens other than those present in serum, and for certain hemopoietic cells this role can be played by IL-3. Therefore, in the presence of v-*raf*, a c-*myc* (or equivalent)–inducing ligand such as IL-3 constitutes the rate-limiting function for growth. Conversely, in cells exposed to and responsive to IL-3, c-*myc* expression is constitutive and late factors (in terms of their need during G_1 phase of the cell cycle) such as perhaps v-*raf*, become limiting.

Using assay conditions which favor the outgrowth of B-lineage lymphoid or erythroid-lineage cells from hemopoietic progenitor cells infected with 3611 MSV, we have recently demonstrated v-*raf* effects in both systems (Klinken et al., in preparation). Our results indicate that in agarose, in the presence of 2-mercaptoethanol (2-ME) 3611 MSV–transformed pre–B cell lines. v-*raf* transformants maintained a stable pre-B phenotype, in contrast to v-*raf*/v-*myc* (J-2 virus)–transformed cells, which spontaneously differentiated into sIg^+ B cells or reverted to pro–B cells and macrophages (see below). In methylcellulose and in the absence of 2ME, 3611 MSV produced colonies of differentiated, hemoglobin-synthesizing erythrocytes, whereas J-2 virus–infected cells had a greater proliferative capacity, but were inhibited from terminally differentiating (Klinken, in preparation). In summary, transformation experiments in cell culture with 3611 MSV demonstrated transforming effects for cells for all lineages that were affected in vivo upon infection of newborn mice with this virus.

Pathogenicity of c-*raf* Retroviruses

Viruses carrying the complete coding sequence of c-*raf*-1 or A-*raf*-1 under the control of their own ATG initiator codon have not yet been tested for transformation in vivo. However, 5′-truncated versions of human c-*raf*-1 fused in frame to a 3′-deleted v-*raf* in 3611 MSV (Bonner et al.,1985; Rapp et al., 1983b) as well as 5′-truncated human (6A, Fig. 1.) or mouse (9IV, Fig. 1) A-*raf* replacing v-*raf* in 3611 MSV have been examined. The target cell range for the transformation in NFS/N mice inoculated intraperitoneally as newborns by any of these viruses was comparable to 3611 MSV.

In culture, retroviruses containing full-length human c-*raf*-1 (EC, Fig. 1) or A-*raf*-1 cDNA initiated from their own ATG in addition to the neomycin resistance gene as a marker did not acutely transform NIH 3T3 cells (Beck et al., unpublished data). However, mutation of conserved region 2 (CR 2) of c-*raf*-1 by linker insertion activated the transforming potential of this gene.

In summary, we conclude that replacement of v-*raf* in 3611 MSV by c-*raf* or A-*raf* homologous cDNA from mouse or man does not appreciably alter its transforming abilities in vivo or in vitro. Thus, point mutations present in v-*raf* are not required for oncogene activation. However, 5′ truncation was required, since retroviruses carrying full-length c-*raf* or A-*raf* under control of their own ATG were nontransforming unless mutated at specific sites.

Pathogenicity of v-*myc* Retroviruses

The roles of v-*myc* viruses in induction of tumors in vivo has been studied by inoculating either newborn, untreated Swiss mice or adult, pristane-primed BALB/c mice with high-titered pseudotypes of the recombinant viruses. Newborn NFS/N mice inoculated with different pseudotypes of J-3 or J-5 died between 6 weeks and 1 year after infection, with the mean latency to death being related to relative abilities of the helper viruses to replicate in tissue of mice infected as newborns (Morse et al., 1986). Thus, the time course of death for mice inoculated with Moloney pseudotypes of J-3 or J-5 ranged from 40 to 120 days, whereas most mice dies more than 150 days after infection with C2S, 4070A, or 1504M pseudotypes of these constructs (Fig. 3; Morse et al., 1986). Similarly, mice inoculated with 4070A pseudotypes of a recombinant virus similar to J-5 died with latencies of 40–160 days (Brightman et al., 1986).

Histopathological, flow cytometry, and molecular genetic studies of the tumors developing in infected animals showed that over 90% of the mice died with lymphoblastic lymphomas representing predominantly T-cell lymphomas, but also including pre–B cell lymphomas (Brightman et al., 1986; Morse et al., 1986). Analyses of these tumors for immunoglobulin (Ig) and T-cell receptor gene organization showed that they were mono- or oligoclonal. Clonal integrations of v-*myc* sequences were also detected in each tumor, associated with high levels of v-*myc* transcription (Brightman et al., 1986; Morse et al., 1986). Continuous in vitro cell lines were readily established from some of these tumors, indicating their malignant nature. These observations of clonality and malignancy strongly suggest that while v-*myc* viruses can initiate transformation of T- and B-lineage cells, additional genetic changes are required for development of fully transformed cells.

The observations that both pre–B and B cells could be transformed by J-3 and J-5 in vivo also indicated that *myc*-related transformation of cells within a particular lineage was not restricted to a single stage of differentiation. The demonstrations that induction of murine plasmacytomas is almost universally associated with deregulated expression of c-*myc* secondary translocations affecting this locus (Adams et al., 1985; Marcu et al., 1983; Mushinski et al., 1983; Shen-Ong et al., 1982) also indicated that aberrant expression of *myc* was probably central to their development. Since plasmacytomas develop only after long latencies in pristine-primed BALB/c mice, it seemed likely that our failure to observed these tumors in

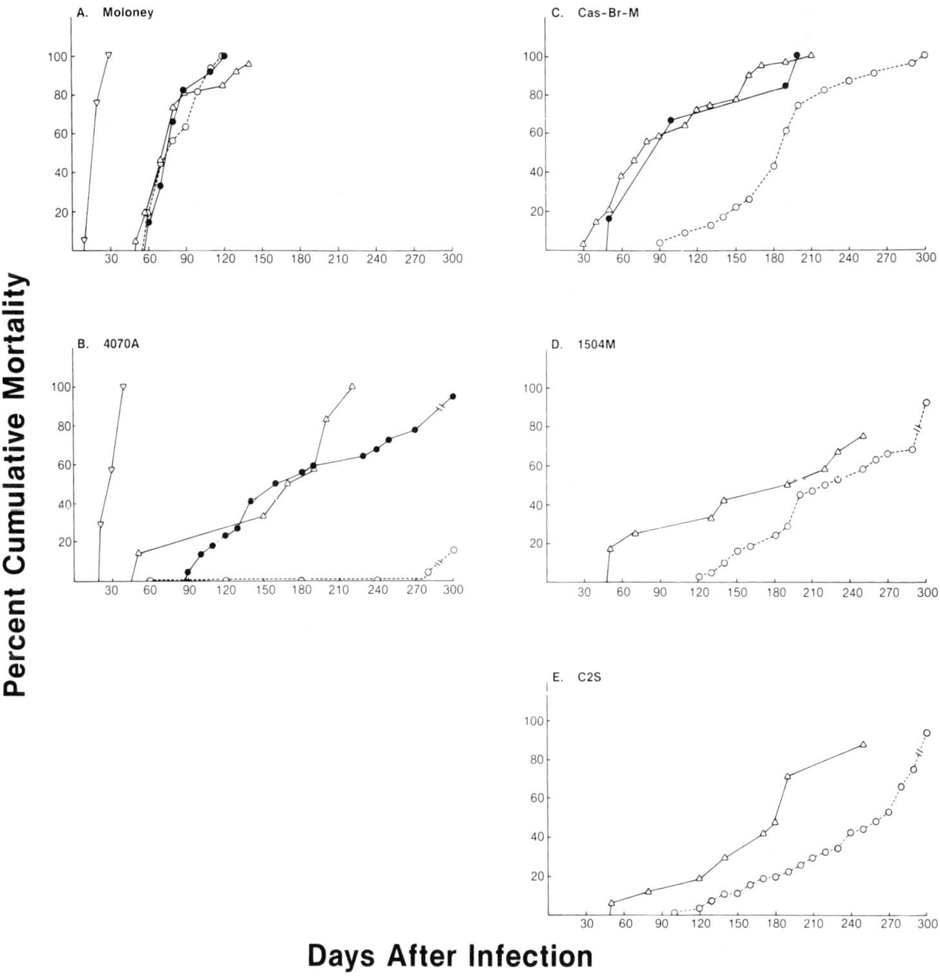

Figure 3 Cumulative mortalities of NFS/N mice inoculated as newborns with Moloney (A), 4070A (B), Cas-Br-M (C), 1504M (D) and C2S (E) pseudotypes of recombinant retroviruses. Data are for mice infected with the helper viruses alone (○—○) or pseudotypes of J-2 (∇—∇), J-3 (●—●), or J-5 (△—△).

the studies cited above could have been due to the use of NFS/N mice that lacked the conditioned environment provided by intraperitoneal inoculation of pristane. To evaluate this possibility, adult, pristane-primed BALB/c mice were inoculated with Moloney pseudotypes of J-3. Approximately 22% of injected mice developed plasmacytomas, with a latency less than half that of mice inoculated with pristane alone (Potter et al., 1987).

In contrast to the tumors induced by pristane alone, the J-3/pristane–induced tumors lacked translocations affecting the c-*myc* locus and instead expressed high levels of v-*myc* from clonally integrated J-3 constructs (Potter et al., 1987). These studies provided direct evidence that deregulated expression of *myc* is crucial to plasmacytoma induction, and indicated that v-*myc* can initiate the translocation of cells at all stages of development within the B-cell pathway. Again, the clear evidence for clonality of these tumors indicated that aberrant expression of *myc* was not sufficient for transformation.

These studies also provided evidence for a more extended range of hematopoietic cells that can be targeted for transformation by v-*myc*. A large number of myeloid tumors with monocyte/macrophage characteristics developed in pristane-primed BALB/c mice infected with J-3 (Potter et al., 1987). In addition, we have found that a high proportion of treated mice infected with J-5 develop monocyte/macrophage tumors, but rarely if ever develop plasmacytomas (Morse, Potter, U. R. Rapp, unpublished observations). The basis for the differences in cell types targeted by J-3 and J-5 is not understood, be the possibilities that they could be due to sequence differences between MC29 and MH2 *myc* genes, levels of v-*myc* expression, or expression of v-*myc* as a spliced gene or a *gag-myc* gene are being investigated.

Evidence for the contribution of v-*myc* sequences to in vivo transformation of nonhematopoietic cells has also been obtained. Studies of newborn NFS/N mice inoculated with J-3 or J-5 showed that approximately 20% of infected animals died with pancreatic acinar adenocarcinomas, and that rare mice (three of 140) developed mammary adenocarcinomas (Morse et al., 1986). Interestingly, two of three mammary tumors developed in male mice and the third in a virgin female. These findings contrast with the mammary tumors of MMTV *myc* transgenic mice (Stewart et al., 1984) which developed in pregnant female mice, indicating a role for hormonal effects in their development. Molecular studies of one of these mammary tumors revealed the presence of two clonal v-*myc* integration sites and abundant v-*myc* transcripts (Morse et al., 1986).

A more detailed analysis of pancreatic acinar cell abnormalities in mice infected with J-2, J-3, or J-5 has recently been completed (T. N. Fredrickson et al., in press). Over 70% of newborn NFS/N mice infected with pseudotypes of J-2 developed foci of dysplastic acinar cells with latencies as short as 15 days. These foci, scattered throughout the pancreatic parenchyma, were composed of large distorted acini surrounded by normal-appearing pancreas. Direct progression of these legions to full-blown tumors in mice infected with J-2 was not observed, most likely owing to accelerated deaths secondary to hematopoietic neoplasms and fibrosarcoma (Rapp et al., 1985).

Mice infected with J-3 or J-5 exhibited more advanced tumors, described as carcinoma in situ, at 40–133 days after inoculation (T. N. Fredrickson et al., in press). These tumors were of intermediate size and consisted of tumor-cell nests containing debris-filled lumina associated with minimal connective tissue stroma or inflammatory cell infiltrates. A high frequency of mitotic figures in these lesions indicated that they were in active growth phase. In spite of this, the lesions remained confined to the body of the pancreas and appeared to be direct expansions of the dysplastic foci noted in mice infected with J-2.

Finally, advanced carcinomas, presenting as large tumors in the pancreas, throughout the abdominal cavity, and with occasional hematogenous spread, were observed in mice infected 115–235 days previously with J-3 or J-5 (T. N. Fredrickson et al., in press). Histologically, these tumors resembled carcinoma in situ, but included variable numbers of acinarlike structures seen in the dysplastic foci. The malignant nature of the advanced carcinomas was demonstrated by their successful transplantation in vivo and the derivation of continuous cell lines from the transplants in vitro (T. N. Fredrickson et al., in press). Analyses of the pancreatic tumors, transplants, and cell lines obtained for J-3 or J-5 integrations showed that the primary tumors were mono- or oligoclonal, and that the integration sites retained in the in vivo and in vitro passages (T. N. Fredrickson et al., in press). It is noteworthy that all of the tumors had multiple (two to eight) clonal v-*myc* integration sites.

We interpret these findings to suggest that v-*myc* is capable of initiating pancreatic acinar carcinomas, and that these tumors progress sequentially from dysplastic foci to carcinoma in situ to advanced clonal carcinomas. While it is not known if the earliest lesions (dysplastic foci) are clonal, the late lesions clearly are. The presence of multiple v-*myc* integrations in these tumors may be analogous to gene amplifications detected in other tumor systems (Klein and Klein, 1985; Kohl et al., 1983; Little et al., 1983; Schwab et al., 1984). Thus, the J-3-and J-5-induced pancreatic tumors may be among a unique set of neoplasms where aberrant expression of a single oncogene may initiate a transformation process that is complicated by amplification of the same gene.

To summarize the observations made with v-*myc* viruses in vivo, we conclude that aberrant expression of *myc* can initiate the transformation of a wide variety of cell types, including T cells, B cells at a variety of stages of differentiation, and monocyte/macrophage-lineage cells as well as mammary adenocarcinomas. Pancreatic acinar cell carcinomas may represent a unique circumstance where v-*myc* can both initiate and complete the transforming process. For the other tumors, additional genetic alterations appear to be required for evolution of the fully transformed state. It should be noted that this range of tumors may not represent the full spectrum of cell types that can be targeted for transformation by v-*myc* (or *raf/myc*). The timing of infection and levels of v-*myc* expression achieved at different stages of differentiation may be crucial to determining if the transformation process is begun within cells of a certain lineage. These variables may be reflected in appearance of very rare tumors in infected mice. Three possible examples of this phenomenon in our series include the appearance of endothelial, pulmonary, and hepatic tumors in mice infected with J-2 (Fig. 4; Fredrickson, Morse, U. R. Rapp, unpublished data.

In vitro analyses of v-*myc* transformation have taken advantage of the effects of these viruses in immortalized, nontransformed cell lines and on explanted bone marrow cells. NRK, SC-1, and NIH 3T3 cells infected with Cas-Br-M or 1504M pseudotypes of J-3 or J-5 resulted in the development of foci with morphological alterations distinct from those induced by *mos, ras,* or *abl*, and extended growth in soft agar (Morse, U. R. Rapp, Yetter, unpublished results). Expanded ring-cloned foci of SC-1 cells also produced large tumors in nude mice within 3 weeks, whereas SC-1 cells infected with the helper viruses alone did not (Morse, U. R. Rapp, Yetter, unpublished observations). Brightman et al. (1986) and Vennström et al. (1984) have also described transformation and growth in soft agar of continuous rat and mouse cell lines infected with retroviral constructs containing MC29 and OK10 v-*myc* genes, respectively. The OK10 construct was also shown to transform fibroblasts from primary cultures of limb bud cells (Vennström et al., 1984).

Transformation of primary hematopoietic cells with J-5 and the MC29 and OK10 constructs has also been achieved (Brightman et al., 1986; Klinken et al., submitted for publication; Vennström et al., 1984; Vogt et al., 1986). Infection of bone marrow cells in vitro using the technique of Rosenberg and Baltimore (1976) resulted in the appearance of foci in soft agar that could be expanded on bone marrow feeder layers and subsequently adapted to feeder layer–independent growth (Klinken et al., submitted for publication). One cell line obtained in this manner has lymphoid morphology and expresses surface markers characteristic of mature B cells, including surface immunoglobulin. In contrast, infection of primary or secondary mouse embryo cultures with the MC29 or OK10 constructs gave rise to continuous lines of macrophages that were initially factor dependent for growth, but later grew as factor-independent cultures (Brightman et al., 1986; Vennström et al., 1984; Vogt et al., 1986). Molecular studies of the J-5–transformed B-cell line showed clonal Ig J_H rearrangements, clonal integration of J-5, and high levels of v-*myc* expression (Klinken et al., in press). A factor-independent macrophage line was also shown to contain

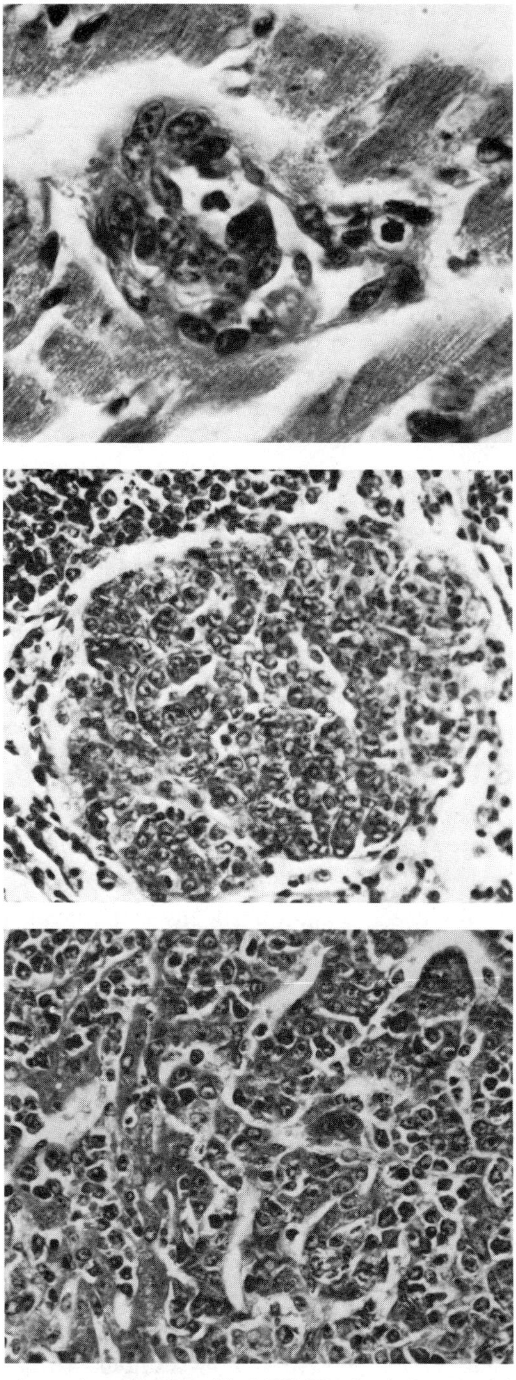

A

B

C

Figure 4 Unusual neoplasms induced in NFS/H mice infected with pseudotypes of J-2. (A) Cardiac capillary endothelioma. (B) Hepatocelluar carcinoma. (C) Pulmonary alveolar carcinoma.

and express v-*myc* (Brightman et al., 1986). These findings indicate that in vitro as well as in vivo v-*myc* can initiate the transformation of primary cells from several hematopoietic lineages.

The mechanisms responsible for v-*myc*–related transformation of hematopoietic cells may be related to the abrogation of growth factor dependence (Rapp et al., 1985). In these studies, it was found that IL-3– or IL-2–dependent cell lines infected with v-*myc*-containing viruses grew in the absence of these factors and became tumorigenic in mice. These results could not be explained by induction of IL-3 or IL-2 production to yield autocrine growth, and was associated with suppression of c-*myc* expression (Rapp et al., 1985). This finding could be related to the studies described above by the following scenario. Infection of bone marrow cells with v-*myc*–containing viruses results in the random chromosomal integrations of the *onc* gene in a polyclonal fashion. Depending on their chromosomal location, some of the integrated viruses will not be expressed, whereas others will be variably expressed at low to high levels. Expression of deregulated v-*myc* at low levels may have two effects—potentiation of growth factor activity (Sorrentino et al., 1986) and suppression of c-*myc* expression (Rapp et al., 1985)–which together can result in increased rounds of proliferation in the face of continued factor dependence. Cells with low expression integrations may, with repeated rounds of division, experience alterations in chromatin structure near these loci, resulting in enhanced expression of *myc* and loss of factor dependence (Cleveland et al., 1987) similar to cells with preferred high expression integrations. The increased growth potential for these cells increases the possibility of genetic errors (Langdon et al., 1986; Vogt et al., 1986) that contribute to evolution of the fully malignant phenotype (Klein and Klein, 1985).

A second approach to studying the role of *myc* in cell transformation has been the development of murine retroviruses containing murine c-*myc* sequences (Keath et al., 1984; Wolff et al., 1986). Fibroblast lines transfected with one of these constructs (Keath et al., 1984), but not the others (Wolff et al., 1986), were found to grow in agar at low efficiency, to proliferate in low serum medium, and to be tumorigenic on inoculation of nude mice (Baumbach et al., 1986).

Bone marrow cells infected with one of these viruses (Baumbach et al., 1986) gave rise to long-term macrophagelike cell lines in cultures supplemented with CSF-1. No lines were obtained in the absence of CSF-1 in contrast to the studies described above for v-*myc* viruses.

Infection of adult pristane-primed BALB/c mice with Moloney pseudotypes of the c-*myc* constructs also resulted in the development of tumors with monocyte-macrophage characteristics (Baumbach et al., 1986;

Wolff et al., 1986). These tumors were readily transplantable to other mice or could be grown in tissue culture without added growth factors, showing they were fully transformed. Similar tumors developed with longer latencies in primed DBA/2 mice (Baumbach et al., 1986). Pristane priming was an absolute requirement for tumor induction with two constructs (Wolff et al., 1986) but not the third (Baumbach et al., 1986). In previous studies of pristane-induced plasmacytomas, it was shown that the priming effect of pristane could be inhibited by treatment of mice with indomethacin (Potter et al., 1985). In contrast, the development of myelomonocytic tumors in pristane-primed mice infected with a c-*myc* virus was not inhibited by treatment with this agent (Wolff et al., submitted for publication). These results suggest important differences in cofactors required for the development of *myc*-dependent tumors in these cell lineages. Nonetheless, the c-*myc*–induced myeloid tumors were found to be clonal, based on the demonstrations of unique proviral integrations (Baumbach et al., 1986; Wolff et al., 1986).

Mechanisms that could contribute to the clonal outgrowth of myelomonocytic lines containing the c-*myc* viruses were described by Baumbach et al (1987). They showed that some of the lines, unlike normal mononuclear phagocytes, produced CSF-1 and occasionally GM-CSF. One of the CSF-1–producing lines was found to respond to this lymphokine and to exhibit a rearrangement of the CSF-1 locus, consistent with an autocrine growth pattern. These results suggest that aberrant expression of CSF-1 and *myc* can complement for transformation of myelomonocytic cells. The role of c-*myc* in this complementation is presumably related to the effects observed for high-level v-*myc* expression on growth factor dependence described before. Similar growth factor abrogation experiments have since been performed with c-*myc*–expressing viruses (Cory et al., 1987; Dean et al., 1987) which showed that constitutive expression of c-*myc* at near normal levels unstably abrogated the requirement of myeloid FDCP-1 cells for interleukin-3 (IL-3).

Interactions Between Oncogenes in Transformation

The paradigm for *onc* gene synergy for transformation in vitro was provided by the studies of Land et al. (1983a,b) and Ruley (1983), who demonstrated a requirement for nuclear and cytoplasmic oncogenes in this process. We and others have reevaluated this process in vivo using mice infected with pairs of oncogenes in a single retrovirus (Blasi et al., 1985; Klinken et al., submitted for publication; Potter et al., 1987; Rapp et al., 1985), or by infecting bone marrow cells in vitro with combinations of retroviruses containing single oncogenes (Vogt et al., 1986; Schwartz et al., 1986).

Our studies of the *raf/myc*-containing J-2 virus showed that newborn inoculated NFS/N mice rapidly developed a variety of neoplasms (Rapp et al., 1985). Within 1–3 weeks of infection, each mouse died with a spectrum of tumors that represented a summation of malignancies induced by v-*raf* alone (erythroblastosis, fibrosarcoma, pancreatic acinar dysplasia) or v-*myc* alone (T- and B-cell lineage lymphomas, pancreatic acinar dysplasia), but appearing in these animals with much longer latencies (4 to >52 weeks). Cell lines from these tumors could be readily established in culture in regular medium in contrast to *raf*-induced tumors that required IL-3 for growth. In contrast, inoculation of adult, pristine-primed BALB/c mice resulted in the development of myelomoncytic tumors as well as T- and B-cell lineage lymphomas (Morse et al., unpublished results; Potter et al., 1987). Plasmacytomas, characteristic of mice inoculated with the J-3 v-*myc* virus, were not detected (Potter et al., 1987).

The in vitro effects of J-2 on bone marrow cells has been examined under two different culture conditions for infected cells. When infected cells were grown in the absence of 2-mercaptoethanol (2-ME), continuous lines with morphological, antigenic, and functional characteristics of bone marrow macrophages were obtained exclusively (Blasi et al., 1985). Under these conditions, the cells proliferated rapidly for 14 days, but then differentiated and stopped proliferating. By adding dextran beads to the quiescent cultures, the macrophages could be induced to proliferate again, indicating that the dominant differentiation process could be reversed, resulting in the establishment of immortalized cell lines (Blasi et al., 1985).

In contrast, inclusion of 2-ME in the medium used to culture infected cells resulted in the outgrowth of lymphoid as well as myeloid colonies in both liquid culture and semisolid agar (Klinken et al., submitted for publication). After expansion of the lymphoid agar colonies in liquid culture, cells adherent to the culture dishes were noted in addition to the predominant nonadherent lymphoid cells. Mutliple single cell clones obtained from these cultures were analyzed for a variety of phenotypic and functional characteristics. Clones with four distinct phenotypes were detected—pro-B cells, pre-B cells, mature surface Ig-positive B cells, and macrophages (Klinken et al., submitted for publication). In spite of this diversity, all the clones were shown to be clonally related, based on common proviral integrations and J_H rearrangements detectable in both the B-cell lineage and macrophage tumors. The results indicate that J-2 had transformed a common precursor to the B-cell and myelomonocytic lineages that we provisionally termed a pro-GMB cell (Davidson et al., 1984; Holmes et al., 1986). They also indicate that high levels of v-*myc* expression are not incompatible with extensive maturation within the B cell and monocyte-macrophages, a conclusion that can also be drawn from the studies of Blasi et al. (1985).

In contrast, J-2 infection of cells in the erythroid lineage was quite different. Whereas cells infected with 3611 MSV showed limited proliferative potential and differentiated into hemoglobinized cells, cells infected with J-2 had an enhanced ability to divide, but had a decreases tendency to differentiate. These findings indicate that the relation of high *myc* expression to differentiation programs varies greatly for cells committed to different hematopoietic lineages (Klinken et al., submitted for publication).

The remarkably strong transforming activity in vivo or in vitro of the combination of *onc* genes in J-2 may be related to the fact that they form part of two different, synergizing signal-transducing pathways controlling cell growth such as a competence (*myc*) and a progression (*raf*) pathway (Cleveland et al., 1986). Alternately, in some cells, both genes might work through a common pathway. The possibility is perhaps best exemplified by studies of B-cell lineage malignancies induced by a wide variety of oncogenes (Morse et al., 1987). These studies showed that a cell surface antigen, termed 6C3 (Tidmarsh et al., 1985), is expressed at high levels on B-lineage cells transformed by *abl*, *ras*, *fes*, *src*, and *erb*B, but not on tumors induced by the *myc*-containing viruses J-3, J-5, or J-2. We concluded that *myc*$^+$ and *myc*$^-$ pathways for B-cell transformation could be distinguished on the basis of 6C3 expression (Morse et al., 1987). A possible relation of *raf* to the hypothetical *myc*$^+$ pathway was suggested by the observation that pre–B cell lymphomas induced in vitro by 3611 MSV are also 6C3$^-$ (Klinken et al., submitted for publication).

Recently, Schwartz et al. (1986) demonstrated synergism between v-*myc* and v-Ha-*ras* coinfections for transformation of murine bone marrow cells in Whitlock-Witte cultures. Infection of the cells with v-*myc* alone had no effect, whereas cells infected with *ras* alone or coinfected with *ras* and *myc* led to the development of clonable B-cell lines. Lines containing both *ras* and *myc* demonstrated increased proliferative activity and cloning ability in soft agar in comparison to lines infected with *ras* alone. Thus, both *ras* and *raf* appear to act synergistically with v-*myc* for transformation of B-lineage cells.

In contrast, bone marrow cells maintained in IL-3–containing medium and coinfected with v-Ha-*ras* and v-*myc* resulted in the development of macrophage lines (Vogt et al., 1986). Cells infected with this combination of viruses initially divided much more rapidly than cells infected with v-*myc* alone. After a crisis phase which was associated with marked karyotypic changes the cells again exhibited high growth factor independence, suggesting that genetic events in addition to aberrant expression of the two *onc* genes is required for full transformation (Vogt et al., 1986).

CONCLUSIONS

Determination of pathogenicity patterns with *raf*- and *myc*-containing retroviruses in vivo and in vitro allows us to draw several major conclusions.

First, the use of the viruses which share their transcription regulatory component made possible for the first time detection of distinct target cell preferences for transformation by either oncogene. *myc* was associated predominantly with lymphoid/myeloid neoplasias, whereas *raf* had a preference for fibroblastic/erythroid cells. However, the observed tissue preference for transformation was fairly broad, since with a lesser frequency *myc* was also able to induce transformation of epithelial cells (pancreas>mammary) and alter the growth potential of fibroblasts as well as chondroblasts in culture (Horton et al., in press; U. R. Rapp et al., in preparation). Similarly, *raf* was also associated with induction of pancreatic acinar dysplasia in vivo and immortalization of mast cells as well as transformation of lymphoid and epithelial cells in culture. Moreover, at least in the case of *raf*, it is likely in light of numerous studies with other mammalian oncogene carrying retroviruses that its range of transformation overlaps with that of many other nonnuclear oncogenes, including several *src* family tyrosine and serine kinase oncogenes as guanosine triphosphate (GTP)–binding *ras* genes (for reviews, see *RNA Tumor Viruses*, 1980). While the contribution of enhancer effects to transformation specificity by the latter viruses specificity cannot yet be rigorously evaluated, indications are that the range of target cells for transformation is similar for many exogenous oncogenes that are neither nuclear nor growth factor derived.

Why are some cells more susceptible to *myc* and others more to *raf* (or equivalent oncogenes) for transformation? We speculate that this may be due to differences in the rate-limiting pathways through which growth is normally controlled in different cell types. The lymphoid system may be harnessed prodominantly through a pathway in which *myc* can function (i.e., by competence class growth factors), and erythroid, fibroblastic cells through a pathway in which *raf* can function (i.e., a progression factor pathway); epithelial cells may be limited in both, since they are susceptible to initiation of transformation in the pancreas by either oncogene.

Second, use of the J series of viruses clearly demonstrated the phenomenon of oncogene synergism for transformation of cells by *raf* and *myc* in vivo and in vitro. Based on growth factor abrogation experiments we speculate that the basis for the observed synergism may be a combination of competence (*myc*) and progression (*raf*) class signals which provide both growth-controlling transcription regulators (*myc* or *myc* induced) and their activating protein kinases (*raf* or *raf* activated). The ability to induce growth in differentiating cells from a variety of cell lineages by somatic gene transfer with dual oncogene-carrying retroviruses in vivo and in culture has made it possible to continuously grow rare stem cells and promises to furnish new insights into processes controlling the branching of related lineages.

Finally, the ability to determine clonality of transformed cells by examining viral integration sites has allowed us to evaluate the role of secondary and later steps in transformation by oncogenes. The phenomenon of oncogene synergism clearly demonstrates the potential contribution of multiple oncogene activations to the acquistion of autonomous growth by tumor cells. The fact that even cells transformed by the dual oncogene carrying J-2 virus in vivo and in culture, were clonal or pauciclonal raises the possibility that even two activated and expressed oncogenes may not suffice. Indeed, it was observed in one instance of fetal liver cell transformation with J-2 virus in culture that an additional cellular proto-oncogene, c-*myb*, was activated by retroviral insertion (Cleveland et al., 1986; Weinstein et al., 1987). This is not to say that secondary and later events necessarily recruit additional oncogenes. One illustration for a second mechanism contributing to the evolution of tumor cells was the finding of multiple copies of J-5 virus in pancreatic epithelial cells transformed in vivo and J-2 virus integrations in B-lymphoid cells transformed in culture (Morse et al., 1986; Klinken et al., 1987). These cases may represent examples for gene amplification as a second step in the completion of the transformation process which was initiated by the same oncogenes in single copy.

Comparison of transformation specificities of different v-*myc* viruses for various lineages of lymphoid/hematopoietic cells has indicated *myc* sequence-specified effects (Potter et al., 1987, and unpublished data). In order to initiate a detailed structure function analysis of the *myc* protein in this system as well as to develop settings for conditional expression of exogeneous *myc*, *raf*, and other oncogenes, we have begun to construct retrovirus vectors of the J series that carry mutant versions of these genes. The adaptability of retrovirus vectors for regulated expression and high-efficiency infection of cells from many species and lineages make them an ideal tool for such somatic gene transfer experiments.

REFERENCES

Adams, J. M., Harris, A. W., Pinkert, C. A., Corcoran, L. M., Alexander, W. S., Cory, S., Palmeter, R. D., and Brinster, R. L. (1985). The c-*myc* oncogene driven by immunoglobulin enhances induces lymphoid malignancy in transgenic mice. *Nature 318*: 533–538.

Adkins, B., Leutz, A., and Graf, T. (1984). Autocrine growth induced by *src*-related oncogenes in transformed chicken myeloid cells. *Cell 39*: 439–445.

Alexander, R. W., Moscovici, C., and Vogt, P. K. (1979). Avian oncovirus mill hill No. 2: Pathogenicity in chickens. *JNCI 62(2)*: 359–366.

Baumbach, W. R., Keath, E. J., and Cole, M. D. (1986). A mouse c-*myc* retrovirus transforms established fibroblast lines *in vitro* and induces monocyte-macrophage tumors *in vivo. J. Virol. 59*: 276–283.

Baumbach, W. R., Stanley, E. R., and Cole, M. D. (1987). Induction of clonal monocyte-macrophage tumors *in vivo* by a mouse c-*myc* retrovirus: Rearrangement of the CSF-1 gene as a secondary transforming event. *Mol. Cell. Biol. 7*: 664–671.

Beard, J. W. (1980). Biology of avian oncoviruses. In *Viral Oncology*. (Klein, G., ed.). New York, Raven Press, pp. 842.

Bechade, C., Calothy, G., Pessac, B., Martin, P., Coll, J., Denhez, F., Saule, S., Ghysdael, J., and Stehelin, D. (1985). Induction of proliferation or transformation of neuroretinal cells by the *mil* and *myc* viral oncogenes. *Nature 316(6028)*: 559–562.

Beck, T. W., Huleihel, N., Gunnell, M., Bonner, T. I., and Rapp, U. R. (1987). The complete sequence of human A-*raf*, a new member of the *raf* family of oncogenes. *Nucleic Acids Res. 15*: 595–609.

Blasi, E., Mathieson, B. J., Varesio, L., Cleveland, J. L., Borchert, P. A., and Rapp, U. R. (1985). Selective immortilization of murine macrophages from fresh bone marrow by a *raf/myc* recombinant murine retrovirus. *Nature 318*: 667–670.

Bonner, T. I., Kerby, S. B., Sutrave, P., Gunnell, M. A., Mark, G., and Rapp, U. R. (1985). Structure and biological activity of human homologs of the *raf/mil* oncogene. *Mol. Cell. Biol. 5*: 1400–1407.

Bonner, T. I., Opperman, H., Seeburg, P., Kerby, S. B., Gunnell, M. A., Young, A. C., and Rapp, U. R. (1986). The complete coding sequence of the human *raf* oncogene and the corresponding structure of the c-*raf*-1 gene. *Nucleic Acids Res. 14*: 1009–1015.

Brightman, B. K., Pattengale, P. K., and Fan, H. (1986). Generation and characterization of a recombinant Moloney murine leukemia virus containing the v-*myc* oncogene in Avian MC29 virus: *In vitro* transformation and *in vivo* pathogenesis. *J. Virol. 60*: 68–81.

Carr, J. G. (1960). Kidney carcinomas of the fowl induced by the MH2 reticuloendothelioma virus. *Brit. J. Cancer 14*: 77–82.

Chida, K., Kato, N., and Kuroki, T. (1986). Down regulation of phorbol diester receptors by proteolytic degradation of protein kinase C in a cultured cell line of fetal rat skin keratinocytes. *J. Biol. Chem. 261*: 13013–13018.

Cleveland, J. L., Jansen, H. W., Bister, K., Fredrickson, T. N., Morse, H. C., III, Ihle, J. N., and Rapp, U. R. (1986a). Interaction between *raf* and *myc* oncogenes in transformation in vivo and in vitro. *J. Cell. Biochem. 30*: 195–218.

Cleveland, J. L., Weinstein, Y., Ihle, J. N., Askew, D. S., and Rapp, U. R. (1986b). Transformation and insertional mutagenesis *in vitro* of primary hematopoietic stem cell cultures. In *Current Topics in Microbiology and Immunology*. (Melchers, F., and Potter, eds.). Springer-Verlag, New York, pp. 44–54.

Cleveland, J. L., Huleihel, M., Storm, S. M., Bressler, P., Siebenlist, U., Eisenman, R., and Rapp, U. R. (1987a). Role of *myc* in tumor induction, growth factor abrogation, and control of c-*myc* expression. *Banbury Conference on Nuclear Oncogenes.* Cold Spring Harbor, New York (in press.)

Cleveland, J. L., Rapp, U. R., and Farrar, W. L. (1987b). Role of c-*myc* and other genes in interleukin 2 regulated CT6 T lymphocytes and other malignant variants. *J. Immunol. 138*: 3495–3504.

Coll, J., Righi, M., de Taisne, C., Dissous, C., Gegonne, A., and Stehelin, D. (1983). Molecular cloning of the avian acute transforming retrovirus MH2 reveals a novel cell-derived sequence (v-*mil*) in addition to the *myc* oncogene. *EMBO J. 2(12)*: 2189–2194.

Cory, S., Bernard, O., Borotell, D., Schrader, S., and Schrader, J. W. (1987). Murine c-*myc* retroviruses alter the growth requirements of myeloid cell lines. *Oncogene Res. 1*: 61–76.

Davidson, W. F., Fredrickson, T. N., Rudikoff, E. K., Coffman, R. L., Hartley, J. W., and Morse, H. C., III. (1984). A unique series of lymphomas related to the Ly-1^+ lineage of B lymphocyte differentiation. *J. Immunol. 133*: 744–753.

Dean, M., Cleveland, J. L., Rapp, U. R., and Ihle, J. N. (1987). Role of *myc* in the abrogation of IL-3 dependence of myeloid FDC-P1 cells. *Oncogene Res. 1*: 279–296.

Fredrickson, T. N., Hartley, J. W., Wolford, N. K., Resau, J. H., Rapp, U. R., and Morse, H. C., III. (198). Histogenesis and clonality of pancreatic tumors induced by v-*myc* and v-*raf* oncogenes in NFS/N mice. *Amer. J. Path.* (in press).

Graf, T., Weizsaecker, F. V., Grieser, S., Coll, J., Stehelin, D., Patschinsky, T., Kister, K., Bechade, C., Calothy, G., and Leutz, A. (1986). v-*mil* induced autocrine growth and enhanced tumorigenicity in v-*myc*-transformed avian macrophages. *Cell 45*: 357–364.

Holmes, K. L., Pierce, J. H., Davidson, W. F., and Morse, H. C., III. (1986). Murine hematopoietic cells with pre-B or pre-B/myeloid characteristics are generated by *in vitro* transformation with retroviruses containing *fes, ras, abl,* and *src* oncogenes. *J. Exp. Med. 164*: 443–457.

Horton, W., Cleveland, T., and Rapp, U. R. (1987). An established rat cell line expressing chondrocyte properties. *Exp. Cell. Res.* (submitted).

Huebner, K., Ar-Rushdi, A., Griffin, C. A., Isobe, M., Kozak, C., Emanuel, B. S., Nagarajan, L., Cleveland, J. L., Bonner, T. I., Goldsborough, M. D., Croce, C. M., and Rapp., U. (1986). Actively transcribed genes in the *raf* oncogene group, located on the X chromosome in mouse and human. *Proc. Natl. Acad. Sci. U.S.A. 83*: 3934–3938.

Huleihel, M., Goldsborough, M., Cleveland, J. L., Gunnell, M., Bonner, T., and Rapp, U. R. (1986). Characterization of murine A-*raf*, a new oncogene related to the v-*raf* oncogene. *Mol. Cell. Biol. 6*: 2655–2662.

Ihle, J. N., Keller, J., Rein, A., Cleveland, J. L., and Rapp, U. R. (1985). Interleukin 3 regulation of the growth of normal and transformed hematopoietic cells. In *Cancer cells 3/Growth Factors and Transformation.* (Feramisco, J., Ozanne, B., and Stiles, C., eds.). New York, Cold Spring Harbor Laboratory, pp. 211–219.

Jansen, H. W., Ruckert, B., Lurz, R., and Bister, K. (1983). Two unrelated cell-derived sequences in the genome of avian leukemia and carcinoma inducing retrovirus MH2. *EMBO J. 2(11)*: 1969–1975.

Jansen, H. W., Lurz, R., Bister, K., Bonner, T., Mark, G., and Rapp, U. R. (1984). Homologous cell-derived oncogenes in avian carcinoma virus MH2 and murine sarcoma virus 3611-MSV. *Nature 307*: 281–284.

Kan, N. C., Flordellis, C. S., Garon, C. F., Duesberg, P. H., and Papas, T. S. (1983). Avian carcinoma virus MH2 contains a transformation-specific sequence, MHT, and shares the *myc* sequence with MC29, CMII, and OK10 viruses. *Proc. Natl. Acad. Sci. U.S.A. 80(21)*: 6566–6570.

Kan, N. C., Flordellis, C. S., Mark, G. E., Duesberg, P. H., and Papas, T. S. (1984). Nucleotide sequence of avian carcinoma virus MH2: Two potential *onc* genes, one related to avian virus MC29 and the other related to murine sarcoma virus 3611. *Proc. Natl. Acad. Sci. U.S.A. 81(10)*: 3000–3004.

Keath, E. J., Caimi, P. G., and Cole, M. D. (1984). Fibroblast lines expressing activated c-*myc* oncogenes are tumorigenic in nude mice and syngeneic animals. *Cell 39*: 339–348.

Keski-Oja, J., Rapp, U. R., and Vaheri, A. (1982). Transformation of mouse epithelial cells by acute murine leukemia virus 3611: Inhibition of collagen synthesis and induction of novel polypeptides. *J. Cell. Biochem. 20*: 139–148.

Klein, G., and Klein, E. (1985). Evolution of tumors and the inpact of molecular oncology. *Nature 315*: 190–195.

Klinkin, S. P., Principato, M. A., Pierce, J. H., Davidson, W. F., Holmes, K. L., Cleveland, J. L., Rapp, U. R., and Morse, H. C., III. (198). Murine lymphocytes transformed by a *raf/myc*-containing retrovirus are able to differentiate along both lymphoid and myeloid pathways (submitted).

Kohl, N. E., Kanda, N., Schreck, R. R., Brums, G., Latt, S. A., Gilbert, F., and Alt, F. W. (1983). Transposition and amplification of oncogene-related sequences in human neuroblastomas. *Cell 35*: 359–367.

Land, H., Parada, L. F., and Weinberg, R. L. (1983a). Tumorigenic conversion of pulmonary embryo fibroblasts requires at least two cooperating oncogenes. *Nature 304*: 596–602.

Land, H., Parada, L. F., and Weinberg, R. A. (1983b). Cellular oncogenes and multistep carcinogenesis. *Science 222*: 771–778.

Langdon, W. Y., Harris, A. W., Cory, S., and Adams, J. M. (1986). The c-*myc* oncogene perturbs B lymphocyte development in Eμ-*myc* transgenic mice. *Cell 47*: 11–18.

Linial, M. (1982). Two retroviruses with similar transforming genes exhibit differences in transforming potential. *Virology 119(2)*: 382–391.

Little, C. D., Nau, M. M., Carney, D. N., Gazdar, A. F., and Minna, J. D. (1983). Amplification and expression of the c-*myc* oncogene in human lung cancer cell lines. *Nature 306*: 194–196.

Marcu, K. B., Harris, L. J., Stanton, L. W., Erickson, J., Watt, R., and Croce, C. M. (1983). Transcriptionally active c-*myc* oncogene is contained within NIARD, a DNA sequence associated with chromosomal translocations in B cell neoplasia. *Proc. Natl. Acad. Sci. U.S.A. 80*: 519–524.

Mark, G. E., and Rapp, U. R. (1984). Primary structure of v-*raf*: Relatedness to the *src* family of oncogenes. *Science 224*: 285–289.

Moelling, K., Heimann, B., Beimling, P., Rapp, U. R., and Sander, T. (1984). Serine-and threonine-specific protein kinase activities of purified gag-*mil* and gag-*raf* proteins. *Nature 312*: 558–561.

Molders, H., Defesche, J., Muller, D., Bonner, T. I., Rapp, U. R., and Muller, R. (1985). Integration of transfected LTR sequences into the c-*raf* proto-oncogene: Activation by promoter insertion. *EMBO J. 4*: 693–698.

Morse, H. C., III, Hartley, J. W., Fredrickson, T. N., Yetter, R. A., Majumdar, C., Cleveland, J. L., and Rapp, U. R. (1986). Recombinant murine retroviruses containing avian v-*myc* induce a wide spectrum of neoplasms in newborn mice. *Proc. Natl. Acad. Sci. U.S.A. 83*: 6868–6872.

Morse, H. C., III, Tidmarsh, G. F., Holmes, K. L., Fredrickson, T. N., Hartley, J. W., Pierce, J. H., Langdon, W. Y., Daily, M. O., and Weissman, I. (1987). Expression of the 6C3 antigen on murine hematopoietic neoplasms. Association with expression of *abl*, *ras*, *fes*, *src*, *erb*B, and Cas NS-1 oncogenes but not with *myc J. Exp. Med. 165*: 920–925.

Mushinski, J. F., Bauer, S. R., Potter, M., and Reddy, E. P. (1983). Increased expression of *myc*-related oncogene mRNA characterizes most BALB/c plasmacytomas induced by pristane or Abelson murine leukemia virus. *Proc. Natl. Acad. Sci. U.S.A. 80*: 1073–1077.

Palmieri, S., and Vogel, M. L. (1987). Fibroblast transformation parameter induced by the avian v-*mil* oncogene. *J. Virol. 61*: 1717–1721.

Parker, P. J., Coussens, L., Totty, N., Rhee, L., Young, S., Chen, E., Stabel, S., Waterfield, M. D., and Ullrich, A. (1986). The complete primary structure of protein kinase C-the major phorbol ester receptor. *Science 233*: 853–866.

Potter, M., Wax, J. S., Anderson, A. O., and Nordon, R. P. (1985). Inhibition of plasmacytoma development in BALB/c mice by indomethacin. *J. Exp. Med. 161*: 996–1012.

Potter, M., Mushinski, J. F., Mushinski, E. B., Brust, S., Wax, J. S., Wiener, F., Bobonits, M., Rapp, U. R., and Morse, H. C., III. (1987). Avian v-*myc* replaces chromosomal translocation in murine plasmacytomagenesis. *Science 235*: 787–789.

Rapp, U. R. (1980). Isolation of leukemia, sarcoma and carcinoma inducing viruses from mouse fibroblast cell lines, chronically infected with endogenous MuLV. In *Viruses in Naturally-Occurring Cancers*, Vol. 7. (Essex, M., Todaro, G., and zur Hausen, H., eds.). New York, Cold Spring Harbor, Cold Spring Harbor Conferences on Cell Proliferation, pp. 1005–1020.

Rapp, U. R. (1984). Die Rolle der Gene bei der Krebsentstehung. In *Fortschritsberichte aus Naturwissenshaft und Medizin.* (Staab, H. A., Gerok, W., Markl, H., Martienssen, W., and Gibian, H., eds.). Shuttgart, Wissenschaftliche Verlagsgesellschaft, pp. 359–369.

Rapp, U. R. (1985). IL-2 and IL-3 regulated growth of lymphoid cells: Abrogation by infection with a *myc/raf* recombinant virus. In *Proceedings of the Third Meeting on "B Cell Neoplasia".* (Melchers, F., and Potter, M. eds.). Basel, Hoffmann-La Roche, pp. 292–301.

Rapp, U. R. (1987). Role of exogeneous *myc* in growth factor abrogation and c-*myc* autoregulation. In *Proceedings of the Third Meeting on "B Cell Neoplasia".* (Melchers, F., and Potter, M. eds.). Basel, Hoffmann-La Roche, (in press.)

Rapp, U. R., and Todaro, G. J. (1978a). Generation of oncogenic type C viruses: Rapid leukemogenic viruses derived from C3H mouse cells *in vivo* and *in vitro*. *Proc. Natl. Acad. Sci. U.S.A. 75*: 2468–2472.

Rapp, U. R., and Todaro, G. J. (1978b). Generation of new mouse sarcoma viruses in cell culture. *Science 201*: 821–824.

Rapp, U. R., and Todaro, G. J. (1980). Generation of oncogenic mouse type C viruses: *In vitro* selection of carcinoma-inducing variants. *Proc. Natl. Acad. Sci. U.S.A. 77*: 624–628.

Rapp, U. R., Nowinski, R. C., Reznikoff, C. A., and Heidelberger, C. (1975). Endogenous oncornaviruses in chemically induced transformation. I. Transformation independent of virus production. *Virology 65*: 392–409.

Rapp, U. R., Reynolds, Jr., F. H., and Stephenson, J. R. (1983a). New mammalian transforming retrovirus: Demonstration of a polyprotein gene product. *J. Virol. 45*: 914–924.

Rapp, U. R., Goldsborough, M. D., Mark, G. E., Bonner, T. I., Groffen, J., Reynolds, Jr., F. H., and Stephenson, J. (1983b). Structure and biological activity of v-*raf*, a unique oncogene transduced by a retrovirus. *Proc. Natl. Acad. Sci. U.S.A. 80*: 4218–4222.

Rapp, U. R., Reynolds, Jr., F. H., and Stephenson, J. R. (1984). Isolation of new mammalian type C transforming viruses. In *Gene Transfer and Cancer. 4th* (Sternberg, N. L., and Pearson, M. L., eds.). New York, Raven Press, pp. 169–178.

Rapp, U. R., Bonner, T. I., Moelling, K., Bister, K., and Ihle, J. (1985a). Genes and gene products involved in growth regulation of tumor cells. In *Recent*

Results in Cancer Research, Vol. 99. (Haveman, K., and Sorenson, G., eds.). New York, pp. 221–236.

Rapp, U. R., Cleveland, J. L., Brightman, K., Scott, A., and Ihle, J. N. (1985b). Abrogation of IL-3 and IL-2 dependence by recombinant murine retroviruses expressing v-*myc* oncogenes. *Nature 317*: 434–438.

Rapp, U. R., Cleveland, J. L., Fredrickson, T. N., Holmes, K. L., Morse, H. C., III, Jansen, H. W., Patschinsky, and Bister, K. (1985c). Rapid induction of hemopoietic neoplasms in newborn mice by a *raf/mil/myc* recombinant murine retrovirus. *J. Virol. 55*: 23–33.

Rapp, U. R., Bonner, T. I., and Cleveland, J. L. (1986). The *raf* oncogene. In *Retroviruses and Human Pathology.* (Gallo, R. C., Stehelin, and Varnier, O. E., eds.). New Jersey, Humana Press, pp. 449–472.

Rapp, U. R., Cleveland, J. L., and Bonner, T. I. (1987). Clinical relevance. *Proceedings from Modern Trends in Human Leukemia VII Hematology and Blood Transfusion* (in press).

Rosenberg, N., and Baltimore, D. (1976). A quantitative assay for transformation of bone marrow cells by Abelson murine leukemia virus. *J. Exp. Med. 143*: 1453–1463.

Ruley, H. E. (1983). Adenovirus early region 1A enables viral and cellular transformining genes to transform pulmonary cells in culture. *Nature 304*: 602–606.

Schultz, A. M., Copeland, T., Oroszlan, S., and Rapp, U. R. Identification and characterization of c-*raf* phosphoproteins from mouse cells . *Oncogene.*

Schwab, M., Ellison, J., Busch, M., Rosenau, W., Varmus, H. E., and Bishop, J. M. (1984). Enhanced expression of the human gene N-*myc* consequent to amplification of DNA may contribute to malignant progression of neuroblastomas. *Proc. Natl. Acad. Sci. U.S.A. 81*: 4940–4944.

Schwartz, R. C., Stanton, L. W., Riley, S. C., Marcu, K. B., and Witte, O. N. (1986). Synergism of N-*myc* and N-Ha-*ras* in the *in vitro* neoplastic progression of murine lymphoid cells. *Mol. Cell. Biol. 6*: 3221–3231.

Shen-Ong, G. L. C., Keath, E. J., Piccoli, S. P., and Cole, M. D. (1982). Novel *myc* oncogene RNA from abortive immunoglobulin gene recombination in murine plasmacytomas. *Cell 31*: 443–452.

Sorrentino, V., Drosdoff, V., McKinney, M. D., Zeitz, L., and Fleissner, E. (1986). Potentiation of growth factor activity by exogenous c-*myc* expression. *Proc. Natl. Acad. Sci. U.S.A. 83*: 8167–8171.

Stewart, T. A., Pattengale, P. K., and Leder, P. (1984). Spontaneous mammary adenocarcinomas in transgenic mice that carry and express MTV/*myc* fusion genes. *Cell 38*: 627–637.

Sutrave, P., Bonner, T. I., Rapp, U. R., Jansen, H. W., and Bister, K. (1984). Nucleotide sequence of avian retroviral oncogene v-*mil*: Homologue of murine retroviral oncogene v-*raf*. *Nature 309*: 85–88.

Tidmarsh, G. F., Daily, M. O., Whitlock, C. A., Pillemer, E., and Weissman, I. L. (1985). Transformed lymphocytes from Abelson-diseased mice express levels of a B lineage transformation associated antigen elevated from that found in normal lymphocytes. *J. Exp. Med. 162*: 1421–1434.

Vennström, B., Kahn, P., Adkins, B., Enrietto, P., Hayman, M. J., Graf, T., and Luciw, P. (1984). Transformation of mammalian fibroblasts and macrophages *in vitro* by a murine retrovirus encoding an avian v-*myc* oncogene. *EMBO J. 3*: 3223–3229.

Vogt, M., Lesley, J., Bogenberger, J., Volkman, S., and Haas, M. (1986). Coinfection with viruses containing the v-Ha-*ras* and N-*myc* oncogenes leads to growth factor independence by a indirect mechanism. *Mol. Cell. Biol. 6*: 3545–3549.

Weinstein, Y., Cleveland, J. L., Askew, D. S., Rapp, U. R., and Ihle, J. N. (1987). Insertion and truncation of c-*myb* by murine leukemia virus in a myeloid cell line derived from cultures of normal hemopoietic cells. *J. Virol. 61*: 2339–2343.

Weiss, R., Teich, N., Varmus, H., and Coffin, J. (eds.). (1982). *RNA Tumor Viruses.* New York, Cold Spring Harbor Laboratory.

Wolff, L., Mushinski, J. F., Gilboa, E., and Morse, H. C., III. (1986). Induction of hematopoietic tumors using a viral construct containing c-*myc* DNA from normal mouse spleen. *Curr. Topics Microbiol. Immunol. 132*: 33–39.

Wolff, L., Mushinski, J. F., Shen-Ong, G. L. C., and Morse, H. C., III. (1987). Contributions of c-*myc* and c-*myb* to myeloid tumors of BALB/c mice: Dependence on the pristane-induced inflammatory response and effects of indomethacin (submitted).

Zhou, R. P., Kan, N., Papas, T., and Duesberg, P. (1985). Mutagenesis of avian carcinoma virus MH2: Only one of two potential transforming genes (Delta *gag/myc*) transforms fibroblasts. *Proc. Natl. Acad. Sci. U.S.A. 82(19)*: 6389–6393.

TWELVE

Consequences of Constitutional Activation of Oncogenes Within Transgenic Mice

Jerry M. Adams
The Walter & Eliza Hall Institute of Medical Research
Melbourne, Australia

INTRODUCTION

A major new avenue for the analysis of oncogenesis has been opened by the creation of transgenic mice carrying specific cancer-promoting genes. These animals bear the introduced oncogene in all their tissues, but its expression can be either widespread or highly restricted, depending upon the attached regulatory sequences. The biological effects of an oncogene on diverse cell types can thus be assessed directly within the living animal. Although the study of transgenic oncogenes is still in its infancy, it seems clear that this new methodology provides the most direct means to demonstrate the tumorigenic potential of presumptive oncogenes. It also opens new avenues for studying the stages in the tumorigenic process, the cooperation between oncogenes, and the biological effects of individual oncogenes upon cellular proliferation and differentiation. This chapter will first sketch how such mice are produced and discuss further their potential for studies on oncogenesis, before describing specific findings. Emphasis will be placed on work with cellular oncogenes, in particular the c-*myc* gene, for which most information is available, but pertinent findings with viral oncogenes will also be surveyed. This topic has also been reviewed by Hanahan (1986) and Cory and Adams (1988).

PRODUCTION OF TRANSGENIC MICE

Transgenic mice, reviewed by Palmiter and Brinster (1986), are generally produced by microinjection of deoxyribonucleic acid (DNA) (Brinster et al., 1984; Gordon et al., 1983; Hogan et al., 1986). A few hundred copies of the gene of interest are injected into one of the pronuclei of a recently fertilized egg, and the injected eggs are then placed within pseudopregnant females and allowed to develop to term. With favorable mouse strains and impeccable technique, some 5–25% of the resulting pups bear the "transgene," which can be detected by hybridization to DNA from tail biopies. A variable proportion of these primary transgenic animals will express the transgene, presumably depending on the position of insertion and the "strength" of the attached regulatory sequences. In any case, on subsequent breeding of these "founders," the transgene behaves like any other mouse allele, being inherited as a simple Mendelian trait. Thus, a new mouse strain can be created bearing a single new character.

A plausible molecular scenario for the integration of the transgene is that random breaks within the mouse chromosomes occur relatively frequently within the egg, and cellular repair mechanisms treat the introduced DNA molecules like chromosome fragments, ligating the ends together. In any case, typically some one to 50 copies of the injected gene is inserted in tandem at a single, seemingly random, position within a mouse chromosome. More rarely, insertion occurs at two positions and these loci segregate among the progeny. If integration occurs after the first cell division, the founder animal is mosaic and less that 50% of its progeny will be transgenic. Such mice may not exhibit phenotypes that appear in their offspring. Usually, however, the transgene is present within all tissues of the primary animal and is inherited in a remarkably consistent manner. Since the transgene is inserted into only one homologue of a given chromosome, the founder mouse will of course be heterozygous at that allele. Subsequently, one can attempt to assess the effects of a double dose of the transgene by making homozygous transgenic mice, although this may not be possible if the insertion has interrupted a gene necessary for development (e.g., see Woychik et al., 1985).

Although most transgenic animals have been made by the microinjection procedure outlined above, there is also interest in introducing genes (including oncogenes) via retroviruses (e.g., see Soriano et al., 1987; Stewart et al., 1985; Van der Putten et al., 1985). A difficulty with that approach is that retroviral transcription, and often also the expression of the attached genes, is silenced as the embryo matures (Jähner et al., 1982).

Another scheme is to introduce the gene as part of an episome. A polyoma-based vector generated an almost quantitative yield of transgenic animals bearing episomes, and the transmission of these to progeny was quantitative (Rassoulzadegen et al., 1986). However, further analysis has revealed that two separate plasmids are required to generate the episomes, and that rearrangement of the sequences is frequent (F. Cuzin, personal communication).

POTENTIAL OF THE TRANSGENIC APPROACH

Direct tests for the action of cellular oncogenes have previously been confined mainly to studies with fibroblasts, largely because most other cell types, particularly primary cells, are recalcitrant to DNA transfection. Although the fibroblast focus assay has been very illuminating, particularly for genes of the *ras* class, a number of oncogenes (indeed even certain mutated *ras* genes) do not give distinct foci (Bos et al., 1985). Moreover, the fibroblast may be inappropriate for assaying certain oncogenes derived from tumors of very different cell types. There is thus a pressing need for new means of delivering putative oncogenes to diverse cell types.

It might be argued that the acutely transforming retroviruses, which have transduced a cellular oncogene, have already told us what those oncogenes do in vivo. While the argument contains a measure of truth, the interpretation of results with the naturally occurring acutely oncogenic retroviruses is much more complex than is often appreciated.

1. The v-*onc* structure usually differs notably from that of its cellular counterpart, involving truncations and/or fusions with the viral genes as well as point mutations.
2. Infectivity may differ widely between cell types, or between cells at different maturation stages within a lineage.
3. The helper virus may sometimes play a critical role in tumorigenesis (e.g., see Shen-Ong et al., 1984).
4. The levels of v-*onc* expression vary depending upon the site of integration.

5. The target cell for viral transformation is often poorly defined. For example, even though pre–B lymphomas are frequently generated by Abelson murine leukemia virus (MuLV), the target cell may only represent a very minor subset of pre–B cells, or even a cell before the pre–B stage. (Whitlock and Witte, 1985).
6. Viral transformation in vivo is frequently oligoclonal owing to continuing virus spread.

The ramifications of transgenic mice for oncogenic studies may well be considerable. First and foremost, the efficacy of a putative oncogene can be tested directly in vivo. Effects can be sought either within a wide spectrum of cell types or, conversely, confined to particular tissues by varying the nature of the attached regulatory sequences. Secondly, once a breeding transgenic line is established, the transgene should behave identically in every animal, and indeed perhaps in every cell of a given type. Thus, a well-characterized transgenic line becomes a permanent resource. Thirdly, the influence of the host genotype on tumor induction can be explored by backcrossing a transgene onto the various genetic backgrounds available as conventional inbred strains. Fourthly, mice bearing certain oncogenes might well provide a ready source of new types of immortal cell lines, not necessarily tumorigenic.

Perhaps the most significant opportunity provided by these transgenic animals is the possibility of exploring the preneoplastic state. One can attempt to assess whether an oncogene has perturbed differentiation within particular lineages. The perturbations may help to delineate early maturation stages and to clarify how differentiation is controlled. Thus, new insights may emerge regarding the normal biological functions of the oncogenes. The rules for oncogene cooperativity can also be evaluated within diverse cell types. For example, one can isolate the relevant cells from a preneoplastic animal bearing an oncogene and attempt to fully transform them in vitro with retroviruses carrying other oncogenes. Alternatively, the second oncogene could be introduced simply by breeding mice of two independent transgenic lines.

VIRAL ONCOGENES

SV40 T-antigen gene

The first oncogenic effects in transgenic animals were detected in mice bearing the SV40 T-antigen genes (Brinster et al., 1984). The constructs initially used included a metallothionein-fusion gene, but the SV40 large T-antigen gene driven by the SV40 enhancer/promoter was later shown to be sufficient (Palmiter et al., 1985). Although the SV40 virus was generally thought to be only very weakly tumorigenic (if at all) in mice, nearly all the transgenic mice died with characteristic brain tumors involving the choroid plexus. The SV40 T antigen was expressed predominantly in affected tumorous tissues, being barely detectable in either unaffected tissues or in susceptible tissues prior to overt pathology. The tumorigenesis is thus thought to depend upon activation of the SV40 DNA locus within the affected tissue. In keeping with that possibility, the foreign DNA was usually amplified or rearranged in the tumors. One explanation for the puzzling restriction of tumorigenesis to the choroid plexus could be that this tissue is more permissive to T-antigen gene activation. The SV40 enhancer is thought to be inactivated during early development, and its reactivation may be a rare event dependent upon cell type. Cell lines derived from several tissues of another T-antigen appeared to express higher levels of the T-antigen gene than the parent tissues and became more tumorigenic on passage in culture (Small et al., 1985).

Nontumorigenic changes noted in the SV40 T-antigen mice included thymic hypertropy and kidney pathology (Brinster et al., 1984). It appears that T-antigen expression does not readily generate tumors in these organs, but transformed stromal cell lines could readily be established in culture from seemingly normal brain and thymic tissues.

Since SV40 T antigen is expressed at the cell surface as well as in the nucleus, immunity is likely to be important in determining whether tumors arise. This possibility was examined by comparing the immune responsiveness of two transgenic strains that express the T-antigen gene but differ greatly in tumor incidence (Faas et al., 1987). Mice of the high-incidence strain (427), which almost invariably succumb to tumors of the choroid plexus before 7 months of age, were found to be tolerant to the antigen. Neither serum antibody to T antigen, nor a cytotoxic lymphocyte response to cells bearing it was detectable, although vaccinia virus–infected cells elicited a robust cytolytic response. On the other hand, with the low incidence strain (419), in which only one of 57 mice developed a choroid plexus tumor within the first year of life, the great majority of mice yielded a strong cytolytic T-cell response to T antigen–bearing cells.

These results suggest that the T antigen expressed in 427 mice, but not that in 419 mice, has been treated as a self-antigen. Likely differences between these two strains are the timing and location of T-antigen expression. Whereas T antigen was detectable within some thymic epithelial cells of 427 mice at 14 days, none has been observed in 419 mice before 32 weeks of age. The thymic expression may be critical because the elimination of self-reactive T-lymphocyte clones is thought to occur in the thymus. Thus, it appears that the high tumor incidence in 427 mice reflects in part their inability to carry out immune surveillance.

It is now clear that the SV40 T-antigen genes can, depending on the attached regulatory sequences, induce a wide spectrum of neoplastic disorders. Under the control of the metallothionein enhancer, hepatocellular carcinomas and islet cell adenomas ensued (Messing et al., 1985). These mice also displayed a demyelinating peripheral neuropathy associated with excessive numbers of abnormal Schwann cells that typically led to hind limb paralysis. Attachment of the SV40 T-antigen genes to the insulin-regulatory region led as expected to expression specifically in pancreatic β cells (Hanahan, 1985). On account of the resulting hyperplasia of the islet cells, many of the first such mice died suddenly owing to hypoglycemia. Those spared by a high sugar diet succumbed later to pancreatic β-cell tumors. Whereas nearly all the islets exhibited hyperplasia, typically only four or five progressed to tumors. Presumably a second genetic alteration has occurred in the tumors, but whether this reflects increased T-antigen expression or an independent change has not been established. Some of the mice develop autoantibodies against T antigen, but it is not clear whether this humoral response reduces the rate of tumor formation (Adams et al., 1987).

The SV40 T antigen appears to be a potent tumorigen in many cell types. The murine α-crystallin enhancer/promoter led to the production of lens tumors, even though no naturally occurring malignancy of the ocular lens has ever been reported (Mahon et al., 1987). The lens tumors were highly invasive and led rapidly to death. In the embryos, differentiation of the lens was clearly affected.

The pancreatic acinar cells were targeted using an elastase promoter region (Ornitz et al., 1987). Karyotypic alterations appear to play a key role in the tumor development within the elastase/T-antigen mice. A marked hyperplasia is evident within the pancreas by day 17 of gestation. In newborn mice, pancreatic function remains intact, and the DNA content is diploid. Remarkably, however, 1 month later the majority of cells are tetraploid. Moreover, between 1 and 4 months of age, hundreds of nodules develop in the pancreas, and death soon ensues. The nodules appear to represent tumorigenic clones, and all appear to be aneuploid, with chromosome numbers between 2n and 4n (e.g., 2.8n and 2.6n for individual nodules). The nodules contain transplantable tumor cells.

These results suggest that SV40 T antigen induces karyotypic instability within these cells. A plausible scenario is that enforced replication promotes tetraploidization and the tetraploid state is unstable, leading to random chromosome loss. The loss of specific chromosomes, or combinations of specific chromosomes, may then trigger tumor onset.

These chromosomes might bear putative recessive oncogenes. Mice like these may thus provide an excellent model for addressing the long-standing issue of the role of chromosome instability in tumor development.

Other Papovaviruses

The early regions of two other papovaviruses, JC and BK, which contain T-antigen genes somewhat related to that of SV40, have also proven to be tumorigenic when incorporated into the mouse genome (Small et al., 1986). Founder mice carrying the JC viral DNA developed adrenal neuroblastomas, whereas one mouse bearing BK DNA developed a renal tumor, and another a hepatocellular carcinoma. The tissue tropism of the pathology was similar to that which the viruses are thought to have in man, suggesting that such mice may provide excellent models for human virus-induced disease. It is interesting that some JC offspring died with a demyelinating syndrome before tumors had time to appear, mimicing a human disease with which JC virus has been associated.

Papillomavirus

The papilloma (wart) viruses are of interest because certain human papillomaviruses are the best-documented viral agents in human cancer. The related bovine papilloma virus (BPV-1), which induces benign skin tumors (fibropapillomas) in cattle, was introduced into the mouse genome as tandem inserts, a form that allows excision of an intact circular genome to generate an episome (Lacey et al., 1986). Starting at about 8 months of age, mice of this line develop multiple skin tumors, particularly in areas of abrasion and wounding. In addition, the skin is abnormally thickened over wide areas. The tumors exhibit disorganized dermal layers. Whereas BPV DNA remained integrated within chromosomal DNA in the young transgenic mice, episomal forms were present in all the tumors as well as amplified integrated copies. Thus, an elevation in copy number may be required for tumor induction.

THE c-*myc* GENE

Mammary Carcinomas

To test the effects of c-*myc* dysregulation in vivo, Stewart et al. (1984) generated mouse lines bearing the human c-*myc* gene linked (within $exon_1$) to the long terminal repeat (LTR) of the mouse mammary tumor virus (MTV). In most of these strains, the female mice developed breast tumors (mammary adenocarcinomas) during their second or third pregnancies. The MTV LTR bears an hormonally inducible enhancer, and it is thought that prolactogenic stimuli trigger its expression in multiparous females. While no consistent pattern of expression was observed, two of 10 founder animals and all their female offspring developed breast tumors, confirming that hormonal induction is involved. No evidence was found for transgene amplification in the tumors. Since the tumors were focal, involving only a single breast region, it was concluded that *myc* expression was not sufficient for tumorigenesis. Presumably a spontaneous mutation occurs in the cell initiating the tumorigenic clone.

Diverse Malignancies

In contrast to the mammary-specific effects just described, one MTV-*myc* lineage (denoted the K strain) proved to express the transgene in a wide variety of tissues, presumably due to some overriding effect of its position of insertion (Leder et al., 1986). Whereas some other strains expressed the transgene only in salivary gland and breast, the K strain also had transcripts in testes, pancreas, lung, spleen, and liver as well as traces in the kidney. This strain thus allowed the range of tissue susceptible to transformation by c-*myc* to be assessed. About half the animals developed one or occasionally even two malignancies, with a mean latency of 14 months. These included testicular tumors, lymphomas of both B- and T-cell origin and mast cell tumors as well as adenocarcinomas of the breast. Thus *myc* is tumorigenic in diverse cells. It is noteworthy, however, that tumors did *not* arise in certain tissues expressing relatively high levels of the transgene (notably lung, pancreas, and salivary gland). This result may mean that c-*myc* does not promote tumorigenesis in all cell types, that the threshold is dependent upon cell type, or that the genetic background of the mice influences the types of tumors that can arise.

Lymphoid Neoplasia

Lymphomagenesis Due to Immunoglobulin Enhancers

In view of the strong association between c-*myc* dysregulation and lymphoid neoplasia (see Chapter 7 by Bornkamm et al.; Cory, 1986), it was of considerable interest to explore transgenic constructs that might promote constitutive expression of c-*myc* within lymphocytes. To that end, a c-*myc* gene was coupled to immunoglobulin enhancers (Adams et al., 1985). One construct was derived from an unusual c-*myc* rearrangement found in a mouse plasmacytoma: Rather than a conventional translocation, a 2.3-kb region bearing the immunoglobulin heavy chain enhancer (Eμ) had inserted just upstream from the c-*myc* promoters (Corcoran et al., 1985). This construct proved remarkably potent as a transgene: 13 of 15 primary mice developed lymphomas within a few months of birth. A construct bearing the kappa light chain enhancer also induced lymphomas, albeit with lower incidence and longer latency. Conjunction of an enhancer and the *myc* gene was required, because neither a normal intact *myc* gene nor one truncated in a fashion like that in most plasmacytomas led to any tumors. The lymphoid specificity can be confidently ascribed to the immunoglobulin enhancers, because other neoplasms arose under control by the SV40 enhancer (Adams et al., 1985) or the MMTV LTR (see above). The remarkably uniform results with the heavy chain enhancer in nearly all primary mice, which presumably bear independent insertions, suggests that this element has a dominant effect in many chromosomal contexts.

The high predisposition to lymphoid malignancy in Eμ-*myc* mice proved highly heritable. The typical pathology is a disseminated lymphoma, usually affecting most lymph nodes, the spleen, and often the thymus. Occasionally other organs, such as the liver and lung, are invaded, and there is usually spillover into the blood, so that the disease can be regarded as a leukemia as well (A. Harris, unpublished results). Despite the frequent thymic involvement, all the tumors so far analyzed (>50) have proven to be of B-lineage origin, as assessed by surface markers, immunoglobin gene rearrangements and expression, and the absence of T-cell receptor gene rearrangements. Some T-cell tumors might have been expected, since a complete immunoglobulin μ transgene is expressed in T as well as B cells (Grosschedl et al., 1984), but the Eμ-*myc* gene does not appear to be expressed in T cells (see below).

The tumors represent more than one stage of B-lymphocyte ontogeny. A minority bear surface immunoglobulin and hence are mature B cells, whereas the rest can be assigned to two pre–B stages, depending upon whether their immunoglobulin gene rearrangements are of DJ or VDJ type. Interestingly, many cell lines derived from the tumors can progress from one stage to another, and may therefore provide useful models for B-cell maturation in culture. Thus, it is clear that *myc*-induced tumorigenesis is not confined to a single stage, and need not "freeze" a cell at one maturation stage. None of the tumors so far studied represents the very early stage lacking any immunoglobulin gene rearrangement. Tumors at that "pro–B" stage would be of great interest, particularly if the cells continue to differentiate in culture because very little is known about the earliest stages of B-cell ontogeny.

Since *myc* translocations are associated with the terminal plasma cell in the mouse, it may appear somewhat paradoxical that plasmacytomas are not among the tumors that normally arise in Eμ-*myc* mice. One explanation might be the genetic background: Plasmacytomas only occur commonly in BALB/c and NZB mice, whereas the Eμ-*myc* mice involve the C57BL and SJL strains (see below). Another possibility is related to the requirement for the mineral oil pristane in conventional plasmacytoma induction. Pristane induces the peritoneal granulomas in which plasmacytomas arise, and this milieu appears to be rich in macrophage-derived factors needed for plasma cell growth. Indeed pristane can encourage plasmacytoma development in Eμ-*myc* mice (A. Harris, unpublished results).

Despite the many similarities between the Eμ-*myc* tumors and B-lymphoid tumors induced by other means, such as by Abelson murine leukemia virus (A-MuLV), there are also notable differences. For example, the frequent generation by Eμ-*myc* mice of tumors at the B-cell stage contrasts with the virtually exclusive pre–B phenotype of those produced by A-MuLV (Rosenberg, 1982). Moreover, all lymphomas generated by A-MuLV, and indeed nearly all those produced by retroviruses bearing several other oncogenes, display the 6C3 surface marker (Morse et al., 1987; Tidmarsh et al., 1985), whereas none of those examined from Eμ-*myc* mice (W. Langdon, unpublished results), or those derived from *myc* retrovirus infection (Morse et al., 1987) bear this marker. 6C3 might correspond to a growth factor or receptor, since it is expressed at high levels on the stromal cells that support pre–B cell proliferation (Whitlock et al., 1987). Whatever its function, its absence from the *myc*-induced tumors suggests either that they derive from a different subset of B-lymphoid cells, or, more likely, that a different pathway to tumorigenesis occurs with *myc* and *abl*. A final noteworthy difference is that most conventional B-lymphoid tumors bear the Ly1 surface antigen, presumably indicating that they derive from the seemingly distinct Ly1$^+$subset of B cells (Hayakawa et al., 1985), whereas most Eμ-*myc* lymphomas lack this marker (W. Langdon, unpublished results). Ly1 is also found on most nontumorigenic B-cell lines derived from normal mice (Braun et al., 1986). This suggests that cells of this minor B-cell lineage can be immortalized more readily that those of the major lineage.

Activation of Transforming Genes

Despite the almost invariant tumorigenicity of the Eμ-*myc* mice, several observations suggest that some critical event(s), almost certainly genetic, precipitate(s) tumor formation. First, the lymphoid tissues of young Eμ-*myc* mice generally lack transplantable tumor cells, whereas cells from the overt tumors are highly transplantable in syngeneic recipients (Langdon et al., 1986). Second, lymphomas appear to rise essentially at random within the cohort of Eμ-*myc* mice, typically at between 1 and 6 months of age (Adams et al., 1985; Harris et al., 1988), whereas the transgene begins to affect the B-lymphoid population even before birth (Langdon et al., 1986). Third, the pattern of immunoglobulin gene rearrangement clearly indicates that nearly all the lymphomas are monoclonal in origin (Adams et al., 1985). Finally, and most definitively, DNA from several of the lymphomas has been found to transform NIH 3T3 fibroblasts (our unpublished results). Since the *myc* gene does not score in this assay, these results indicate that an independent oncogene has been activated spontaneously in each tumor, presumably an oncogene that can collaborate with c-*myc*. The nature of the transforming genes is presently under study.

Influence of Genetic Background

The rate of lymphoma formation in the Eμ-*myc* mice may be governed by the genetic background of the mice. Because transgenic mice can be created more efficiently from hybrid eggs (Brinster et al., 1984), each founder was an F_2 derived from the C57BL and SJL strains, and most of the Eμ-*myc* mice have been maintained an an F_2 pool. It is interesting that a minority of these transgenic mice initiate tumor formation at a much slower rate than the rest. Since at any locus, a quarter of these transgenic mice will be homozygous for the allele of a particular parent strain, a plausible interpretation of this result is that C57BL and SJL differ at a tumor susceptibility locus. It appears relevant that old SJL mice develop a malignancy that appears to be lymphoid in character (Morse et al., 1985). This SJL predisposition may reflect the presence of a single recessive trait (Bubbers, 1984). Backcross experiments with Eμ-*myc* mice support the notion that the background influences the rate of lymphoma formation (A. Harris, unpublished results). Nevertheless, all the Eμ-*myc* mice eventually succumb to lymphomas.

The Preneoplastic State in Eμ-*myc* Mice

The absence of malignant cells in young Eμ-*myc* mice provided a unique opportunity to examine the consequences of constitutive c-*myc* expression upon B-lymphocyte development (Langdon et al., 1986). The bone marrow, which is the site of postnatal lymphopoiesis, was found to be markedly altered by a greatly expanded population of pre–B cells. The accelerated production of pre–B cells commences in the fetal liver by 18 days of gestation and finally reaches a plateau level representing about 65% of the bone marrow cells at 3–4 weeks of age. In contrast of the tumors, this population is polyclonal, and it appears to comprise several early stages of B-cell development. The pre–B cells are also found in the spleen, which is not the case in normal mice. Curiously, they are not found in the lymph nodes of Eμ-*myc* mice even though the lymph nodes (and thymus) are the most common sites of tumor expansion (see above). Thus, the ability to invade the lymph nodes and thymus may be a critical step toward malignancy.

Both the Eμ-*myc* pre–B and B cells were found to be notably larger than most of their normal counterparts. This increase of size is suggestive of proliferative activity, and indeed more than twice as many of the pre–B cells and the B cells are in replicative cycle. In fact, all these cells may be proliferating, since the analysis did not distinguish between noncycling cells and those traversing G_1. In view of this high replicative fraction, it seems evident that a large proportion of the Eμ-*myc* bone marrow cells must continually die to account for the steady-state level found in adult Eμ-*myc* mice. How this plateau is set is unclear, but one obvious possibility is that the cells proliferate until they exhaust the available supply of the requisite growth factor.

Since lymphocyte activation is associated with a marked transient rise in c-*myc* expression (Kelly et al., 1983), intriguing questions arise regarding the immunological competence of B cells subjected to continual *myc* expression (Vaux et al., 1987). Analysis of the function of Eμ-*myc* B cells in vitro revealed that their stimulation with either mitogens or antigens did lead to proliferation and antibody formation. The frequency of responsive B cells from Eμ-*myc* mice, however, was only 30% that of B cells from normal littermates. Thus, enforced *myc* expression is not sufficient to block the differentiation of all B cells, but a much larger fraction of the immunoglobulin-bearing cells from Eμ-*myc* mice are not immunologically competent. In vivo the responses were sometimes delayed but reached normal final levels, and switching from IgM to IgG production occurred. Thus, the constitutive expression of the c-*myc* gene appears to retard B-cell differentiation, but does not grossly impair immunological function in vivo.

myc Autoregulation

All the effects noted to date in the Eμ-*myc* mice appear to reflect alterations within their B-lymphoid compartment. This is consistent with evidence that the transgene is expressed almost exclusively within those cells (Alexander et al., 1987). It is interesting to note that the level of transgene expression is comparable to that in activated normal lymphocytes. Thus, constitutive expression at physiological levels of a normal cellular gene can elicit all the profound biological effects cited above.

How is this potent tumorigenic agent normally held in check? A striking feature of every Eμ-*myc* tumor examined, including those at both the pre–B and the B-cell stage, is that the endogeneous *myc* alleles are transcriptionally silent (Adams et al., 1985; Alexander et al., 1987). This finding clearly mirrors earlier observations regarding the untranslocated *myc* allele in plasmacytomas and Burkitt's lymphomas (e.g., see Bernard et al., 1983). This apparent "suppression" of the unaffected *myc* allele cannot be merely an indirect consequence of the tumorigenesis because a similar conclusion holds for the preneoplastic pre–B cells in the transgenic bone marrow, and the splenic B cells (Alexander et al., 1987; Vaux et al., 1987). These results strongly support a negative feedback model for control of *myc* expression (Leder et al., 1983; Rabbitts et al., 1984). In such models, a *myc* polypeptide level above a threshold level normally leads to repression of further *myc* transcription. Presumably a translocated *myc* allele, or the Eμ-*myc* transgene, is recalcitrant to this repression.

Steps Toward Tumorigenesis *in Vitro*

Since an immortalizing role has often been ascribed to c-*myc*, the behavior of the preneoplastic Eμ-*myc* bone marrow cells was investigated in culture (Langdon et al., 1988). In view of claims that v-*myc* can abrogate the factor dependence of hemopoietic cell lines (Rapp et al., 1985), it is noteworthy that Eμ-*myc* B-lymphoid cells cultured in normal medium without a source of growth factors died rapidly, indeed sooner than their normal counterparts. Thus, no evidence was found that c-*myc* had abolished factor requirements, but more subtle alterations, such as the apparently increased sensitivity to growth factors displayed by some hematopoietic cell lines infected with *myc* retroviruses (Cory et al,. 1987), would not have been detectable. Moreover, B cells from transgenic spleen did not display unlimited proliferative capacity, even in the presence of mitogens and rich sources of growth factor (Vaux et al., 1987). Thus, the description of c-*myc* as an immortalizing gene may not be generally appropriate.

At present, the Eμ-*myc* pre–B cells can only be maintained in vitro within Whitlock-Witte cultures (Langdon et al., 1988), in which bone marrow adherent cells provide the unidentified growth factors needed by pre–B cells (Whitlock et al., 1985). In such cultures, the transgenic cells display the same elevated cycling behavior as they do in vivo, but they reach steady-state levels no more than twice that of normal pre–B cells, presumably because growth factor is limiting. Interestingly, after several months of growth, several transgenic cultures began to reach much higher saturation densities, although the layer was still required and one culture finially became factor independent. Thus, steps toward the tumorigenic state can be observed in vitro.

It would be interesting to reconstruct the entire tumorigenic process in vitro with known oncogenes. Preliminary results indicate that infection of Eμ-*myc* B-lymphoid cells with retroviruses bearing either a v-*ras* or v-*raf* gene enhances their growth properties in vitro, but does not always give fully tumorigenic clones (W. Alexander, unpublished results). Hence, both these classes of cytoplasmic oncogene products appear to be able to cooperate with *myc* in progression toward lymphoid neoplasia, but even a *ras-myc* or *raf-myc* combination may not always be sufficient. Thus, some lymphoid malignancies may involve more than two activated oncogenes.

N-*myc*

Several genes with sequences related to that of c-*myc* have been identified. The best studied of these is N-*myc*, which is amplified in many neuroblastomas (Schwab et al., 1983) as well as in some small cell lung carcinomas (Nau et al., 1986). N-*myc* has not been implicated in lymphoid malignancy, but the gene is expressed within lymphocytes at an early stage of their maturation (Zimmerman et al., 1986). To determine how N-*myc* affects lymphocytes, the gene coupled to Eμ has been introduced into mice (our unpublished results). Interestingly, several such mice have developed a lymphoid malignancy. It will be interesting to determine whether these tumors are equivalent to those induced by c-*myc* and whether N-*myc* has perturbed B-cell development.

Why Does Constitutive c-*myc* Expression Establish a High Predisposition to Malignancy?

The results summarized above provide a few clues as to why dysregulated *myc* creates tumor-prone mice. The total number of B-lymphoid cells in the Eμ-*myc* is elevated about fourfold, and more than twice as many of the cells are replicating. Hence, the total number of B-lineage cell divisions has been increased by an order of magnitude. Since the risk of genetic accident is generally assumed to be proportional to the number of cell divisions, this marked increase may be a significant part of the answer. It is also conceivable that the immunoglobulin rearrangement machinery is an added risk factor in lymphocytes. Nevertheless, it is difficult to accept that these factors fully account for the very high frequency of the tumors. Perhaps the c-*myc* level in the Eμ-*myc* mice is high enough to increase the mutation frequency.

ras GENES

Pancreatic Expression

Transgenic mice were constructed in which either a normal c-H-*ras* gene or an oncogenic derivative having valine at position 12 is driven by the elastase promoter (Quaife et al., 1987). This promoter directs expression to pancreatic acinar cells, commencing at 14 days of gestation. Although the elastase promoter is powerful, the level of expression of the elastase-*ras* genes typically was only a few fold higher than that of the endogenous *ras* gene.

The normal c-H-*ras* driven by elastase did not cause tumors or early death. Nevertheless, anaplastic changes were observed. As well as altered cellular morphology and hyperplasia, the pancreas contained many areas that lacked normal acinar structure.

With the mutant *ras* gene, the results were particularly dramatic. Of 19 transgenic pups, 14 were dead or moribund at birth, and the others probably survived because they were mosaic. Development of the pancreas was grossly disrupted, dysplasia being observable even at 14 days of gestation. By day 20, there was large-scale disruption of the pancreatic architecture; islets were no longer recognizable, and insulin-containing cells were scattered throughout the cellular mass. Thus changes in the acinar cells may have indirectly affected the endocrine cells. The acinar cells appeared to be blocked in differentiation, as they did not undergo the morphological changes in size and staining pattern normally seen late in their maturation.

Thus, the acinar cells within a week of their generation had proliferated to a huge, often necrotic mass with the appearance of a carcinoma. These results provide direct evidence for a single-step model for tumorigenesis. Whether the acinar cells were truly malignant is problematical, however, since there was no evidence of aneuploidy, invasiveness, or metastasis. Furthermore, preliminary results indicated that they did not initiate tumors in syngenetic or nude mice. Thus rather than a malignancy, these tumors may be more akin to the polyclonal cell proliferation observed in the erythroblastosis induced in mice by Friend murine leukemia virus, or in some of the retrovirus-induced diseases of the chicken (Graf, 1986).

Curiously, a few mosaic elastase/*ras* mice remained free of disease for several months but then developed pancreatic carcinomas. One might have expected that even a few transgenic cells would have initiated neonatal tumors. One explanation considered was that a mutation might have increased the level of transgene expression in the initiating cell. An intriguing alternative suggestion was that the presence of normal cells may have suppressed the transformed phenotype (Land et al., 1986). If such suppression exists, clarifying how it operates may be of profound importance to understanding tumorigenesis. A third interpretation is that *ras* has a much more profound effect in embryonic than adult cells.

Mammary Expression

An activated H-*ras* gene was subjected to the promoter region of the murine whey acidic protein (*Wap*) gene, which is expressed in mammary epithelial cells in response to lactogenic hormones (Andres et al., 1987). A low level of *Wap-ras* expression was observed in the mammary glands (and brain) of lactating females in two of four lines derived from female founders. No expression was observed after lactation terminated. A tumor emerged after 11 months in one lactating founder female. The *Wap-ras* RNA level was greatly elevated in the tumor.

In one male founder, the transgene had inserted into the Y chromosome, and expression unexpectedly ensued in the salivary gland. As a consequence, five animals developed tumors of that gland (adenocarcinomas), at 9 months of age. Again *Wap-ras* RNA levels were greatly elevated in the tumors compared to that in a corresponding nonmalignant salivary gland from the same individual. In neither the mammary nor salivary gland tumor was there evidence of amplification or rearrangement of the tansgene. Since the level of expression of the endogenous *Wap* gene was not increased in the tumor examined, a *trans*-acting factor stimulating *Wap-ras* transcription seems unlikely. Other explanations, such as a factor that promotes *ras* mRNA stability or a mutation within the promoter, cannot be ruled out.

THE *fos* GENE

The c-*fos* proto-oncogene, which encodes a nuclear polypeptide, has been implicated in control of cell proliferation, since growth factor stimulation of many cell types leads to a transient burst of c-*fos* synthesis. The gene may also have other roles, however, since high constitutive levels have been found in extraembryonic tissues and in macrophages. The two versions of v-*fos*, on the other hand, are associated with osteosarcomalike tumors.

Transgenic mice were produced bearing a murine c-*fos* gene under the direction of the human metallothionein promoter/enhancer (Rüther et al., 1987). The constructs had the natural 3′ end of the c-*fos* gene, a prominent site of posttranscriptional regulation for c-*fos*, or a 3′ end contributed by a retroviral LTR. In eight transgenic lines involving the natural c-*fos* 3′ terminus, only traces of RNA were detected except in the presence of cycloheximide, which is thought to prevent degradation of c-*fos* mRNA. In two of five transgenic lines involving the 3′ LTR, however, high levels of expression were obtained in pancreas, kidney, brain, heart, and muscle. This pattern differs from that expected with the murine metallothionein control region, which usually promotes high expression in liver.

The most striking effect noted in the c-*fos* mice is a marked abnormality in bone formation, most often observed as swollen tibiae. Curiously, visible hind limb swellings, which were detectable 2–3 weeks after birth, only occurred in a proportion of animals, 40% of males and 20% of females, but bone lesions were detectable by x-ray analysis in the others. The swellings did not increase after 4 weeks of age, and no tumors emerged during the observation period of 8–11 months.

Histological analysis of the swollen bones indicated that the normal processes of bone remodeling were disturbed, with much more bone formation than bone resorption. Such lesions were found in almost all mice of the two lineages expressing the transgene. Hence, one normal function of the proto-oncogene may be to regulate bone morphogenesis. It is interesting to note that no abnormalities were noted in several other tissues expressing the transgene. Thus, in contrast to c-*myc* and c-*ras*, the oncogenic potential of c-*fos* may be restricted to a very few tissues.

There are intriguing similarities between these bone lesions and the osteosarcomas induced by v-*fos*. Rüther et al. (1987) suggest that both the virally induced tumors and the bone lesions arise from a multipotent bone precursor cell. If so, the bone lesions might be regarded as a hyperplastic state from which tumors might arise. The absence of overt tumors might reflect structural differences between v-*fos* and c-*fos*, a higher level of v-*fos* expression, or helper virus effects.

The level of c-*fos* expression may well determine the degree of hyperplasia because a c-*fos* gene linked to the H-2k^b promoter induced multiple swellings in all leg bones, but only when the 3′ LTR modification was present. As would be expected with the H-2 promoter, the H-2-c-*fos* gene appears to be expressed in multiple cell type, in particular within hemopoietic tissues, and perturbations of lymphopoiesis have been observed (E. Wagner, personal comm).

ONCOGENE COOPERATIVITY

The combination of activated *myc* and *ras* genes has been shown to convert primary fibroblasts to the fully tumorigenic phenotype (Land et al.,

1983). Such observations have led to the notion that oncogenes fall into two complementary classes (Land et al., 1983; Ruley, 1983). The generality of this important notion, however, requires its test in diverse cell types.

A dramatic illustration of *myc/ras* cooperativity in breast epithelial cells has been obtained by breeding an MTV-*ras* transgenic mouse with an MTV-*myc* mouse (Sinn et al., 1987). Whereas tumors in the MTV-*myc* strain arise sporatically with a long latency (see above), the *myc/ras* mice develop tumors that encompass the entire breast, and these emerge concomittantly with the development of breast tissue.

Myc and *ras* appear to collaborate also in B-lymphoid neoplasia. The introduction of an activated *ras* oncogene via a helper-free retrovirus into neonatal Eμ-*myc* mice greatly accelerates lymphoma induction (our unpublished results). Thus, it appears that some of the rules for oncogene collaboration will be similar in diverse cell types. However, it remains to be determined whether *myc* plus *ras* is sufficient to generate a lymphoma.

CONCLUSIONS AND FUTURE PROSPECTS

It seems clear that transgenic mice are having a significant impact on the analysis of the genes that promote neoplasia. Already the efficacy of several cellular oncogenes (*myc*, *ras*, *fos*) as tumor-promoting agents has been demonstrated conclusively in the living animal. With the apparent exception of embryonic pancreatic cells expressing an activated *ras* gene (see above), the emergence of a tumorigenic clone has required other genetic events. The existence of the pretumorous state in these animals is of particular importance because it provides a new avenue for studying the biological effects of individual oncogenes upon the development of tissues and organs as well as upon the proliferation and maturation of diverse individual cell types. As more types of oncogenes are introduced into the mouse germ line, studies on how oncogenes interact will become feasible for many kinds of tissues, as already illustrated by the demonstration of *myc/ras* cooperativity.

As it is now possible to target oncogene expression to a number of tissues or specific cell types, it will be of considerable interest to compare the biological effects of different oncogenes within the same cell type. An example of such studies is the comparison of the effects of *myc* and *ras* within mammary epithelium (Sinn et al., 1987; Stewart et al., 1984). For the analysis of lymphoid neoplasia, several different oncogenes have been coupled to an immunoglobulin enhancer (our published results). These include not only N-*myc* and N-*ras* (see above), but also v-*myc*, v-*abl*, and *bcr*/v-*abl*, a construct mimicking the hybrid oncogene thought to play a central role in chronic myeloid leukemia. Transgenic mice bearing most of these constructs appear to be prone to lymphoid neoplasia. Interestingly, among the tumors already observed are not only pre–B and B-cell tumors but also plasmacytomas and T lymphomas, tumors not previously observed among Eμ-*myc* mice. The analysis of these new transgenic lines should provide new insights into the basis of lymphoid neoplasia and the control of lymphoid ontogeny.

Because certain proto-oncogenes, such as *int*-1 and *int*-2, appear to be expressed preferentially or exclusively at certain early stages of mouse development (Jakobovits et al., 1986), it is tempting to think that such genes have a normal role in the control of early development. For example, *int*-2 may be an embryonic growth factor (Dickson and Peters, 1987). Transgenic mice may thus provide an effective approach for determining the normal biological function of these genes irrespective of their role in tumorigenesis.

The relationship between oncogenes and growth factors is a continuing saga, and it will be very interesting to determine the effects, particularly on oncogenesis, of introducing deregulated factor genes into mice. Autocrine production may well lead to an elevated tumor incidence. Transgenic production of a hemopoietic colony-stimulating factor has led to a gross overproduction of macrophages, but as yet no tumors have emerged (R. Lang et al., personal communication).

Although the transgenic studies to date have for obvious reasons involved the dominant-acting oncogenes, there is increasing interest in recessive oncogenes; i.e., genes encoding products that normally *prevent* the emergence of a tumorgenic state. A strong candidate for the recessive retinoblastoma-susceptibility gene has been cloned recently (Lee et al., 1987). It is conceivable that high-level expression of an antisense copy of this gene in transgenic mice would mimic loss of the gene and thereby induce retinoblastomas. Such mice would provide a definitive identification of the cloned gene and establish a important animal model for this malignancy of childhood.

REFERENCES

Adams, J. R., Harris, A. W., Pinkert, C. A., Corcoran, L. M., Alexander, W. A., Cory, S., Palmiter, R. D., and Brinster, R. L. (1985). The c-*myc* oncogene driven by immunoglobulin enhancers induces lymphoid malignancy in transgenic mice. *Nature 318*: 533–538.

Adams, T. E., Alpert, S., and Hanahan, D. (1987). Non-tolerance and autoantibodies to a transgenic self antigen expressed in pancreatic β cells. *Nature 325*: 223–228.

Alexander, W. S., Schrader, J. W. and Adams, J. M. (1987). Expression of the c-*myc* oncogene under control of an immunoglobulin enhancer in Eμ-*myc* transgenic mice. *Molec. Cell. Biol. 7*: 1436–1444.

Andres, A. C., Schonenberger, C. A., Groner, B., Henninghausen, L., LeMeur, M., and Gerlinger, P. (1987). Ha-*ras* oncogene expression directed by a milk protein gene promoter: Tissue specificity, hormonal regulation, and tumor induction in transgenic mice. *Proc. Natl. Acad. Sci. U.S.A. 84*: 1299–1303.

Bernard, O., Cory, S., Gerondakis, S., Webb, E., and Adams, J. M. (1983). Sequence of the murine and human cellular *myc* oncogenes and two modes of *myc* transcription resulting from chromosome translocation in B lymphoid tumors. *EMBO J. 2*: 2375–2383.

Bos, J., Toksoz, D., Marshall, C., Verlaan-de Vries, M., Veeneman, G., Van der Eb, A., Van Boom, J., Janssen, J., and Steenvoorden, A. (1985). Amino-acid substitutions at codon 13 of the N-*ras* oncogene in human acute myeloid leukemia. *Nature 315*: 726–730.

Braun, J., Forouzanpour, F., King, L., Teheranizadeh, T., Bray, M., and Kliewer, S. (1986). B-Ly1 cells: Immortal Ly-1$^+$ B lymphocyte cell lines spontaneously arising in mature splenic cultures. *Immunological Rev. 93*: 5–21.

Brinster, R. L., Chen, H. Y., Messing, A., Van Dyke, T., Levine, A. J., and Palmiter, R. D. (1984). Transgenic mice harboring SV40 T-antigen genes develop characteristic brain tumors. *Cell 37*: 367–379.

Brinster, R. L., Chen, H. Y., Trumbauer, M. E., Yagle, M. K., and Palmiter, R. D. (1985). Factors affecting the efficiency of introducing foreign DNA into mice by microinjecting eggs. *Proc. Natl. Acad. Sci. U.S.A. 82*: 4438–4442.

Bubbers, J. E. (1984). Identification and linkage analysis of a gene, Rcs-1, suppressing spontaneous SJL/J lymphoma expression. *J. Natl. Cancer. Inst. 72*: 441–446.

Corcoran, L. M., Cory, S., and Adams, J. A. (1985). Transposition of the immunoglobulin heavy chain enhancer to the *myc* oncogene in a murine plasmacytoma. *Cell 40*: 71–79.

Cory, S. (1986). Activation of cellular oncogenes in haemopoietic cells by chromosome translocation. *Adv. Cancer Res. 47*: 189–234.

Cory, S., Bernard, O., Bowtell, D., and Schrader, J. W. (1987). Murine c-*myc* retroviruses alter the growth requirements of myeloid cell lines. *Oncogene Res. 1*: 61–76.

Cory, S. and Adams, J. M. (1988). Transgenic mice and oncogenesis. *Adv. Immunol.*, in press.

Dickson, C., and Peters, G. (1987). Potential oncogene product related to growth factors. *Nature 326*: 833.

Faas, S., Pan, S., Pinkert, C., Brinster, R., and Knowles, B. (1987). Simian virus 40 (SV40)—transgenic mice that develop tumours are specifically tolerant to SV40 T antigen. *J. Exp. Med. 165*: 417–427.

Gordon, J. W., and Ruddle, F. H. (1983). Gene transfer into mouse embryos: Production of transgenic mice by pronuclear injection. *Methods Enzymol. 101*: 411-433.

Graf, T. (1986). Co-operation of viral oncogenes in the induction of avian leukemia. In *Cell Receptors and Tumor Markers.* (Hubner, ed.). *Verh. Dtsch. Ges. Path. 70*: 1.

Grosschedl, R., Weaver, D., Baltimore, D., and Costantini, F. (1984). Introduction of a μ immunoglobulin gene into the mouse germ line: Specific expression in lymphoid cells and synthesis of functional antibody. *Cell 38*: 647–658.

Hanahan, D. (1985). Heritable formation of pancreatic β-cell tumours in transgenic mice expressing recombinant insulin/simian virus 40 oncogenes. *Nature 315*: 115–122.

Hanahan, D. (1986). Oncogenesis in transgenic mice. In *Oncogenes and Growth Control.* (Kahn and Graf, ed.) Springer-Verlag pp 349–363.

Harris, A. W., Pinkert, C. A., Crawford, M., Langdon, W. Y., Brinster, R. L. and Adams, J. M. (1988). The Eμ-*myc* transgenic mouse: a model for high incidence spontaneous lymphoma and leukemia of early B cells. *J. Expt. Med. 167*: 353-371.

Hayakawa, K., Hardy, R., Herzenberg, L. A., and Herzenberg, L. A. (1985). Progenitors for Ly-1 B cells are distinct from progenitors for other B cells. *J. Exp. Med. 161*: 1554-1568.

Hogan, B., Costantini, F., and Lacy, E. (1986). *Manipulating the mouse embryo: A laboratory manual.* Cold Spring Harbor Laboratory Press.

Jähner, D., Stuhlmann, H., Stewart, C. L., Harbers, K., Löhler, J., Simon, I., and Jaenisch, R. (1982). *De novo* methylation and expression of retroviral genomes during mouse embryogenesis. *Nature 298*: 623–628.

Jakobovits, A., Shackleford, G. M., Varmus, H. E., and Martin, G. R. (1986). Two proto-oncogenes implicated in mammary carcinogenesis, *int*-1 and *int*-2, are independently regulated during mouse development. *Proc. Natl. Acad. Sci. U.S.A. 83*: 7806–7810.

Kelly, K., Cochran, B., Stiles, C., and Leder, P. (1983). Cell-specific regulation of the c-*myc* by lymphocyte mitogens and platelet-derived growth factor. *Cell 35*: 603–610.

Lacey, M., Alpert, S., and Hanahan, D. (1986). Bovine papillomavirus genome elicits skin tumours in transgenic mice. *Nature 322*: 609–612.

Land, H., Parada, L., and Weinberg, R. A. (1983). Tumorigenic conversion of primary embryo fibroblasts requires at least two co-operating oncogenes. *Nature 304*: 596–600.

Land, H., Chen, A. C., Morgenstern, J. P., Parada, L. F., and Weinberg, R. A. (1986). Behavior of *myc* and *ras* oncogenes in transformation of rat embryo fibroblasts. *Mol. Cell. Biol. 6*: 1917–1925.

Langdon, W. Y., Harris, A. W., Cory, S., and Adams, J. A. (1986). The c-*myc* oncogene perturbs B lymphocyte development in Eμ-*myc* transgenic mice. *Cell 47*: 11–18.

Langdon, W. Y., Harris, A. W. and Cory, S. (1988). Growth of Eμ-*myc* transgenic B-lymphoid cells *in vitro* and their evolution towards autonomy. *Oncogene Res.*, in press.

Leder, P., Battey, J., Lenoir, G., Moulding, L., Murphy, W., Potter, H., Stewart, T., and Taub, R. (1983). Translocations among antibody genes in human cancer. *Science 222*: 765–771.

Leder, A., Pattengale, K., Kuo, A., Stewart, T. A., and Leder, P. (1986). Consequence of widespread deregulation of the c-*myc* gene in transgenic mice: Multiple neoplasms and normal development. *Cell 45*: 485–495.

Lee, W-H., Bookstein, R., Hong, F., Young, L.-J., Shew, J.-Y., and Lee, E. Y.-H. P. (1987). Human retinoblastoma susceptibility gene: Cloning, identification and sequence. *Science 235*: 1394–1399.

Mahon, K. A., Chepelinsky, A. B., Khillian, J. S., Overbeek, P. A., Piatigorsky, J., and Westphal, H. (1987). Oncogenesis of the lens in transgenic mice. *Science 235*: 1622–1628.

Messing, A., Chen, H. Y., Palmiter, R. D., and Brinster, R. L. (1985). Peripheral neuropathies, hepatocellular carcinomas and islet cell adenomas in transgenic mice. *Nature 316*: 461–463.

Morse, H. C., Roths, J. B., Davidson, W., Langdon, W. Y., Fredrickson, T., and Hartley, J. (1985). Abnormalities induced by the mutant gene, *1pr*: Patterns of disease and expression of murine leukemia viruses in SJL/J mice homozygous and hetrozygous for *1pr*. *J. Exp. Med. 161*: 602–616.

Morse, H. C., Tidmarsh, G. F., Holmes, K. L., Fredrickson, T., Hartley, J., Pierce, J., Langdon, W. Y., Dailey, M., and Weissman, I. L. (1987). Expression of the 6C3 antigen on murine hematopoietic neoplasms. *J. Exp. Med. 165*: 920–925.

Nau, M., Brooks, B., Carney, D., Gazdar, A., Battey, J., Sausville, E., and Minna, J. (1986). Human small cell lung carcinomas show amplification and expression of the N-*myc* gene. *Proc. Natl. Acad. Sci. U.S.A. 83*: 1092–1096.

Ornitz, D., Hammer, R., Messing, A., Palmiter, R., and Brinster, R. (1987). *Science* (in press).

Palmiter, R. D., and Brinster, R. L. (1986). Germline transformation of mice. *Ann. Rev. Genet. 20*: 465–499.

Palmiter, R. D., Chen, H. Y., Messing, A., and Brinster, R. L. (1985). SV40 enhancer and large-T antigen are instrumental in development of choroid plexus tumors in transgenic mice. *Nature 316*: 457–460.

Quaife, C. J., Pinkert, C. A., Ornitz, D. M., Palmiter, R. D., and Brinster, R. L. (1987). Pancreatic neoplasia induced by *ras* expression in acinar cells of transgenic mice. *Cell 48*: 1023–1034.

Rabbits, T., Forster, A., Hamlyn, P., and Baer. (1984). Effect of somatic mutation within translocated c-*myc* genes in Burkitt's lymphoma. *Nature 309*: 592–597.

Rapp, U., Cleveland, J., Brightman, K., Scott, A., and Ihle, J. (1985). Abrogation of IL-3 and IL-2 dependence by recombinant murine retroviruses expressing v-*myc* oncogene. *Nature 317*: 434–438.

Rassoulzadegan, M., Léopold, P., Vailly, J., and Cuzin, F. (1986). Germline transmission of autonomous genetic elements in transgenic mouse strains. *Cell 46*: 513–519.

Rosenberg, N. (1982). Abelson leukemia virus. *Curr. Topics Microbiol. Immunol. 101*: 95–126.

Ruley, E. (1983). Adenovirus early region 1A enables viral and cellular transforming genes to transform primary cells in culture. *Nature 304*: 503–507.

Rüther, U., Garber, C., Komitowski, D., Muller, R., and Wagner, E. F. (1987). Deregulated c-*fos* expression interferes with normal bone development in transgenic mice. *Nature 325*: 412–416.

Schwab, M., Alitalo, K., Klempnauer, K.-H., Varmus, H., Bishop, J. M., Gilbert, F., Brodeur, G., Goldstein, M., and Trent, J. (1983). Amplified DNA with limited homology to *myc* cellular oncogene is shared by human neuroblastoma cell lines and a neuroblastoma tumor. *Nature 305*: 245–248.

Shen-Ong, G., Potter, M., Mushinski, J. F., Lavu, S., and Reddy, E. P. (1984). Activation of the c-*myc* locus by viral insertional mutagenesis in plasmacytoid lymphosarcomas. *Science 226*: 1077–1080.

Sinn, E., Muller, W., Pattengale, P., Tepler, I., Wallace, R. and Leder, P. (1987). Coexpression of MMTV/v-Ha-*ras* and MMTV/c-*myc* genes in transgenic mice: synergistic action of oncogenes in vivo. *Cell 49*: 465–475.

Small, J. A., Blair, D. G., Showalter, S. D., and Scangos, G. A. (1985). Analysis of a transgenic mouse containing simian virus 40 and v-*myc* sequences. *Mol. Cell. Biol. 5*: 642–648.

Small, J. A., Khoury, G., Jay, G., Howley, P. M., and Scangos, G. A. (1986). Early regions of JC virus and BK virus induce distinct and tissue-specific tumors in transgenic mice. *Proc. Natl. Acad. Sci. U.S.A. 83*: 8288–8292.

Soriano, P., Cone, R., Mulligan, R., and Jaenisch, R. (1987). Tissue-specific and ectopic expression of genes introduced into transgenic mice by retroviruses. *Science 234*: 1409–1413.

Stewart, T. A., Pattengale, P. K., and Leder, P. (1984). Spontaneous mammary adenocarcinomas in transgenic mice that carry and express MTV/*myc* fusion genes. *Cell 38*: 627–637.

Stewart, L., Vanek, M., and Wagner, E. F. (1985). Expression of foreign genes from retroviral vectors in mouse teratocarcinoma chimaeras. *EMBO J. 4*: 3701–3709.

Tidmarsh, G., Dailey, M., Whitlock, C., Pillemer, E., and Weissman, I. L. (1985). Transformed lymphocytes from Abelson-derived mice express levels of a B lineage transformation associated antigen elevated from that found on normal lymphocytes. *J. Exp. Med. 162*: 1421–1430.

Van der Putten, H., Botteri, F., Miller, A. D., Rosenfeld, M., Fan, H., Evans, R., and Verma, I. (1985). Efficient insertion of genes into the mouse germ line via retroviral vectors. *Proc. Natl. Acad. Sci. U.S.A. 82*: 6148–6152.

Vaux, D. L., Adams, J. M., Alexander, W. S., and Pike, B. L. (1987). Immunological competence of B cells subjected to constitutive c-*myc* oncogene expression in Eμ-*myc* transgenic mice. *J. Immunol. 139*: 3854–3860.

Whitlock, C. A., and Witte, O. M. (1985). The complexity of virus-cell interactions in Abelson virus infection of lymphoid and other hematopoietic cells. *Adv. Immunol. 37*: 77–98.

Whitlock, C. A., Denis, K., Robertson, D., and Witte, O. (1985). In vitro analysis of murine B-cell development. *Ann. Rev. Immunol. 3*: 213–235.

Whitlock, C. A., Tidmarsh, G. F., Muller-Sieburg, C., and Weissman, I. L. (1987). Bone marrow stromal cell lines with lymphopoietic activity express high levels of a pre-B neoplasia-associated molecule. *Cell 48*: 1009–1021.

Woychik, R. P., Stewart, T. A., Davis, L., D'Eustachio, P., and Leder, P. (1985). An inherited limb deformity created by insertional mutagenesis in a transgenic mouse. *Nature 318*: 36–41.

Zimmerman, K., Yancopoulos, G., Collam, R., Smith, R., Kohl, N., Denis, K., Nau, M., Witte, O., Toran-Allerand, D., Gee, C., Minna, J., and Alt, F. (1986). Differential expression of *myc* family genes during murine development. *Nature 319*: 780–783.

Index

O

P

R